T0289916

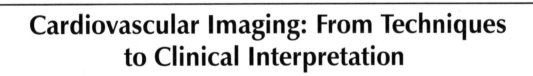

Cardiovascular Imaging: From Techniques to Clinical Interpretation

Cardiovascular Imaging: From Techniques to Clinical Interpretation

Editor: Aaron Jackson

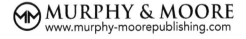
MURPHY & MOORE
www.murphy-moorepublishing.com

www.murphy-moorepublishing.com

ⓂMURPHY & MOORE

Cataloging-in-Publication Data

Cardiovascular imaging : from techniques to clinical interpretation / edited by Aaron Jackson.
    p. cm.
Includes bibliographical references and index.
ISBN 978-1-63987-784-3
1. Cardiovascular system--Imaging. 2. Heart--Imaging. 3. Cardiovascular system--Diseases--Diagnosis.
4. Diagnostic imaging. I. Jackson, Aaron.
RC683.5.I42 C37 2023
616.107 54--dc23

Murphy & Moore Publishing
1 Rockefeller Plaza,
New York City,
NY 10020, USA

ISBN 978-1-63987-784-3

Contents

Preface

This book has been an outcome of determined endeavour from a group of educationists in the field. The primary objective was to involve a broad spectrum of professionals from diverse cultural background involved in the field for developing new researches. The book not only targets students but also scholars pursuing higher research for further enhancement of the theoretical and practical applications of the subject.

Cardiovascular imaging encompasses cardiac imaging and vascular imaging. Cardiac imaging focuses on the non-invasive imaging of the heart through techniques such as MRI, CT scan and ultrasound. Vascular imaging refers to a set of diagnostic procedures used to evaluate the condition of the blood vessels. There are several techniques that are used to generate the images of the blood vessels. Carotid duplex ultrasound is a type of vascular imaging tool that evaluates the neck's carotid arteries which supply blood to the brain. It helps to evaluate the blood flow in the arteries. This book traces some of the recent advancements in cardiovascular imaging methods that are used to diagnose different diseases. With state-of-the-art inputs by acclaimed experts of this medical field, it covers techniques and clinical interpretations of cardiovascular imaging. This book is meant for students who are looking for an elaborate reference text on this topic.

It was an honour to edit such a profound book and also a challenging task to compile and examine all the relevant data for accuracy and originality. I wish to acknowledge the efforts of the contributors for submitting such brilliant and diverse chapters in the field and for endlessly working for the completion of the book. Last, but not the least; I thank my family for being a constant source of support in all my research endeavours.

Editor

Red Blood Cells and Hemoglobin in Human Atherosclerosis and Related Arterial Diseases

Jean-Baptiste Michel [1,*] **and José Luis Martin-Ventura** [2,*]

[1]   UMR 1148, Inserm & Paris University, X. Bichat University Hospital, 75018 Paris, France
[2]   IIS-Fundation Jimenez-Diaz, Autonoma University of Madrid and CIBERCV, 28040 Madrid, Spain
*   Correspondence: Jean-Baptiste.Michel@inserm.fr (J.-B.M.); JLMartin@fjd.es (J.L.M.-V.)

Abstract: As the main particulate component of the circulating blood, RBCs play major roles in physiological hemodynamics and impact all arterial wall pathologies. RBCs are the main determinant of blood viscosity, defining the frictional forces exerted by the blood on the arterial wall. This function is used in phylogeny and ontogeny of the cardiovascular (CV) system, allowing the acquisition of vasomotricity adapted to local metabolic demands, and systemic arterial pressure after birth. In pathology, RBCs collide with the arterial wall, inducing both local retention of their membranous lipids and local hemolysis, releasing heme-Fe^{++} with a high toxicity for arterial cells: endothelial and smooth muscle cells (SMCs) cardiomyocytes, neurons, etc. Specifically, overloading of cells by Fe^{++} promotes cell death. This local hemolysis is an event associated with early and advanced stages of human atherosclerosis. Similarly, the permanent renewal of mural RBC clotting is the major support of oxidation in abdominal aortic aneurysm. In parallel, calcifications promote intramural hemorrhages, and hemorrhages promote an osteoblastic phenotypic shift of arterial wall cells. Different plasma or tissue systems are able, at least in part, to limit this injury by acting at the different levels of this system.

Keywords: evolution; iron; oxidation; frictional forces; atheroma; intraplaque hemorrhages; clotting; aneurysm; calcification; infarction; stroke; senescence; inhibitors; anti-oxidant

---

1. Introduction

On the one hand, red blood cells (RBCs) or erythrocytes are the most abundant ($4.5 \ 10^6/mm^3$) circulating cells (90%). Platelets are the second most abundant ($300,000/mm^3$), and polymorpho-nuclear leucocytes (PMNs, $<8000/mm^3$) are the third. On the other hand, the arterial structures are permanently submitted to mechanical, biochemical and cellular stress, always initiated by hemodynamics, responsible for repeated wall injuries [1]. The purpose of the present synthesis is to describe the physiology and pathologies of the human arterial wall, directly involving RBCs and their derived membranous and cytosolic products. Therefore, we review observational data in humans, focusing on the presence of RBCs, hemoglobin and redox-active iron, and try to explain how RBCs, and particularly intratissue hemolysis and Fe^{++}-derived oxidative stress, are cytotoxic and directly participate in these human pathologies. Finally, RBCs and their derivatives are omnipresent in all cardiovascular (CV) and neurovascular (NV) pathologies.

2. How Phylogeny and Ontogeny Define Red Blood Cells (RBCs) in the Human Circulation

The circulation in invertebrates is composed of a myoepithelial tube (heart) generating motion of the hemolymph in an archaic circulatory system, directly open to the extracellular fluid. Hemolymph is composed of a fluid phase (plasma and interstitial fluid) and a cellular phase: hemocytes. Hemocytes are nucleated cells, mainly involved in innate immunity [2] and coagulation in invertebrates.

Oxygen transport is carried out more by plasma proteins such as hemocyanin (a blue copper-protein) than by hemocytes, which contain only a small quantity of hemoglobin (a red ferrous iron-protein). For instance, the ability of the horseshoe crab amoebocyte to clot (Limulus test), used for the sensitive detection of liposaccharides of bacterial origin [3], provides evidence of the role of amoebocytes in innate immunity and its mediation by clotting in invertebrates.

In fish (lower vertebrates), erythrocytes are nucleated, containing cytosolic organelles, carrying hemoglobin (Hb) and distributing oxygen to the body. However, they also actively participate in immunity, being involved in pathogen recognition, binding and clearance, particularly in antiviral defense [4], as an imprinting of the invertebrate stage.

In mammalian embryos, nucleated erythroblasts appear at three weeks and are produced by the yolk sac. During fetal life, the initial liver production shifts to bone-marrow, from five months until birth. After birth, the bone marrow remains the only site of hematopoiesis. Nucleated erythroblasts are derived from pluripotent hematopoietic progenitor cells [5], which are progressively loaded by synthesis of globin and iron recycling. Finally, the nucleus is expelled by an actin-dependent mechanism. Each erythrocyte is loaded with 30 pg of Hb. Besides RBC hemoglobin, other tissue goblins exist such as myoglobin, neuroglobin and cytoglobin, genetically derived from ancient hemoglobin. They predominantly serve for tissue oxygen storage, particularly in marine mammals. The mean life of erythrocytes is 120 days. In laminar rheology, RBCs flow in the center of the blood stream at a distance from the wall, whereas low-mass platelets flow in the periphery, close to the endothelium [6,7]. RBCs (8-μm diameter) are highly deformable, allowing them to penetrate very small channels, such as the 0.5-μm-wide slits in the reticulo-endothelial system of the spleen red pulp, and adapt their form to the circulating shear rate [8]. This property is linked, at least in part, to the enrichment of the RBC membrane in cholesterol with a high ratio of cholesterol to phospholipids. Non-laminar flow causes loss of this property and brings the RBCs close to the arterial wall.

With time, anucleate erythrocytes progressively expose phosphatidylserine (PS) on their external membrane, as a signal of senescence recognition. Fluorescent Annexin V binding in flow cytometry can be used to quantify this senescence [9]. Senescent RBC clearance [10] by phagocytes (spleen macrophages) is dependent on PS exposure and physiologically takes place in the red pulp of the spleen (for details, see Section: Clearance of senescent RBC physiology/pathology). In this context, transfusion experiments with fresh or conserved old blood provide an informative lesson about the relationship between RBC/Hb and the arterial tissue. There is evidence that blood submitted to a long storage before transfusion is not well supported in humans [11]. Experimental models of long versus short storage confirmed and extended these observational data. Baek and coworkers [12] performed an outstanding study comparing 2-day to 21- and 28-day RBC storage in guinea-pigs. The animals perfused with "senescent blood" presented a higher level of hemolysis with free hemoglobin within plasma, an acute hypertension mainly related to NO inhibition by free Hb, a decrease in RBC deformability, an increase in methemoglobin (Fe^{+++} Hb) and kidney and arterial injury (necrotic localized lesions). Finally, ferrous (Fe^{++}) redox-active iron accumulates in liver and spleen, as well as in the aortic wall. A majority of these detrimental effects are prevented by the co-administration of haptoglobin (Hp). Sickle cell anemia and malaria attacks share some similarities with this pathophysiology. These data demonstrate that senescent RBCs are frail and more sensitive to hemolysis and that their detrimental cytotoxicity on the arterial wall is mainly mediated by hemolysis and the powerful oxidative capacity of heme-ferrous iron. For instance, the focal external application of $FeCl_3$ is a usual model to induce experimental clotting in arteries. This model involves the inward cellular transport of $FeCl_3$ towards the endothelium and is dependent on local hemolysis of circulating RBCs [13]. Formation of endothelial RBC aggregates, hemolysis and loss of endothelium precede platelet activation and thrombus formation in this model [14]. This model underlines the importance of the interaction between redox-active iron, de-endothelialization and clotting in the CV system. Therefore, it is necessary to detect redox-active Fe^{++} in tissue submitted to local hemolysis.

3. Frictional Forces Involve RBCs and Interact with Nitric Oxide (NO)

Blood is a viscous fluid moving in the circulation due to the kinetic energy generated by the heart's pumping ability. Due to its high viscosity (51 ± 15 mPa), blood motion along the arterial tree generates frictional forces, which can transform kinetic energy (flow and shear stress) into potential energy (pressure), by the law of mechanical energy conservation in a closed homeothermic system (Bernoulli's principle) and dissipation of both kinetic and potential mechanical energy upstream to the capillary capacitive compartment. The first experimental description of frictional forces in the dog mesenteric arteries was made by Stephen Hale (1677–1761, Statical Essays containing haemostaticks; London 1733). The relationship among pressure, flow velocity, viscosity and arterial radius is defined by the Hagen–Poiseuille law in which peripheral resistance to flow is directly proportional to viscosity (1/1) and inversely proportional $(1/r^4)$ to the fourth power of the radius [1]. Therefore, changes in the radius are the most important determinants of variations in frictional forces, responsible for blood pressure, in association with viscosity. Blood viscosity components are dependent on both circulating cell density and plasma protein concentration. Since RBCs represent 90% of the circulating cells, in physiological conditions, the hematocrit is classically considered as the main determinant of blood viscosity.

Viscosity-dependent shear stress is also the main physiological activator of endothelial NO synthase. NO promotes smooth muscle cell (SMC) relaxation by inhibition of vasomotor tone, inducing functional dilation of the artery (local regulation of vasomotricity). Free Hb or heme are potent local or systemic chelators of NO, enhancing SMC contraction and arterial vasomotor tone within tissue (vasospasm), or systemic hypertension [15]. Heme from free Hb scavenges NO and forms nitrosoHb, promoting the shift of Fe^{++} (ferrous) to Fe^{+++} (ferric), forming metHb, which cannot bind oxygen, and nitrite release as an intermediate metastable metabolite rapidly converted to nitrate as the definitive stable metabolite [16]. However, NO can also be stored and transported by binding to cysteine 93 of the globin β−chain (SNOHb). NitrosoHb predominates. Moreover, nitrite can be reconverted to NO [17] by mitochondrial nitrite reductase in relation to hypoxia [18]. These NO pathways in interaction with Hb are mainly involved in hypoxia-induced vasodilation [18], but not in physiological shear endothelium-dependent vasodilation in which the inhibitory role of free Hb and nitrate formation predominates. Moreover, cytoglobin (Cygb), an ancient hemoglobin isoform, plays also a major role in the modulation of NO activity [19]. Cygb is the predominant globin in arterial SMCs. It has a powerful ability to metabolize NO due to its dioxygenase activity [20]. When NO reacts with the oxygen bound to Cygb-heme, it produces nitrate and the oxidative shift from the Fe^{++} to the Ferric Fe^{+++} reduced state, bound to ferritin (storage and recycling). Cygb has the capacity to act both functionally, by limiting in part the SMC relaxation caused by endothelial NO, and structurally. Cygb suppression in mouse inhibits SMC intimal proliferation in vivo and promotes SMC apoptosis in vitro [21].

In parallel, free Hb is highly toxic for endothelial cells [22]. Important frictional forces, involving RBCs colliding with endothelial cells are also, with time, the main determinant of endothelial abrasion in conductance arteries [23]. Exposure of circulating blood to subendothelial glyco-aminoglycans [24,25] and collagen promotes platelet activation and aggregation and finally RBC clotting. Erosion is relatively specific of the coronary circulation (not observed in carotid arteries for instance) and predominates in epicardial conductance arteries, since shear stress is high in protodiastole, when the left ventricle relaxes, and flow abruptly invades the myocardium. These cyclic transitory high frictional forces occur around 3.10^9 times during a lifespan of 80 years [1] and are responsible for endothelial abrasion. Erosion can cause localized de-endothelization and potentially acute coronary syndrome. This specific pathology predominates in women [26], potentially linked to the hormonal environment [27] and/or a high coronary flow rate during pregnancy and preeclampsia [28].

4. RBCs Colliding with the Arterial Wall

The relationship of atherosclerosis to arterial wall RBC accumulation, membrane cholesterol release forming cholesterol crystals [29], in situ hemolysis and powerful oxidative stress [30] are now well established. As described above, the evolution of the circulation from an "in series" closed system to an "in-parallel" system, with numerous changes in arterial wall geometry, has caused impingements of flow [1]. These changes in geometry induce loss in flow laminarity and an increased entropy (internal energy instability and dissipation) of the particulate part of the blood, promoting collision of blood cells with the wall and between themselves. The impact of colliding blood cells on the wall is mainly determined by the angulation of the bifurcation and luminal narrowing, but also depends on the hemorheology of circulating cells. The forces of collision impacting the wall are proportional to the mass (m) of the interacting RBCs and the velocity (v) at each point, corresponding to the mechanical quantity of movement (F = m.v). RBCs collide with the irregular geometry of the wall in participation or association with other biomechanical forces operating on the wall and drive intimal tears, micro-fissures and the formation of small mural hematomas. Collision of circulating cells among themselves is usually related to luminal dilation, associated with blood stagnation and vortices promoting endovascular clotting [31].

As proposed above, the phylogeny of circulating cells, involving hemocytes, innate immunity and clot formation, potentially imprints the behavior of these cells and the role of fibrinogen in mammals. In vivo, pure intra-tissue bleeding and the formation of mural hematoma without fibrin processing and coagulation does not exist. This is due to coagulation factor III (usually tissue factor, TF), a cell transmembrane protein, predominantly present on SMCs and on adventitial fibroblasts, in the arterial wall. TF initiates the extrinsic pathway of the coagulation [32]. This pathway leads to conversion of plasma prothrombin into active thrombin and finally to fibrin reticulation. These tissue and plasma cascades actively participate in physiological hemostasis, causing RBC clotting.

Conversely, thrombus formation without RBC entrapping within the fibrin network can occur in vivo (white clots including platelets, leukocytes and fibrin formation), but is unusual and a very large majority of thrombi are red (cruoric), due to the presence of RBCs within the fibrin network. Initial clotting is frequent in CV pathologies, due the platelet activation by the wall structural components (mainly collagen), including both plaque fissuration [33] and erosion [34]. The secondary fibrin reticulation entraps RBCs within the thrombi. Clotting can also be the consequence of blood stagnation and collision between circulating cells, related to dilation of the wall and hemodynamic vortices (aneurysm).

Therefore, the roles of RBCs in human atherosclerosis and related diseases are always intricately related with fibrin formation, fibrinolysis, platelet activation and fibrin entrapping of other circulating cells, mainly neutrophils [35]. Clotting of RBCs causes delayed hemolysis and release of membranes and Hb. Then, constituted clot evolves from red to brown and yellow, reflecting the transformation of hemoglobin, its oxidation and degradation. Until now, the relationship of RBCs to atherosclerosis was focused on tissue cholesterol enrichment by RBC membranes [29,36] in relation to intraplaque hemorrhages and plaque vulnerability [37]. In the present synthesis we focus on hemolysis occurring within tissues, associating extra and/or intracellular release of free hemoglobin and heme, which catalyze oxidative reactions by Fe^{++} as an electron donor. This pro-oxidant effect is not limited to the late stages (vulnerable plaque) [38] but also includes the initial stages of human atheroma and other associated acquired diseases.

In contrast, ferric iron (Fe^{+++}), the ferritin-bound storage form of iron, is essentially neutral, without direct oxidative capacity. This contrast between heminic (ferrous) and ferric iron is exemplified by hemochromatosis in human. Hemochromatosis is a disease due to an increase in ferric iron intestinal absorption, leading to important iron storages in the liver, pancreas, spleen and myocardium [39,40]. Absorbed iron under the control of hepcidin is intracellularly transported by ferritin and extracellularly by transferrin, maintaining its redox-inactivity. Contrasting with hemolysis, hemochromatosis does not injure the arterial wall, and hemochromatosis is not an independent risk factor for atherosclerosis [41–43]. These observational data in human highlight that the behavior of Fe^{++} and Fe^{+++} is quite different in living tissues.

5. Presence of RBCs and Redox-Active Ferrous Iron in Different Human Arterial Pathologies

5.1. Methods for Ionized iron Detection in CV Tissues

Because RBCs contain Fe^{++}-rich hemoglobin, fresh RBCs are able, in the presence of hydrogen peroxide (H_2O_2, Haber–Weiss and Fenton reactions), to produce free radicals and to oxidatively polymerize diaminobenzidine (DAB) into polybenzimidazole, forming a stable brown colored fiber, which precipitates within the tissue. This capacity disappears with ex-vivo time. In contrast, ferric iron (Fe^{+++}) usually chelated by ferritin in vivo (redox inactive) is not directly able to polymerize DAB, but reacts with ferrocyanide, which precipitates as ferricyanide (Prussian blue, Perl's reaction). The double reaction, first with ferricyanide and secondly, DAB polymerization in the presence of H_2O_2, is able to stain the redox-active Fe^{++}, reflecting the oxidative imprinting of heme within the arterial tissue. It can also be revealed by ferricyanide in the presence of H_2O_2 (Turnbull reaction) [44]. The oxidative power of Fe^{++} is directly linked to its ability to promote electron transfer to superoxide anions or hydroxyl radicals ($O_2 \cdot^-$ and $OH \cdot +$ Haber–Weiss and Fenton reactions). In these two reactions, redox-active Fe^{++} is the electron donor, catalyzing numerous oxidations of organic compounds such as lipids, proteins and DNA. Glycophorin A, a specific protein of the RBC, could also be used for detection or imprinting of cholesterol-rich RBC membranes within tissues. On histological sections, the co-localization of glycophorin A staining with cholesterol clefts (cholesterol crystals) suggests that these cholesterol clefts come from RBC membrane compaction within the vascular tissue.

In this tissue context, the formation of autofluorescent ceroids are markers of the ability of free heme to promote oxidation of lipids and proteins, forming an insoluble precipitate within the tissue. Since heme and hemoglobin spontaneously auto-fluoresce at 550 nm, ceroids are easily detected at this wavelength without staining. Ceroids can appear as punctiform cellular or extracellular autofluorescence, or as rings, reflecting a more advanced stage. For instance, ceroids can directly polymerize and precipitate DAB, providing evidence of heme-dependent oxidation. They can be also stained by oil red O on deparaffined sections, providing evidence of lipid entrapping in these insoluble aggregates.

5.2. Early Stages of Atheroma

Classically, the first step of human atherosclerosis is the deposit of lipids (fatty streaks, FS) in the most luminal subendothelial layer, where circulating plasma apolipoproteins (apo), involving apo B, low density lipoproteins (LDL) and lipoprotein, Lp(a), directly interact with the hydrophilic GlycosAmino Glycans [45] synthesized by the intimal SMCs. In this lipid environment, SMCs are able to engulf LDL forming foam cells that accumulate lipid vesicles. The mass transport of lipoproteins from plasma to the wall is dependent on the outward hydraulic advective conductance driven by the pressure gradient between the circulating blood (80–120 mmHg) and adventitial interstitium (10–40 mmHg). This is why atherosclerosis is specific to the arterial part of the circulation, depending on the arterial hemodynamics, and is not observed in the venous system [46]. In the aorta, FS develop preferentially in the near proximity of intercostal or lumbar ostia, where the subendothelial lipid deposits lift up the endothelial layer creating irregularities. Early on, it was proposed that free heme has a detrimental effect on endothelial cells via its oxidant capacity [47,48] and catalyzes the peroxidase activity of neutrophils. This small enhancement of the endothelial layer is potentially enough to induce collision of RBCs with the wall (Figure 1A). In parallel, the first hematomas also appear in the angulation of these ostia (Figure 1B), providing evidence of the importance of specific local hemodynamics in the development of atherosclerosis by both increasing outward transport of plasma lipoproteins to the wall and promoting localized RBC collisions and hemolysis. These FS and early hematomas are progressively covered over by migrating SMCs that proliferate and synthesize extracellular matrix (ECM), producing the fibro-cellular cap. This healing process defines the second step in atheroma progression, plaques of fibro-atheroma (FA) with a lipid core and the cap. The lipid core is mainly acellular, due to the death of the SMCs. At this stage, whatever the source of lipids, lipoproteins or RBC membranes, the high density of tissue cholesterol forms crystals, liquid crystals which predominate in fatty streaks, progressing towards solid crystals which predominate in FA [49]. A similar process has been observed in coronary arteries.

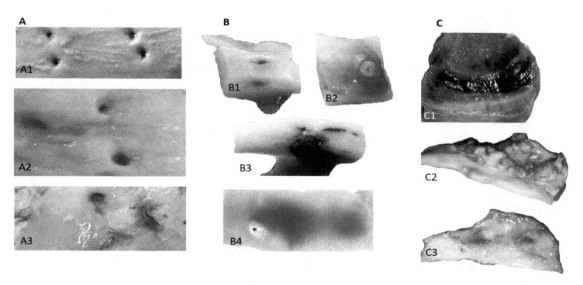

Figure 1. Macroscopic view of hemorrhages in human arterial lesions: (**A**) involvement of RBCs in the initial stages of human atherosclerotic lesions ((**A1**) aortic fatty streaks in human aorta and their relationship to intercostal ostia; (**A2**) fibro-atheroma with limited subintimal bleeding; (**A3**) more advanced lesions with numerous small hemorrhages and intimal breaches); (**B**) 0stial hematoma ((**B1**) ostial luminal view; (**B2**) outside collateral view; (**B3**) longitudinal trans-ostial section showing the local diffusion of the hematoma; and (**B4**) whole-mount immunostaining of Glycophorin A in peri-ostial clarified aortic tissue showing the hematoma diffusion from the ostia (*)); and (**C**) ILT in AAA and aortic valve; (**C1**) the multilayered intraluminal thrombus (ILT) of human AAA, where the most luminal layer (red) is extremely rich in RBCs and the subjacent layers are yellow/brown, demonstrating the release of heme and ferrous iron, and the metabolism of hemoglobin into bilirubin; (**C2**) aortic view of a calcified aortic valve, with peri-calcification hemorrhages (red), where the macro-crystallized calcifications protrude from the fibrosa; and (**C3**) view of the ventricularis of the same valve where the ventricularis surface is smoother than that of the fibrosa and the neo-angiogenesis network is visible (red)).

The constitution of a biobank of healthy and early or late pathological human cardiovascular tissues, provides opportunities to compare advanced pathologies to early stages and healthy arterial walls and hearts, including coronary arteries (PFS 09-007, BRIF BB-0033-00029; BBMRI-EU/infrastructure BIOBANK). Using this original and rare human material resource, Delbosc and coworkers [9] observed the presence and demonstrated the role of RBCs and ferrous iron release in the initial stages of atheroma in human aorta. Using ferrocyanide, H_2O_2 + DAB polymerization (see above), they revealed the presence of redox-active Fe^{++} mainly present in foam cells, whereas the redox inactive, ferritin-stored, Fe^{+++} was detectable by the Perl's reaction alone in these tissues and also in foam cells. The redox active Fe^{++} was associated with the presence of Hb, which colocalized with SMC myosin, suggesting that SMCs could endocytose hemoglobin or phagocytose RBCs. This process was associated with the presence of lipids (Oil Red O), autofluorescent (550 nm) red granules and small rings (ceroids) and glyphorin A (RBC membranes), providing evidence that RBCs penetrate early into the aortic intima and release hemoglobin and heme-iron (Figure 2). The quantity of iron present in the intimal tissue significantly increased with the progression from FS to FA. These foam SMCs were CD68 positive, showing activation of their phagolysosome. In this context, tissue redox-active iron and hemoglobin was increased in FS as compared to healthy aorta, but less than in FA, providing evidence that RBC-dependent release of redox-active iron is associated with the progression of the atheroma.

As a consequence of this iron-dependent oxidative injury, the level of oxidized lipids and proteins were significantly increased in the intima of early stages of atheroma. Conversely, an increased tissue expression of natural resistance-associated macrophage protein (NRAMP), ferritin, ferroportin, hepcidin, heme-oxygenase (HO-1) and mannose receptor was associated with this hemolytic oxidative injury. This human tissue approach was completed by a cellular one in which human SMCs were cultured in the presence of fresh or senescent (PS-exposing) RBCs (Figure 3). Similar tissue observations were made in early stages of atherosclerosis in human coronary arteries. These data extend preceding data showing the presence of transition metal ions, mainly iron, in FS and their correlation to cholesterol accumulation [50]. In this context, redox-active iron could play a major role in the early oxidation of LDL [51]. These data are also important because the passage of a lipid into a necrotic core, involving cell death, is an important step in the evolution of atheroma towards the clinical expression of the disease. The cytotoxicity of free hemoglobin, releasing redox-active Fe^{++}, promoting endoplasmic reticulum stress and oxidation of lipids, proteins and DNA, is now well established [52].

A specific iron-dependent, non-apoptotic process of cell death, named ferroptosis, has been described in cancer cells [53]. Ferroptosis involves the presence of redox-active iron, lipid peroxidation, mitochondrial fission and cell detachment, and it is largely dependent of non-enzymatic reactions [54]. This process was rescued by iron chelation (deferoxamine) and anti-oxidants [55]. This cytotoxic pathway could also be induced by ferric iron. It necessitates the entrance into the cell of the Fe^{+++}/transferrin complex via the transferrin receptor and its reduction in Fe^{++} by endosomal ferric reductase at pH 5.2–5.6. It was recently shown that smoking-induced SMC toxicity in the CV system is mediated by ferroptosis [56]. Therefore, both SMCs and endothelial cells could be targets for ferroptosis [57]. To the best of our knowledge, the role of ferroptosis in the impact of hemoglobin-generated ferrous iron on the arterial wall remains to be explored.

5.3. Neo-Angiogenesis and Intraplaque Hemorrhages

Physiologically, the arterial media and intima are avascular; only the adventitia, the external layer of the wall, is vascularized (vasa vasorum). Thus, transport of soluble molecules and diapedesis of circulating cells are quite different between the arterial wall and the capillaries. In the capillaries, where pressure and velocity are low, oxygen and glucose transport is mainly due to diffusion, in which the concentration gradients are the driving force. In contrast, this transport is advective (convection) in the arterial wall, due to the hydraulic conductance driven by a pressure gradient that is more efficient than diffusion. Therefore, there is no phylogenic and developmental need for the presence of capillaries to ensure the energetic support of the wall media [1], and circulating cell diapedesis essentially occurs in the adventitia. Neo-angiogenesis within the wall is essentially associated with pathology. Due to the metabolism of retained phospholipids by phospholipase A_2 (PLA_2) in fatty streaks and fibroatheroma, arachidonic acid is generated and the cyclo-oxygenase pathway activated. This pathway produces prostanoids, including prostaglandin J2, which activate the expression of vascular endothelial growth factor (VEGF) by subjacent SMCs (growth factor gradient and outward convection) [58]. SMC-VEGF initiates neo-angiogenesis from the adventitia towards the plaque [59]. However, these neo-vessels remain frail because of the proteolytic micro-environment within the advanced plaques [60]. This neo-angiogenesis allows diapedesis of RBCs throughout the neo-endothelium toward the medial tissue. It is the main source of bleeding when neo-vessels reach the plaque core. These intraplaque hemorrhages also lead to clotting including fibrin formation and leukocyte retention, which increase both the proteolytic [61] and the oxidant activities of MPO by Fe^{++} [62] within the core, promoting plaque vulnerability [38]. These events are one of the most important causes of the evolution of atherothrombotic diseases towards clinical expression [63,64]. These intraplaque hemorrhages have been described in culprit plaques of different localizations: coronary arteries [29], carotid arteries [65] and infrarenal aorta (see below AAA).

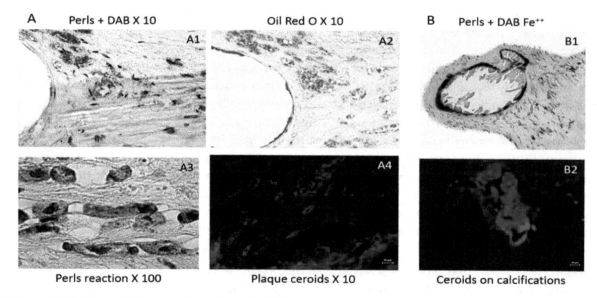

Figure 2. Histological views of tissue hemolysis in human aortic plaques and valves: (**A**) atherosclerosis ((**A1**) Perl's + DAB staining of redox-active Fe^{++} in the shoulder of an atherosclerotic plaque; (**A2**) ORO lipid staining, colocalizing with Fe^{++} on a serial section; (**A3**) high magnification of foam SMCs by Prussian blue precipitation, showing the presence of Fe^{+++}, potentially linked to ferritin (redox-inactive); and (**A4**) autofluorescent (550-nm wavelength, red) ceroid rings in an atherosclerotic plaque); and (**B**) calcified aortic valves ((**B1**) a crown of ferrous iron around calcification in an aortic valve, suggesting a compliant mismatch between the solid calcification and the soft elastic valve tissue; and (**B2**) red autofluorescence (550-nm wavelength) directly associated with aortic valve calcification).

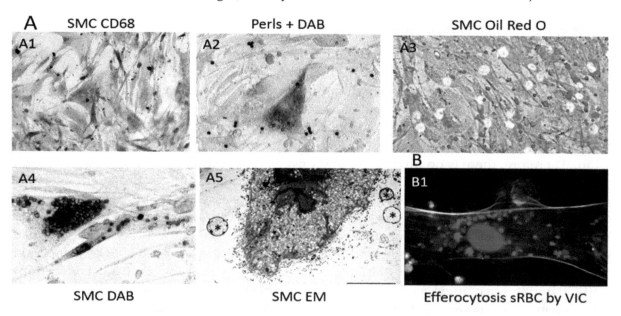

Figure 3. Phagocytosis of senescent RBCs by cultured human SMCs: (**A**) SMCs exposed to senescent sRBCs ((**A1**) acquisition of CD68, the phagolysosome functional marker of phagocytosis activity by cultured SMCs, usually used as a marker of macrophages, but not lineage-specific; (**A2**) acquisition of intracellular Fe^{++} staining; (**A3**) acquisition of lipid staining from sRBC membranes within SMCs; (**A4**) early phagocytosis of intact sRBCs, stained by DAB alone (pseudo-peroxidase activity); and (**A5**) electron microscopic view of efferocytosis of sRBCs by cultured human SMCs with the presence of extracellular RBC skeletons (*), containing hyperdense bodies, potentially iron and extracellular release of numerous micro-vesicles and exosomes by the sRBC-phagocytic SMCs); and (**B**) valvular Interstitial Cell (VIC) ((**B1**) efferocytosis of sRBCs (red) by human VIC).

5.4. In-Stent Neoatherosclerosis

Currently used drug-eluting stents (DESs), despite preventing SMC proliferation-induced restenosis, promote the development of in-stent neoatherosclerosis [66]. We recently observed that peri-strut micro-hemorrhages were the main pathological phenomenon associated the long-term implantation of DES [67], leading to the development of late in-stent vulnerable plaques and finally to delayed thrombosis [68,69]. These hemorrhages are mainly related to the mechanical mismatch between the elastic behavior of the arterial wall (pulsation) and the unalterable rigid property of the metal stent, acting at each systolo/diastolic motion (see below calcifications).

5.5. Consequences of Clot Integration

Besides bleeding, the integration of a clot within the arterial wall is a historic observational paradigm in human atherothrombotic disease. The famous Austrian pathologist C. Rokitansky (1804–1878) described the arterial atheromatous process as evolutive intimal blood deposits, including advective insudation of plasma proteins (convection) [70] and blood cell deposits and their integration within the intima [71]. In this context, the integration of RBC clotting is one of the main pathological phenomena [72] associating, as usual, RBC membrane release participating (not exclusively, as platelet membranes may also play a role [73]) in tissue enrichment in cholesterol and its crystallization, and associated oxidative processes due to hemoglobin and Fe^{++} release [47]. These early observations were reinforced by the study of E. Arbustini [36] showing that atherosclerotic fatty plaques can develop in pulmonary arteries only in cases of pulmonary artery hypertension (PAH) secondary to pulmonary embolism but not in cases of primary PAH. The observed pultaceous plaques consist of organizing thrombi, foam cells, cholesterol clefts, vascular angiogenesis, RBCs and sometimes calcifications, usually incorporated into the pulmonary arterial wall from the embolism.

Whatever the source, bleeding or thrombus integration, RBC retention within the wall and intratissue hemolysis participate actively in oxidation. High Density Lipoproteins (HDL) also transit through the wall, potentially more than LDL, but do not interfere with the early stages of human atherosclerosis. In advanced stages of atherothrombosis, the association of redox-active hemoglobin with neutrophil MPO is so powerfully oxidative that it oxidizes ApoA1 (the main apo of HDL) and separates it from its lipid cargo [74] in the arterial wall [75]. In this context, free oxidized ApoA1 (MW 30,000 Da) is filtrated by the glomerulus and metabolized in the proximal tubule via cubulin, decreasing the plasma bio-availability of ApoA1. This mural oxidative pathway potentially explains the observed decrease in HDL associated with the progression of oxidation, and atherothrombosis in human [76]. Conversely the observed decrease in tissue HDL is a biomarker of arterial wall oxidation due to the additional interaction of hemolysis with MPO release.

5.6. RBC Clotting in Aneurysms of the Abdominal Aorta

As described by S. Glagov in human autopsy studies [63], the infrarenal aorta is a privileged site for atherothrombotic disease. Arterial modeling during the fetal life in mammals is mainly adapted to frictional forces due to flow [1]. The heart and aorta are submitted to a high flow load during fetal life because they support both the vascularization of the fetal body (60%) and the placental circulation (40%). Therefore, the aortic diameter remains abnormally large after birth, with a low shear rate ($16 \, \text{s}^{-1}$ in the aorta, ten times less as compared to $160 \, \text{s}^{-1}$ in common carotid artery) and a high tensional stress as the product of pressure multiplied by radius [1]. Therefore, the infrarenal aorta is highly sensitive to atherothrombosis including clotting, plaque hemorrhages and calcifications. However, due to the wide aortic diameter, these acquired pathologies can remain asymptomatic at this site, for long periods.

They may specifically and frequently evolve toward aneurysmal lesions (AAA), which are characterized by the development of luminal clotting (intraluminal thrombus, ILT), permanently renewed by the circulation [77]. RBC trapping and hemolysis are the most important components of the ILT in association with fibrin formation and neutrophil trapping [78]. We observed first the predominant role of RBC trapping by the ILT and the bipolar pro-oxidative role of this process, involving both the oxidation in the ILT, but also the outward transport of ferrous iron and associated oxidative reaction toward adventitia [79], able to initiate and promote adaptive immune response in the adventitia [80,81]. In these seminal studies, we observed the ability of luminal RBC entrapping to oxidatively precipitate DAB (Fe^{++}), but also retention of cholesterol-rich membrane promoting cholesterol crystal cleft formation. In this context, iron is outwardly transported to adventitia and storage of Fe^{+++} (Perl's) was observed at the interface with adventitia [79] (Figure 4). Thiobarbituric acid reactive substances (TBARS) markers of lipid oxidation, advanced oxidation protein product (AOPP) and 8-hydroxy-deoxyguanosine (8-OH-dG) products of DNA oxidation were intensively release by all AAA wall, including adventitia. Moreover, conditioned media of the most luminal layer of the ILT provoked a high level of ROS production and SMC apoptosis when incubated with cultured SMC, a process which was significantly rescued by Hb depletion or iron chelation (Deferoxamine). Moreover, the ILT has renewal and lytic dynamics, consumptive of platelets and fibrinogen, but also of circulating RBCs causing hemolysis and relative anemia [82]. This consumptive anemia is characterized by a decrease in RBC count and blood hemoglobin, associated with low circulating iron and transferrin, but high iron retention and hepcidin concentration, leading to altered iron recycling. Such consumptive anemia is predictive of poor patient outcome, and, in association with neutrophil MPO, of intensive oxidation dynamics [83]. As described above for advanced atherosclerosis, ApoA-1 is highly sensitive to oxidation and the ILT of AAA induces this oxidation [84] rendering HDL less protective for vascular tissue. Therefore, AAA evolution in humans is characterized by consumption of HDL by ILT oxidative dynamics, correlated with the decrease in plasma ApoA-1 and inversely correlated with AAA size and ILT volume [85]. HDL consumption by ILT oxidative dynamics is predictive of AAA growth, and HDL plasma levels were shown to be inversely associated with the need of surgical repair. Moreover, the HDL decrease observed in AAA patients is more intense than the decrease observed in patients with aorto-iliac atherosclerosis. These data are impressive, showing how much the constant renewal of the ILT with new RBCs and, potentially, neutrophils is redox-active, generating anemia with iron retention and further HDL degradation and ApoA-1 dysfunction. Therefore, the decrease in HDL associated with different localizations and forms of atherothrombosis provides evidence of heme-dependent oxidation during HDL transport through the wall [75]. In this context, magnetic resonance imaging (MRI) can detect iron as a black signal in the most luminal part of the ILT and at the wall/adventitia interface, both sites where ferric iron accumulates within phagocytes. This spontaneous signal can be enhanced by superparamagnetic status of ultra-small particle iron oxide (USPIO) [86,87].

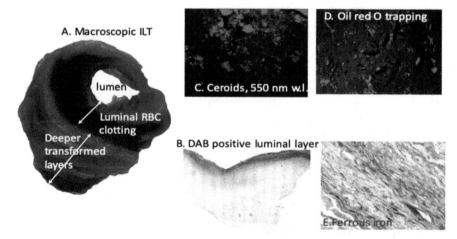

Figure 4. RBC-dependent oxidative stress in AAA: (**A**) macroscopic luminal view of the thrombus, with a predominant RBC fresh clotting at the interface with circulating blood; (**B**) diaminobenzidin (DAB) staining of RBC in the most luminal layer; (**C**) autofluorescent ceroids (550 nm), the wavelength of Hb; (**D**) oil red O staining of lipids (orange color); and (**E**) Perl's blue staining of Fe^{+++}, the storage redox inactive form of iron, bound to ferritin and transported by transferrin (recycling).

5.7. RBCs and Vascular Calcifications

The relationship between valvular and arterial calcifications [88] and RBCs or Hb are bidirectional: calcifications promote hemorrhages and hemoglobin release promotes calcifications of elastic vascular tissues. The initiation of calcifications in soft vascular tissues is directly related to extracellular exposure of tissue-cell-derived anionic phosphates (PO_4^{3-}) on which the ionized soluble cationic calcium (Ca^{++}) precipitates. This reaction leads to the formation of calcium-phosphate [$Ca_3(PO_4)_2$], which polymerizes into solid hydroxyapatite crystals (mineralization). This passive process rapidly initiates a phenotypic switch of SMCs towards an osteoblastic phenotype [89]. In the context of soft viscoelastic tissues such as arterial and valvular walls, calcifications promote a mechanical mismatch between the high strain of the elastic tissue, measured by finite element analysis, and the solid crystals, inducing a distortion energy at the interface between solid calcifications and elastic tissues (von Mises stress) [90]. This distortion causes fatigue-like repeated microdamage such as microscopic tears or macroscopic hemorrhages at the interface between calcifications and elastic tissue where the distortion shear is maximal. When microcalcifications develop in the intima, they can cause some breaches, which may sensitize to plaque rupture [91,92]. If the calcifications develop deeper in the media, distortion forces can induce tears of the neo-vascularization (see above) and peri-calcification hemorrhages [67]. A similar scenario develops in the aortic valves (Figure 1(C2) and Figure 2B). Aortic valve diseases are initiated by transvalvular transport of plasma lipoproteins, mainly LDL and Lp(a), during diastole, due to the pressure gradient between the aorta and the intraventricular diastolic pressure. This is why the lesions always develop in the fibrosa of the aortic valve (ventricularis for the mitral valve). Similar to healthy arterial media, healthy valves are avascular tissues [93]. As in the early stages of atheroma, lipid accumulation in the fibrosa can promote the development of angiogenesis within the valves, a process always associated with aortic valve diseases. In this context, microcalcifications develop in the fibrosa and could cause neovascularization tears and hemorrhages, which accelerate the calcification process [94], because hemoglobin and its derivatives (heme, ferrous iron, free radicals and NF-kB activation) promote the release of exosomes and the osteoblastic differentiation of valvular interstitial cells [95] as well as of SMCs in the arterial wall [96]. Therefore, there is a vicious circle between calcifications and RBC/iron which promotes exponential development of both valvular and vascular calcifications in association with CV risk factors: aging, tobacco, dyslipidemia, etc. These data suggest that membrane-associated release of NO promotes an osteoblastic shift in SMCs [97]. In this study, the authors showed that, besides phospholipids, isolated RBC membranes are able to promote vascular calcifications, independently of hemoglobin and depending on NO release by membranes. Membranes from RBCs deficient in NO synthase have limited procalcifying effects. These data suggest that, besides phospholipid support associated of RBC membranes, NO release complementarily promotes an osteoblastic shift in SMCs [97]. SMCs phagocytosing RBCs release numerous microvesicles and exosomes exposing the amphiphilic pole of phospholipids [9].

5.8. Myocardial Infarction (MI)

Heme-iron homeostasis is paradoxical in cardiac diseases, depending on the environmental conditions: local myocardial iron retention and tissue toxicity in MI [98] and systemic anemia in heart failure (HF) [99]. The frequency of anemia is around 30% in HF patients and hemoglobin is inversely correlated to left ventricle ejection fraction. The pathophysiology of anemia is multifactorial and heterogenous [100], but associated with inadequate erythropoietin [101], a decline in circulating hepcidin and an iron deficit [100]. Low hepcidin independently relates to unfavorable outcome.

There are two sources of heme-iron within the heart: hemoglobin of circulating RBCs in the coronary circulation and myoglobin, a hemoprotein for oxygen storage within cardiomyocytes, which is released into the plasma during MI. MI is always variably associated with erythrodiapedesis and hemorrhagic transformation, leading to tissue iron retention. The importance of iron retention, detected by MRI, has a predictive value for adverse remodeling of the LV and evolution toward HF [102]. As reported above for arteries, this detrimental effect is directly related to the cytotoxicity of heme-iron and catalysis of free radical release. Beside the ischemic death of cardiomyocytes, ferroptosis (see above) is certainly an aggravating factor of cell loss, extending the dysfunctional area and promoting detrimental evolution toward congestive HF [103].

5.9. Stroke

The neurotoxicity of free hemoglobin is well known. Neurons do not survive more than 24 h of exposure to hemoglobin. Therefore, erythrodiapedesis and hemolysis in the brain tissue, hemorrhages and hemorrhagic transformation of ischemic stroke are highly aggravating. It has been recently demonstrated that secondary vasospasm (due to NO inhibition by Hb) and neurotoxicity (due to subarachnoid hemorrhage) were rescued by the infusion of Hp in the cerebral spinal fluid, by a direct inhibition and sequestration of Hb-Hp complexes (m.w. > 100 kD) [104]. With regard to intact RBCs, erythrophagocytosis by microglia [105] is usually insufficient to prevent free hemoglobin release and neurotoxicity. Similar to myoglobin in muscles, neuroglobin is a reserve form of hemoprotein able to store oxygen and protect the brain, at least in part, from hypoxic/ischemic insults [106]. Ferroptosis also plays a role in secondary cell death in hemorrhagic stroke [107,108] and selenium loading can partially prevent ferroptosis in experimental strokes [109].

6. Protection from RBC Injury: From Cells, Plasma and Antioxidant Molecules

6.1. Clearance of Senescent RBC Physiology/Pathology

Clearance by phagocytosis is the physiological mechanism by which spleen macrophages remove senescent (s)RBCs, allowing the renewal of circulating RBCs. Erythrocytes pass through the cords of Billroth and reticular cell-rich sinusoids in the red pulp (reticulo-endothelial system), which contains a large population of monocytes and macrophages (professional phagocytes). sRBC exposing PS are engulfed by these macrophages and metabolized, allowing iron transport by transferrin and recycling within bone marrow. However, this physiological system corresponds to a systemic homeostasis of blood RBCs. In contrast, tissue stromal cells, including arterial wall SMCs [110], valvular interstitial cells (VIC) in cardiac valves [95], interstitial fibroblasts in the myocardium, glial cells [105] in the brain and epithelial cells [111], are also capable of local tissue RBC efferocytosis. Many data exist showing that non-professional phagocytosis, involved in efferocytosis, is a general feature of cells in most tissues [112]. This point is important in pathophysiology, because it suggests that professional phagocytes, macrophages for instance, are not mandatory for tissue debridement by efferocytosis [113]. Primary cultures of arterial SMCs are able to clear (and metabolize) a load of 10^6 senescent RBCs in five days, whereas fresh RBCs remained intact. Senescent RBCs were phagocytosed by SMCs [110], whereas fresh RBCs were not (Figure 3). This phagocytic capacity of SMCs confirmed previous results, showing that this SMC phagocytosis is dependent on PS exposure [114]. SMC phagocytosis of RBCs causes accumulation of lipids (from membranes) and ferrous iron, and it increases their production of ROS. RBC phagocytosis also induces expression of CD68 (phagolysosome) and the synthesis of HO-1 and ferritin. After RBC intracellular hemolysis, lipid and hemoglobin metabolisms completely diverge. Heme, having gotten rid of globin, is metabolized by HO-1 into biliverdin, CO and Fe^{++}, which is oxidized into redox-inactive Fe^{+++}. Ferric iron binds to ferritin and can be exported, stored or recycled under the control of hepcidin. Similar capacities of efferocytosis were observed with cultured VIC (Figure 3(B1))

6.2. Haptoglobin, CD 163, Hemopexin, Deferoxamine

Haptoglobin (Hp, liver synthesis and secretion) is the endogenous direct ligand-inhibitor of free Hb [115]. The complex can be measured in the plasma as a marker of hemolysis. Hp structure and functions is genetically determined. The Hp/Hb complex binds the scavenger receptor CD163 present on numerous cells, physiologically including the spleen reticulo-endothelial system, but also SMCs of the pulmonary artery [116]. To the best of our knowledge, the ability of the arterial wall, particularly SMCs, to clear Hp/Hb complexes has not yet been explored.

Hemopexin is the endogenous ligand-inhibitor of free heme [117]. The heme/hemopexin complex is endocytosed by low density related protein-1 (LRP-1), a poorly selective scavenger receptor [118] highly present in SMCs. LRP-1 is able to engulf numerous complexes, such as LDL, protease/antiprotease complexes, heme/hemopexin, etc. More than 40 possible ligands have been identified [2].

Deferoxamine is a pharmacological iron chelator able to enter the cell, bind free iron and remove it via excretion in urine and feces [119]. By this direct effect on iron, chelators are capable of limiting iron-dependent oxidative stress within tissues and cells [120].

6.3. Anti-Oxidants: Glutathione, Thioredoxin, Peroxiredoxin, SOD, Glutathione Peroxidases, Catalase, Paraoxonase

Redox imbalance in the arterial wall could be the result of high ROS production but also of decreased/altered antioxidant systems. The main antioxidants comprise catalase, paraoxonase (PON), superoxide dismutase (SOD), glutathione (GSH) and glutathione peroxidases (GPX) and proteins of the thioredoxin (TRX) family, including TRX, TRX-reductase and peroxiredoxins (PRDXs) [121]. The role of these proteins in chronic vascular diseases has been previously reviewed [122]. Hydrogen peroxide (H_2O_2) produced by autoxidation of Hb is a predominant ROS in RBCs [123]. While intracellular ROS are neutralized by the highly abundant cytosolic antioxidant systems in RBCs (catalase, GPX and PRDX), ROS associated with Hb oxidation (among them, heme degradation products) are mainly located on the membrane [123]. An increase in heme products has been found in the membrane fraction of sRBCs and of pathological RBCs (with less stable Hb) [124]. In this respect, we previously showed that both catalase and PRDX-2 are decreased in the membrane of RBCs from AAA patients [125]. Moreover, a decreased activity of membrane bound antioxidant systems has been suggested to potentially decrease RBC lifespan [126], which could lead to anemia. Moreover, a low level of GPX-1 activity in RBCs is associated with increased cardiovascular risk and with future cardiovascular events [127,128]. Moreover, other cells with high pro-oxidant content such as neutrophils also contain antioxidant enzymes, such as catalase and SOD. Interestingly, both enzymes were decreased in neutrophils from AAA patients [129].

Finally, antioxidants could also have a non-cellular source such as those present in plasma (vitamins) or associated with plasma components (e.g., lipoproteins). The role of vitamins in preventing CVD is still a matter of debate, but new data support the importance of the correct identification of a specific target population for this treatment, such as patients with diabetes mellitus (DM) and the Hp genotype 2-2 [130]. Interestingly, Hp-Hb deficient clearance in Hp 2-2 DM individuals results in increased Hp-Hb binding to ApoA1 on HDL, thereby tethering the pro-oxidative heme moiety to HDL [131]. In addition, the activity of PON-1, the main antioxidant enzyme associated with HDL, is decreased in both atherosclerosis and AAA patients [131,132]. Thus, all these data strongly support the hypothesis that redox imbalance in chronic vascular remodeling could be derived, at least in part, from reduced antioxidant activities of both cell and plasma sources.

7. Conclusions

Because of their abundance, blood RBCs maintain permanent physiological and/or pathological interference with CV tissues, mainly the arterial wall, cardiac valves, kidneys, myocardium and brain tissues. Physiologically, RBCs are the main determinant of blood viscosity and, therefore, of the frictional forces exerted by the circulating blood on the arterial wall. In pathology, acute and chronic local colliding of RBCs with the wall, causing tissue hemolysis, is a major source of redox-active iron. Fe^{++} is the major catalyzer of all the oxidative reactions in living cells and tissues. In this pathological context, the main future challenge is to explore how to protect SMC, the stromal cell of the arterial wall, against iron-dependent oxidative stress in conjunction with biomechanical stress.

Acknowledgments: I would like to thank Mary Osborne-Pellegrin for English editing of the review, Jamila Laschet and Marion Morvan for their help with the figures.

References

1. Michel, J.B. Phylogenic determinants of cardiovascular frailty, focus on hemodynamics and arterial smooth muscle cells. *Physiol. Rev.* **2020**, *100*, 1779–1837. [CrossRef] [PubMed]
2. Buchmann, K. Evolution of innate immunity: Clues from invertebrates via fish to mammals. *Front. Immunol.* **2014**, *5*, 459. [CrossRef]
3. Iwanaga, S. Biochemical principle of Limulus test for detecting bacterial endotoxins. *Proc. Jpn. Acad. Ser. B Phys. Biol. Sci.* **2007**, *83*, 110–119. [CrossRef] [PubMed]
4. Chico, V.; Salvador-Mira, M.E.; Nombela, I.; Puente-Marin, S.; Ciordia, S.; Mena, M.C.; Perez, L.; Coll, J.; Guzman, F.; Encinar, J.A.; et al. IFIT5 Participates in the Antiviral Mechanisms of Rainbow Trout Red Blood Cells. *Front. Immunol.* **2019**, *10*, 613. [CrossRef]
5. Ogawa, M. Hematopoiesis. *J. Allergy Clin. Immunol.* **1994**, *94*, 645–650. [CrossRef]
6. Aarts, P.A.; van den Broek, S.A.; Prins, G.W.; Kuiken, G.D.; Sixma, J.J.; Heethaar, R.M. Blood platelets are concentrated near the wall and red blood cells, in the center in flowing blood. *Arteriosclerosis* **1988**, *8*, 819–824. [CrossRef]
7. Uijttewaal, W.S.; Nijhof, E.J.; Bronkhorst, P.J.; Den Hartog, E.; Heethaar, R.M. Near-wall excess of platelets induced by lateral migration of erythrocytes in flowing blood. *Am. J. Physiol.* **1993**, *264*, H1239–H1244. [CrossRef] [PubMed]
8. Viallat, A.; Abkarian, M. Red blood cell: From its mechanics to its motion in shear flow. *Int. J. Lab. Hematol.* **2014**, *36*, 237–243. [CrossRef]
9. Delbosc, S.; Bayles, R.G.; Laschet, J.; Ollivier, V.; Ho-Tin-Noe, B.; Touat, Z.; Deschildre, C.; Morvan, M.; Louedec, L.; Gouya, L.; et al. Erythrocyte efferocytosis by the arterial wall promotes oxidation in early-stage atheroma in humans. *Front. Cardiovasc. Med.* **2017**, *4*, 43. [CrossRef]
10. Lutz, H.U.; Bogdanova, A. Mechanisms tagging senescent red blood cells for clearance in healthy humans. *Front. Physiol.* **2013**, *4*, 387. [CrossRef] [PubMed]
11. McQuilten, Z.K.; French, C.J.; Nichol, A.; Higgins, A.; Cooper, D.J. Effect of age of red cells for transfusion on patient outcomes: A systematic review and meta-analysis. *Transfus. Med. Rev.* **2018**, *32*, 77–88. [CrossRef]
12. Baek, J.H.; D'Agnillo, F.; Vallelian, F.; Pereira, C.P.; Williams, M.C.; Jia, Y.; Schaer, D.J.; Buehler, P.W. Hemoglobin-driven pathophysiology is an in vivo consequence of the red blood cell storage lesion that can be attenuated in guinea pigs by haptoglobin therapy. *J. Clin. Invest.* **2012**, *122*, 1444–1458. [CrossRef] [PubMed]
13. Woollard, K.J.; Sturgeon, S.; Chin-Dusting, J.P.; Salem, H.H.; Jackson, S.P. Erythrocyte hemolysis and hemoglobin oxidation promote ferric chloride-induced vascular injury. *J. Biol. Chem.* **2009**, *284*, 13110–13118. [CrossRef] [PubMed]
14. Barr, J.D.; Chauhan, A.K.; Schaeffer, G.V.; Hansen, J.K.; Motto, D.G. Red blood cells mediate the onset of thrombosis in the ferric chloride murine model. *Blood* **2013**, *121*, 3733–3741. [CrossRef] [PubMed]
15. Helms, C.C.; Gladwin, M.T.; Kim-Shapiro, D.B. Erythrocytes and vascular function: Oxygen and nitric oxide. *Front. Physiol.* **2018**, *9*, 125. [CrossRef]
16. Gladwin, M.T.; Ognibene, F.P.; Pannell, L.K.; Nichols, J.S.; Pease-Fye, M.E.; Shelhamer, J.H.; Schechter, A.N. Relative role of heme nitrosylation and beta-cysteine 93 nitrosation in the transport and metabolism of nitric oxide by hemoglobin in the human circulation. *Proc. Natl. Acad. Sci. USA* **2000**, *97*, 9943–9948. [CrossRef]
17. van Faassen, E.E.; Bahrami, S.; Feelisch, M.; Hogg, N.; Kelm, M.; Kim-Shapiro, D.B.; Kozlov, A.V.; Li, H.; Lundberg, J.O.; Mason, R.; et al. Nitrite as regulator of hypoxic signaling in mammalian physiology. *Med. Res. Rev.* **2009**, *29*, 683–741. [CrossRef]
18. Dungel, P.; Penzenstadler, C.; Ashmwe, M.; Dumitrescu, S.; Stoegerer, T.; Redl, H.; Bahrami, S.; Kozlov, A.V. Impact of mitochondrial nitrite reductase on hemodynamics and myocardial contractility. *Sci. Rep.* **2017**, *7*, 12092. [CrossRef]
19. Mathai, C.; Jourd'heuil, F.L.; Lopez-Soler, R.I.; Jourd'heuil, D. Emerging perspectives on cytoglobin, beyond NO dioxygenase and peroxidase. *Redox Biol.* **2020**, *32*, 101468. [CrossRef]
20. Zweier, J.L.; Ilangovan, G. Regulation of nitric oxide metabolism and vascular tone by cytoglobin. *Antioxid. Redox Signal.* **2020**, *32*, 1172–1187. [CrossRef]

21. Jourd'heuil, F.L.; Xu, H.; Reilly, T.; McKellar, K.; El Alaoui, C.; Steppich, J.; Liu, Y.F.; Zhao, W.; Ginnan, R.; Conti, D.; et al. The hemoglobin homolog cytoglobin in smooth muscle inhibits apoptosis and regulates vascular remodeling. *Arter. Thromb. Vasc. Biol.* **2017**, *37*, 1944–1955. [CrossRef] [PubMed]

22. Frimat, M.; Boudhabhay, I.; Roumenina, L.T. Hemolysis derived products toxicity and endothelium: Model of the second hit. *Toxins* **2019**, *11*. [CrossRef] [PubMed]

23. Falk, E.; Nakano, M.; Bentzon, J.F.; Finn, A.V.; Virmani, R. Update on acute coronary syndromes: The pathologists' view. *Eur. Heart J.* **2013**, *34*, 719–728. [CrossRef]

24. Kolodgie, F.D.; Burke, A.P.; Farb, A.; Weber, D.K.; Kutys, R.; Wight, T.N.; Virmani, R. Differential accumulation of proteoglycans and hyaluronan in culprit lesions: Insights into plaque erosion. *Arter. Thromb. Vasc. Biol.* **2002**, *22*, 1642–1648. [CrossRef]

25. Kolodgie, F.D.; Burke, A.P.; Wight, T.N.; Virmani, R. The accumulation of specific types of proteoglycans in eroded plaques: A role in coronary thrombosis in the absence of rupture. *Curr. Opin. Lipidol.* **2004**, *15*, 575–582. [CrossRef] [PubMed]

26. Yahagi, K.; Davis, H.R.; Arbustini, E.; Virmani, R. Sex differences in coronary artery disease: Pathological observations. *Atherosclerosis* **2015**, *239*, 260–267. [CrossRef]

27. Tarhouni, K.; Freidja, M.L.; Guihot, A.L.; Vessieres, E.; Grimaud, L.; Toutain, B.; Lenfant, F.; Arnal, J.F.; Loufrani, L.; Henrion, D. Role of estrogens and age in flow-mediated outward remodeling of rat mesenteric resistance arteries. *Am. J. Physiol. Heart Circ. Physiol.* **2014**, *307*, H504–H514. [CrossRef]

28. de Jager, S.C.A.; Meeuwsen, J.A.L.; van Pijpen, F.M.; Zoet, G.A.; Barendrecht, A.D.; Franx, A.; Pasterkamp, G.; van Rijn, B.B.; Goumans, M.J.; den Ruijter, H.M. Preeclampsia and coronary plaque erosion: Manifestations of endothelial dysfunction resulting in cardiovascular events in women. *Eur. J. Pharmacol.* **2017**, *816*, 129–137. [CrossRef] [PubMed]

29. Kolodgie, F.D.; Gold, H.K.; Burke, A.P.; Fowler, D.R.; Kruth, H.S.; Weber, D.K.; Farb, A.; Guerrero, L.J.; Hayase, M.; Kutys, R.; et al. Intraplaque hemorrhage and progression of coronary atheroma. *N. Engl. J. Med.* **2003**, *349*, 2316–2325. [CrossRef] [PubMed]

30. Jeney, V.; Balla, G.; Balla, J. Red blood cell, hemoglobin and heme in the progression of atherosclerosis. *Front. Physiol.* **2014**, *5*, 379. [CrossRef] [PubMed]

31. Zahid, M.; Mangin, P.; Loyau, S.; Hechler, B.; Billiald, P.; Gachet, C.; Jandrot-Perrus, M. The future of glycoprotein VI as an antithrombotic target. *J. Thromb. Haemost.* **2012**, *10*, 2418–2427. [CrossRef] [PubMed]

32. Tatsumi, K.; Mackman, N. Tissue factor and atherothrombosis. *J. Atheroscler. Thromb.* **2015**, *22*, 543–549. [CrossRef] [PubMed]

33. Mann, J.; Davies, M.J. Mechanisms of progression in native coronary artery disease: Role of healed plaque disruption. *Heart* **1999**, *82*, 265–268. [CrossRef] [PubMed]

34. Virmani, R.; Burke, A.P.; Farb, A. Plaque rupture and plaque erosion. *Thromb. Haemost.* **1999**, *82*, 1–3. [PubMed]

35. Engelmann, B.; Massberg, S. Thrombosis as an intravascular effector of innate immunity. *Nat. Rev. Immunol.* **2013**, *13*, 34–45. [CrossRef] [PubMed]

36. Arbustini, E.; Morbini, P.; D'Armini, A.M.; Repetto, A.; Minzioni, G.; Piovella, F.; Vigano, M.; Tavazzi, L. Plaque composition in plexogenic and thromboembolic pulmonary hypertension: The critical role of thrombotic material in pultaceous core formation. *Heart* **2002**, *88*, 177–182. [CrossRef]

37. Michel, J.B.; Martin-Ventura, J.L.; Nicoletti, A.; Ho-Tin-Noe, B. Pathology of human plaque vulnerability: Mechanisms and consequences of intraplaque haemorrhages. *Atherosclerosis* **2014**, *234*, 311–319. [CrossRef]

38. Michel, J.B.; Virmani, R.; Arbustini, E.; Pasterkamp, G. Intraplaque haemorrhages as the trigger of plaque vulnerability. *Eur. Heart J.* **2011**, *32*, 1977–1985, 1985a, 1985b, 1985c. [CrossRef]

39. Porter, J.L.; Rawla, P. Hemochromatosis. In *StatPearls*; StatPearls Publishing: Treasure Island, FL, USA, 2020.

40. Diez-Lopez, C.; Comin-Colet, J.; Gonzalez-Costello, J. Iron overload cardiomyopathy: From diagnosis to management. *Curr. Opin. Cardiol.* **2018**, *33*, 334–340. [CrossRef]

41. Ellervik, C.; Tybjaerg-Hansen, A.; Grande, P.; Appleyard, M.; Nordestgaard, B.G. Hereditary hemochromatosis and risk of ischemic heart disease: A prospective study and a case-control study. *Circulation* **2005**, *112*, 185–193. [CrossRef]

42. van der, A.D.; Rovers, M.M.; Grobbee, D.E.; Marx, J.J.; Waalen, J.; Ellervik, C.; Nordestgaard, B.G.; Olynyk, J.K.; Mills, P.R.; Shepherd, J.; et al. Mutations in the HFE gene and cardiovascular disease risk: An individual patient data meta-analysis of 53 880 subjects. *Circ. Cardiovasc. Genet.* **2008**, *1*, 43–50. [CrossRef] [PubMed]

43. Sullivan, J.L. Do hemochromatosis mutations protect against iron-mediated atherogenesis? *Circ. Cardiovasc. Genet.* **2009**, *2*, 652–657. [CrossRef]

44. Meguro, R.; Asano, Y.; Odagiri, S.; Li, C.; Iwatsuki, H.; Shoumura, K. Nonheme-iron histochemistry for light and electron microscopy: A historical, theoretical and technical review. *Arch. Histol. Cytol.* **2007**, *70*, 1–19. [CrossRef] [PubMed]

45. Tabas, I.; Garcia-Cardena, G.; Owens, G.K. Recent insights into the cellular biology of atherosclerosis. *J. Cell. Biol.* **2015**, *209*, 13–22. [CrossRef] [PubMed]

46. Anitschkow, N.; Chalatow, S. Ueber experimentelle cholesterinsteatose und ihre bedeutungfur die entstchung einiger pathologischer prozesse. *Zentralbl. Allg. Pathol.* **1313**, *24*, 1–9.

47. Balla, G.; Jacob, H.S.; Eaton, J.W.; Belcher, J.D.; Vercellotti, G.M. Hemin: A possible physiological mediator of low density lipoprotein oxidation and endothelial injury. *Arter. Thromb.* **1991**, *11*, 1700–1711. [CrossRef]

48. Balla, G.; Vercellotti, G.M.; Muller-Eberhard, U.; Eaton, J.; Jacob, H.S. Exposure of endothelial cells to free heme potentiates damage mediated by granulocytes and toxic oxygen species. *Lab. Invest.* **1991**, *64*, 648–655.

49. Ho-Tin-Noe, B.; Vo, S.; Bayles, R.; Ferriere, S.; Ladjal, H.; Toumi, S.; Deschildre, C.; Ollivier, V.; Michel, J.B. Cholesterol crystallization in human atherosclerosis is triggered in smooth muscle cells during the transition from fatty streak to fibroatheroma. *J. Pathol.* **2017**, *241*, 671–682. [CrossRef]

50. Stadler, N.; Lindner, R.A.; Davies, M.J. Direct detection and quantification of transition metal ions in human atherosclerotic plaques: Evidence for the presence of elevated levels of iron and copper. *Arter. Thromb. Vasc. Biol.* **2004**, *24*, 949–954. [CrossRef]

51. Yoshida, H.; Kisugi, R. Mechanisms of LDL oxidation. *Clin. Chim. Acta* **2010**, *411*, 1875–1882. [CrossRef]

52. Gall, T.; Balla, G.; Balla, J. Heme, heme oxygenase, and endoplasmic reticulum stress-a new insight into the pathophysiology of vascular diseases. *Int. J. Mol. Sci.* **2019**, *20*. [CrossRef] [PubMed]

53. Dixon, S.J.; Lemberg, K.M.; Lamprecht, M.R.; Skouta, R.; Zaitsev, E.M.; Gleason, C.E.; Patel, D.N.; Bauer, A.J.; Cantley, A.M.; Yang, W.S.; et al. Ferroptosis: An iron-dependent form of nonapoptotic cell death. *Cell* **2012**, *149*, 1060–1072. [CrossRef] [PubMed]

54. Conrad, M.; Pratt, D.A. The chemical basis of ferroptosis. *Nat. Chem. Biol.* **2019**, *15*, 1137–1147. [CrossRef]

55. Hirschhorn, T.; Stockwell, B.R. The development of the concept of ferroptosis. *Free Radic. Biol. Med.* **2019**, *133*, 130–143. [CrossRef] [PubMed]

56. Sampilvanjil, A.; Karasawa, T.; Yamada, N.; Komada, T.; Higashi, T.; Baatarjav, C.; Watanabe, S.; Kamata, R.; Ohno, N.; Takahashi, M. Cigarette smoke extract induces ferroptosis in vascular smooth muscle cells. *Am. J. Physiol. Heart Circ. Physiol.* **2020**, *318*, H508–H518. [CrossRef] [PubMed]

57. Xiao, F.J.; Zhang, D.; Wu, Y.; Jia, Q.H.; Zhang, L.; Li, Y.X.; Yang, Y.F.; Wang, H.; Wu, C.T.; Wang, L.S. miRNA-17-92 protects endothelial cells from erastin-induced ferroptosis through targeting the A20-ACSL4 axis. *Biochem. Biophys. Res. Commun.* **2019**, *515*, 448–454. [CrossRef] [PubMed]

58. Patsch, C.; Challet-Meylan, L.; Thoma, E.C.; Urich, E.; Heckel, T.; O'Sullivan, J.F.; Grainger, S.J.; Kapp, F.G.; Sun, L.; Christensen, K.; et al. Generation of vascular endothelial and smooth muscle cells from human pluripotent stem cells. *Nat. Cell. Biol.* **2015**, *17*, 994–1003. [CrossRef]

59. Ho-Tin-Noe, B.; Michel, J.B. Initiation of angiogenesis in atherosclerosis: Smooth muscle cells as mediators of the angiogenic response to atheroma formation. *Trends Cardiovasc. Med.* **2011**, *21*, 183–187. [CrossRef]

60. Le Dall, J.; Ho-Tin-Noe, B.; Louedec, L.; Meilhac, O.; Roncal, C.; Carmeliet, P.; Germain, S.; Michel, J.B.; Houard, X. Immaturity of microvessels in haemorrhagic plaques is associated with proteolytic degradation of angiogenic factors. *Cardiovasc. Res.* **2009**. [CrossRef]

61. Leclercq, A.; Houard, X.; Loyau, S.; Philippe, M.; Sebbag, U.; Meilhac, O.; Michel, J.B. Topology of protease activities reflects atherothrombotic plaque complexity. *Atherosclerosis* **2007**, *191*, 1–10. [CrossRef]

62. Xiao, X.; Saha, P.; Yeoh, B.S.; Hipp, J.A.; Singh, V.; Vijay-Kumar, M. Myeloperoxidase deficiency attenuates systemic and dietary iron-induced adverse effects. *J. Nutr. Biochem.* **2018**, *62*, 28–34. [CrossRef] [PubMed]

63. Glagov, S.; Zarins, C.; Giddens, D.P.; Ku, D.N. Hemodynamics and atherosclerosis. Insights and perspectives gained from studies of human arteries. *Arch. Pathol. Lab. Med.* **1988**, *112*, 1018–1031. [PubMed]

64. Bassiouny, H.S.; Zarins, C.K.; Kadowaki, M.H.; Glagov, S. Hemodynamic stress and experimental aortoiliac atherosclerosis. *J. Vasc. Surg.* **1994**, *19*, 426–434. [CrossRef]

65. Leclercq, A.; Houard, X.; Philippe, M.; Ollivier, V.; Sebbag, U.; Meilhac, O.; Michel, J.B. Involvement of intraplaque hemorrhage in atherothrombosis evolution via neutrophil protease enrichment. *J. Leukoc. Biol.* **2007**, *82*, 1420–1429. [CrossRef]

66. Nakazawa, G.; Otsuka, F.; Nakano, M.; Vorpahl, M.; Yazdani, S.K.; Ladich, E.; Kolodgie, F.D.; Finn, A.V.; Virmani, R. The pathology of neoatherosclerosis in human coronary implants bare-metal and drug-eluting stents. *J. Am. Coll. Cardiol.* **2011**, *57*, 1314–1322. [CrossRef]

67. Terzian, Z.; Gasser, T.C.; Blackwell, F.; Hyafil, F.; Louedec, L.; Deschildre, C.; Ghodbane, W.; Dorent, R.; Nicoletti, A.; Morvan, M.; et al. Peristrut microhemorrhages: A possible cause of in-stent neoatherosclerosis? *Cardiovasc. Pathol.* **2017**, *26*, 30–38. [CrossRef] [PubMed]

68. Otsuka, F.; Nakano, M.; Ladich, E.; Kolodgie, F.D.; Virmani, R. Pathologic etiologies of late and very late stent thrombosis following first-generation drug-eluting stent placement. *Thrombosis* **2012**, *2012*, 608593. [CrossRef] [PubMed]

69. Alfonso, F.; Fernandez-Vina, F.; Medina, M.; Hernandez, R. Neoatherosclerosis: The missing link between very late stent thrombosis and very late in-stent restenosis. *J. Am. Coll. Cardiol.* **2013**, *61*, e155. [CrossRef]

70. Zhang, Y.; Cliff, W.J.; Schoefl, G.I.; Higgins, G. Plasma protein insudation as an index of early coronary atherogenesis. *Am. J. Pathol.* **1993**, *143*, 496–506.

71. Rokitansky, C.V. *A Manual of Pathological Anatomy*; Sydenham Society: London, UK, 1855.

72. Duguid, J.B. The thrombogenic hypothesis and its implications. *Postgrad. Med. J.* **1960**, *36*, 226–229. [CrossRef]

73. Chandler, A.B.; Hand, R.A. Phagocytized platelets: A source of lipids in human thrombi and atherosclerotic plaques. *Science* **1961**, *134*, 946–947. [CrossRef] [PubMed]

74. Huang, Y.; DiDonato, J.A.; Levison, B.S.; Schmitt, D.; Li, L.; Wu, Y.; Buffa, J.; Kim, T.; Gerstenecker, G.S.; Gu, X.; et al. An abundant dysfunctional apolipoprotein A1 in human atheroma. *Nat. Med.* **2014**, *20*, 193–203. [CrossRef] [PubMed]

75. DiDonato, J.A.; Huang, Y.; Aulak, K.S.; Even-Or, O.; Gerstenecker, G.; Gogonea, V.; Wu, Y.; Fox, P.L.; Tang, W.H.; Plow, E.F.; et al. Function and distribution of apolipoprotein A1 in the artery wall are markedly distinct from those in plasma. *Circulation* **2013**, *128*, 1644–1655. [CrossRef] [PubMed]

76. Ouimet, M.; Barrett, T.J.; Fisher, E.A. HDL and Reverse Cholesterol Transport. *Circ. Res.* **2019**, *124*, 1505–1518. [CrossRef] [PubMed]

77. Michel, J.B.; Martin-Ventura, J.L.; Egido, J.; Sakalihasan, N.; Treska, V.; Lindholt, J.; Allaire, E.; Thorsteinsdottir, U.; Cockerill, G.; Swedenborg, J.; et al. Novel aspects of the pathogenesis of aneurysms of the abdominal aorta in humans. *Cardiovasc. Res.* **2011**, *90*, 18–27. [CrossRef]

78. Houard, X.; Leclercq, A.; Fontaine, V.; Coutard, M.; Martin-Ventura, J.L.; Ho-Tin-Noe, B.; Touat, Z.; Meilhac, O.; Michel, J.B. Retention and activation of blood-borne proteases in the arterial wall implications for atherothrombosis. *J. Am. Coll. Cardiol.* **2006**, *48*, A3–A9. [CrossRef]

79. Delbosc, S.; Diallo, D.; Dejouvencel, T.; Lamiral, Z.; Louedec, L.; Martin-Ventura, J.L.; Rossignol, P.; Leseche, G.; Michel, J.B.; Meilhac, O. Impaired high-density lipoprotein anti-oxidant capacity in human abdominal aortic aneurysm. *Cardiovasc. Res.* **2013**, *100*, 307–315. [CrossRef]

80. Dutertre, C.A.; Clement, M.; Morvan, M.; Schakel, K.; Castier, Y.; Alsac, J.M.; Michel, J.B.; Nicoletti, A. Deciphering the stromal and hematopoietic cell network of the adventitia from non-aneurysmal and aneurysmal human aorta. *PLoS ONE* **2014**, *9*, e89983. [CrossRef]

81. Clement, M.; Guedj, K.; Andreata, F.; Morvan, M.; Bey, L.; Khallou-Laschet, J.; Gaston, A.T.; Delbosc, S.; Alsac, J.M.; Bruneval, P.; et al. Control of the T follicular helper-germinal center B-cell axis by CD8(+) regulatory T cells limits atherosclerosis and tertiary lymphoid organ development. *Circulation* **2015**, *131*, 560–570. [CrossRef]

82. Martinez-Pinna, R.; Lindholt, J.S.; Madrigal-Matute, J.; Blanco-Colio, L.M.; Esteban-Salan, M.; Torres-Fonseca, M.M.; Lefebvre, T.; Delbosc, S.; Laustsen, J.; Driss, F.; et al. From tissue iron retention to low systemic haemoglobin levels, new pathophysiological biomarkers of human abdominal aortic aneurysm. *Thromb. Haemost.* **2014**, *112*, 87–95. [CrossRef]

83. Sakalihasan, N.; Michel, J.B.; Katsargyris, A.; Kuivaniemi, H.; Defraigne, J.O.; Nchimi, A.; Powell, J.T.; Yoshimura, K.; Hultgren, R. Abdominal aortic aneurysms. *Nat. Rev. Dis. Primers* **2018**, *4*, 34. [CrossRef]

84. Martinez-Lopez, D.; Camafeita, E.; Cedo, L.; Roldan-Montero, R.; Jorge, I.; Garcia-Marques, F.; Gomez-Serrano, M.; Bonzon-Kulichenko, E.; Blanco-Vaca, F.; Blanco-Colio, L.M.; et al. APOA1 oxidation is associated to dysfunctional high-density lipoproteins in human abdominal aortic aneurysm. *EBioMedicine* **2019**, *43*, 43–53. [CrossRef]

85. Burillo, E.; Lindholt, J.S.; Molina-Sanchez, P.; Jorge, I.; Martinez-Pinna, R.; Blanco-Colio, L.M.; Tarin, C.;

Torres-Fonseca, M.M.; Esteban, M.; Laustsen, J.; et al. ApoA-I/HDL-C levels are inversely associated with abdominal aortic aneurysm progression. *Thromb. Haemost.* **2015**, *113*, 1335–1346. [CrossRef]

86. Nchimi, A.; Defawe, O.; Brisbois, D.; Broussaud, T.K.; Defraigne, J.O.; Magotteaux, P.; Massart, B.; Serfaty, J.M.; Houard, X.; Michel, J.B.; et al. MR imaging of iron phagocytosis in intraluminal thrombi of abdominal aortic aneurysms in humans. *Radiology* **2010**, *254*, 973–981. [CrossRef]

87. Nchimi, A.; Courtois, A.; El Hachemi, M.; Touat, Z.; Drion, P.; Withofs, N.; Warnock, G.; Bahri, M.A.; Dogne, J.M.; Cheramy-Bien, J.P.; et al. Multimodality imaging assessment of the deleterious role of the intraluminal thrombus on the growth of abdominal aortic aneurysm in a rat model. *Eur. Radiol.* **2015**. [CrossRef] [PubMed]

88. Gomel, M.A.; Lee, R.; Grande-Allen, K.J. Comparing the role of mechanical forces in vascular and valvular calcification progression. *Front. Cardiovasc. Med.* **2018**, *5*, 197. [CrossRef]

89. Voelkl, J.; Lang, F.; Eckardt, K.U.; Amann, K.; Kuro, O.M.; Pasch, A.; Pieske, B.; Alesutan, I. Signaling pathways involved in vascular smooth muscle cell calcification during hyperphosphatemia. *Cell. Mol. Life Sci.* **2019**, *76*, 2077–2091. [CrossRef] [PubMed]

90. Liang, L.; Liu, M.; Martin, C.; Sun, W. A deep learning approach to estimate stress distribution: A fast and accurate surrogate of finite-element analysis. *J. R. Soc. Interface* **2018**, *15*. [CrossRef] [PubMed]

91. Li, Z.Y.; Howarth, S.; Tang, T.; Graves, M.; Jean, U.K.-I.; Gillard, J.H. Does calcium deposition play a role in the stability of atheroma? Location may be the key. *Cerebrovasc. Dis.* **2007**, *24*, 452–459. [CrossRef] [PubMed]

92. Fitzgerald, P.J.; Ports, T.A.; Yock, P.G. Contribution of localized calcium deposits to dissection after angioplasty. An observational study using intravascular ultrasound. *Circulation* **1992**, *86*, 64–70. [CrossRef] [PubMed]

93. Akahori, H.; Tsujino, T.; Masuyama, T.; Ishihara, M. Mechanisms of aortic stenosis. *J. Cardiol.* **2018**, *71*, 215–220. [CrossRef] [PubMed]

94. Akahori, H.; Tsujino, T.; Naito, Y.; Matsumoto, M.; Lee-Kawabata, M.; Ohyanagi, M.; Mitsuno, M.; Miyamoto, Y.; Daimon, T.; Hao, H.; et al. Intraleaflet haemorrhage is associated with rapid progression of degenerative aortic valve stenosis. *Eur. Heart J.* **2011**, *32*, 888–896. [CrossRef] [PubMed]

95. Morvan, M.; Arangalage, D.; Franck, G.; Perez, F.; Cattan-Levy, L.; Codogno, I.; Jacob-Lenet, M.P.; Deschildre, C.; Choqueux, C.; Even, G.; et al. Relationship of Iron Deposition to Calcium Deposition in Human Aortic Valve Leaflets. *J. Am. Coll. Cardiol.* **2019**, *73*, 1043–1054. [CrossRef] [PubMed]

96. Kawada, S.; Nagasawa, Y.; Kawabe, M.; Ohyama, H.; Kida, A.; Kato-Kogoe, N.; Nanami, M.; Hasuike, Y.; Kuragano, T.; Kishimoto, H.; et al. Iron-induced calcification in human aortic vascular smooth muscle cells through interleukin-24 (IL-24), with/without TNF-alpha. *Sci. Rep.* **2018**, *8*, 658. [CrossRef]

97. Tziakas, D.N.; Chalikias, G.; Pavlaki, M.; Kareli, D.; Gogiraju, R.; Hubert, A.; Bohm, E.; Stamoulis, P.; Drosos, I.; Kikas, P.; et al. Lysed erythrocyte membranes promote vascular calcification. *Circulation* **2019**, *139*, 2032–2048. [CrossRef] [PubMed]

98. Kobayashi, M.; Suhara, T.; Baba, Y.; Kawasaki, N.K.; Higa, J.K.; Matsui, T. Pathological roles of iron in cardiovascular disease. *Curr. Drug. Targets* **2018**, *19*, 1068–1076. [CrossRef]

99. Jankowska, E.A.; Malyszko, J.; Ardehali, H.; Koc-Zorawska, E.; Banasiak, W.; von Haehling, S.; Macdougall, I.C.; Weiss, G.; McMurray, J.J.; Anker, S.D.; et al. Iron status in patients with chronic heart failure. *Eur. Heart J.* **2013**, *34*, 827–834. [CrossRef]

100. Anand, I.S.; Gupta, P. Anemia and iron deficiency in heart failure: Current concepts and emerging therapies. *Circulation* **2018**, *138*, 80–98. [CrossRef]

101. Grote Beverborg, N.; van Veldhuisen, D.J.; van der Meer, P. Anemia in Heart Failure: Still Relevant? *JACC Heart Fail.* **2018**, *6*, 201–208. [CrossRef]

102. Carberry, J.; Carrick, D.; Haig, C.; Ahmed, N.; Mordi, I.; McEntegart, M.; Petrie, M.C.; Eteiba, H.; Hood, S.; Watkins, S.; et al. Persistent iron within the infarct core after ST-segment elevation myocardial infarction: Implications for left ventricular remodeling and health outcomes. *JACC Cardiovasc. Imaging* **2018**, *11*, 1248–1256. [CrossRef]

103. Baba, Y.; Higa, J.K.; Shimada, B.K.; Horiuchi, K.M.; Suhara, T.; Kobayashi, M.; Woo, J.D.; Aoyagi, H.; Marh, K.S.; Kitaoka, H.; et al. Protective effects of the mechanistic target of rapamycin against excess iron and ferroptosis in cardiomyocytes. *Am. J. Physiol. Heart Circ. Physiol.* **2018**, *314*, H659–H668. [CrossRef]

104. Hugelshofer, M.; Buzzi, R.M.; Schaer, C.A.; Richter, H.; Akeret, K.; Anagnostakou, V.; Mahmoudi, L.; Vaccani, R.; Vallelian, F.; Deuel, J.W.; et al. Haptoglobin administration into the subarachnoid space prevents hemoglobin-induced cerebral vasospasm. *J. Clin. Invest.* **2019**, *129*, 5219–5235. [CrossRef] [PubMed]

105. Marquez-Ropero, M.; Benito, E.; Plaza-Zabala, A.; Sierra, A. Microglial corpse clearance: Lessons from macrophages. *Front. Immunol.* **2020**, *11*, 506. [CrossRef]

106. Van Acker, Z.P.; Luyckx, E.; Dewilde, S. Neuroglobin expression in the brain: A story of tissue homeostasis preservation. *Mol. Neurobiol.* **2019**, *56*, 2101–2122. [CrossRef] [PubMed]

107. Gregson, J.M.; Freitag, D.F.; Surendran, P.; Stitziel, N.O.; Chowdhury, R.; Burgess, S.; Kaptoge, S.; Gao, P.; Staley, J.R.; Willeit, P.; et al. Genetic invalidation of Lp-PLA$_2$ as a therapeutic target: Large-scale study of five functional Lp-PLA$_2$-lowering alleles. *Eur. J. Prev. Cardiol.* **2017**, *24*, 492–504. [CrossRef] [PubMed]

108. Zille, M.; Kumar, A.; Kundu, N.; Bourassa, M.W.; Wong, V.S.C.; Willis, D.; Karuppagounder, S.S.; Ratan, R.R. Ferroptosis in neurons and cancer cells is similar but differentially regulated by histone deacetylase inhibitors. *eNeuro* **2019**, *6*. [CrossRef]

109. Alim, I.; Caulfield, J.T.; Chen, Y.; Swarup, V.; Geschwind, D.H.; Ivanova, E.; Seravalli, J.; Ai, Y.; Sansing, L.H.; Ste Marie, E.J.; et al. Selenium drives a transcriptional adaptive program to block ferroptosis and treat stroke. *Cell* **2019**, *177*, 1262–1279.e1225. [CrossRef] [PubMed]

110. Kolb, S.; Vranckx, R.; Huisse, M.G.; Michel, J.B.; Meilhac, O. The phosphatidylserine receptor mediates phagocytosis by vascular smooth muscle cells. *J. Pathol.* **2007**, *212*, 249–259. [CrossRef] [PubMed]

111. Mesa, K.R.; Rompolas, P.; Zito, G.; Myung, P.; Sun, T.Y.; Brown, S.; Gonzalez, D.G.; Blagoev, K.B.; Haberman, A.M.; Greco, V. Niche-induced cell death and epithelial phagocytosis regulate hair follicle stem cell pool. *Nature* **2015**, *522*, 94–97. [CrossRef] [PubMed]

112. Seeberg, J.C.; Loibl, M.; Moser, F.; Schwegler, M.; Buttner-Herold, M.; Daniel, C.; Engel, F.B.; Hartmann, A.; Schlotzer-Schrehardt, U.; Goppelt-Struebe, M.; et al. Non-professional phagocytosis: A general feature of normal tissue cells. *Sci. Rep.* **2019**, *9*, 11875. [CrossRef] [PubMed]

113. Morioka, S.; Maueroder, C.; Ravichandran, K.S. Living on the edge: Efferocytosis at the interface of homeostasis and pathology. *Immunity* **2019**, *50*, 1149–1162. [CrossRef] [PubMed]

114. Bennett, M.R.; Gibson, D.F.; Schwartz, S.M.; Tait, J.F. Binding and phagocytosis of apoptotic vascular smooth muscle cells is mediated in part by exposure of phosphatidylserine. *Circ. Res.* **1995**, *77*, 1136–1142. [CrossRef] [PubMed]

115. Andersen, C.B.F.; Stodkilde, K.; Saederup, K.L.; Kuhlee, A.; Raunser, S.; Graversen, J.H.; Moestrup, S.K. Haptoglobin. *Antioxid. Redox Signal.* **2017**, *26*, 814–831. [CrossRef] [PubMed]

116. Ramakrishnan, L.; Pedersen, S.L.; Toe, Q.K.; West, L.E.; Mumby, S.; Casbolt, H.; Issitt, T.; Garfield, B.; Lawrie, A.; Wort, S.J.; et al. The hepcidin/ferroportin axis modulates proliferation of pulmonary artery smooth muscle cells. *Sci. Rep.* **2018**, *8*, 12972. [CrossRef]

117. Vanacore, R.; Eskew, J.D.; Sung, L.; Davis, T.; Smith, A. Safe coordinated trafficking of heme and iron with copper maintain cell homeostasis: Modules from the hemopexin system. *Biometals* **2019**, *32*, 355–367. [CrossRef]

118. Etique, N.; Verzeaux, L.; Dedieu, S.; Emonard, H. LRP-1: A checkpoint for the extracellular matrix proteolysis. *Biomed. Res. Int.* **2013**, *2013*, 152163. [CrossRef]

119. Fibach, E.; Rachmilewitz, E.A. Iron overload in hematological disorders. *Presse. Med.* **2017**, *46*, e296–e305. [CrossRef]

120. Bennett, C.; Mohammed, F.; Alvarez-Ciara, A.; Nguyen, M.A.; Dietrich, W.D.; Rajguru, S.M.; Streit, W.J.; Prasad, A. Neuroinflammation, oxidative stress, and blood-brain barrier (BBB) disruption in acute Utah electrode array implants and the effect of deferoxamine as an iron chelator on acute foreign body response. *Biomaterials* **2019**, *188*, 144–159. [CrossRef]

121. Martin-Ventura, J.L.; Rodrigues-Diez, R.; Martinez-Lopez, D.; Salaices, M.; Blanco-Colio, L.M.; Briones, A.M. Oxidative stress in human atherothrombosis: Sources, markers and therapeutic targets. *Int. J. Mol. Sci.* **2017**, *18*. [CrossRef]

122. Martin-Ventura, J.L.; Madrigal-Matute, J.; Martinez-Pinna, R.; Ramos-Mozo, P.; Blanco-Colio, L.M.; Moreno, J.A.; Tarin, C.; Burillo, E.; Fernandez-Garcia, C.E.; Egido, J.; et al. Erythrocytes, leukocytes and platelets as a source of oxidative stress in chronic vascular diseases: Detoxifying mechanisms and potential therapeutic options. *Thromb. Haemost.* **2012**, *108*, 435–442. [CrossRef]

123. Mohanty, J.G.; Nagababu, E.; Rifkind, J.M. Red blood cell oxidative stress impairs oxygen delivery and induces red blood cell aging. *Front. Physiol.* **2014**, *5*, 84. [CrossRef] [PubMed]

124. Nagababu, E.; Mohanty, J.G.; Bhamidipaty, S.; Ostera, G.R.; Rifkind, J.M. Role of the membrane in the formation of heme degradation products in red blood cells. *Life Sci.* **2010**, *86*, 133–138. [CrossRef] [PubMed]

125. Martinez-Pinna, R.; Burillo, E.; Madrigal-Matute, J.; Lopez, J.A.; Camafeita, E.; Torres-Fonseca, M.M.; Llamas-Granda, P.; Egido, J.; Michel, J.B.; Blanco-Colio, L.M.; et al. Label-free proteomic analysis of red blood cell membrane fractions from abdominal aortic aneurysm patients. *Proteomics Clin. Appl.* **2014**, *8*, 626–630. [CrossRef] [PubMed]

126. Tsantes, A.E.; Bonovas, S.; Travlou, A.; Sitaras, N.M. Redox imbalance, macrocytosis, and RBC homeostasis. *Antioxid. Redox Signal.* **2006**, *8*, 1205–1216. [CrossRef]

127. Blankenberg, S.; Rupprecht, H.J.; Bickel, C.; Torzewski, M.; Hafner, G.; Tiret, L.; Smieja, M.; Cambien, F.; Meyer, J.; Lackner, K.J.; et al. Glutathione peroxidase 1 activity and cardiovascular events in patients with coronary artery disease. *N. Engl. J. Med.* **2003**, *349*, 1605–1613. [CrossRef]

128. Espinola-Klein, C.; Rupprecht, H.J.; Bickel, C.; Schnabel, R.; Genth-Zotz, S.; Torzewski, M.; Lackner, K.; Munzel, T.; Blankenberg, S.; AtheroGene, I. Glutathione peroxidase-1 activity, atherosclerotic burden, and cardiovascular prognosis. *Am. J. Cardiol.* **2007**, *99*, 808–812. [CrossRef]

129. Ramos-Mozo, P.; Madrigal-Matute, J.; Martinez-Pinna, R.; Blanco-Colio, L.M.; Lopez, J.A.; Camafeita, E.; Meilhac, O.; Michel, J.B.; Aparicio, C.; Vega de Ceniga, M.; et al. Proteomic analysis of polymorphonuclear neutrophils identifies catalase as a novel biomarker of abdominal aortic aneurysm: Potential implication of oxidative stress in abdominal aortic aneurysm progression. *Arter. Thromb. Vasc. Biol.* **2011**, *31*, 3011–3019. [CrossRef]

130. Vardi, M.; Levy, N.S.; Levy, A.P. Vitamin E in the prevention of cardiovascular disease: The importance of proper patient selection. *J. Lipid Res.* **2013**, *54*, 2307–2314. [CrossRef]

131. Bamm, V.V.; Tsemakhovich, V.A.; Shaklai, M.; Shaklai, N. Haptoglobin phenotypes differ in their ability to inhibit heme transfer from hemoglobin to LDL. *Biochemistry* **2004**, *43*, 3899–3906. [CrossRef]

132. Burillo, E.; Tarin, C.; Torres-Fonseca, M.M.; Fernandez-Garcia, C.E.; Martinez-Pinna, R.; Martinez-Lopez, D.; Llamas-Granda, P.; Camafeita, E.; Lopez, J.A.; Vega de Ceniga, M.; et al. Paraoxonase-1 overexpression prevents experimental abdominal aortic aneurysm progression. *Clin. Sci.* **2016**, *130*, 1027–1038. [CrossRef]

Targeting Platelet in Atherosclerosis Plaque Formation: Current Knowledge and Future Perspectives

Lei Wang [1] and Chaojun Tang [1,2,3,*]

1   Cyrus Tang Hematology Center, Cyrus Tang Medical Institute, Soochow University, Suzhou 215123, China; lwangLeiW@stu.suda.edu.cn
2   Collaborative Innovation Center of Hematology of Jiangsu Province, Soochow University, Suzhou 215123, China
3   National Clinical Research Center for Hematologic Diseases, the First Affiliated Hospital of Soochow University, Suzhou 215123, China
*   Correspondence: zjtang@suda.edu.cn

Abstract: Besides their role in hemostasis and thrombosis, it has become increasingly clear that platelets are also involved in many other pathological processes of the vascular system, such as atherosclerotic plaque formation. Atherosclerosis is a chronic vascular inflammatory disease, which preferentially develops at sites under disturbed blood flow with low speeds and chaotic directions. Hyperglycemia, hyperlipidemia, and hypertension are all risk factors for atherosclerosis. When the vascular microenvironment changes, platelets can respond quickly to interact with endothelial cells and leukocytes, participating in atherosclerosis. This review discusses the important roles of platelets in the plaque formation under pro-atherogenic factors. Specifically, we discussed the platelet behaviors under disturbed flow, hyperglycemia, and hyperlipidemia conditions. We also summarized the molecular mechanisms involved in vascular inflammation during atherogenesis based on platelet receptors and secretion of inflammatory factors. Finally, we highlighted the studies of platelet migration in atherogenesis. In general, we elaborated an atherogenic role of platelets and the aspects that should be further studied in the future.

Keywords: platelet; atherogenesis; disturbed flow; hyperglycemia; hyperlipidemia; inflammation; platelet migration

1. Introduction

Atherosclerosis (AS) is a chronic inflammatory disease induced by multiple factors, involving a complex series of circulating blood cells (e.g., platelets and monocytes) and plasma components (e.g., lipoproteins), which interact with vascular cells and initiate atherosclerosis [1–3]. AS lesions often occur at the bifurcation or curvature of the large- and medium-sized arteries (e.g., aorta, carotid arteries), where disturbed flow (d-flow) occurs. In addition, a change of the microenvironment in circulation like hypertension, hyperglycemia, or hyperlipidemia can accelerate the formation of atherosclerosis [4–6]. When plaques are formed, changes in hemodynamics will exacerbate the tendency to increase plaque in an arterial stenosis environment, making it unstable and causing rupture. Once the plaque ruptures, platelets-rich blood clots are immediately formed to block blood vessels, and ischemic thrombotic events occur.

Platelets are the key mediator of plaque rupture and atherothrombosis. In recent years, many studies have shown that platelets play an inflammatory role as an immune cell and participate in the development of atherosclerosis [7,8]. When the shear stress of the blood flow changes sharply or the vascular microenvironment alters, the platelets circulating in the blood can quickly perceive these signals and respond. Subsequently, they are activated rapidly during endothelial dysfunction and then they adhere to damaged blood vessels to maintain blood vessel integrity [1,9]. Further, activated platelets recruit immune cells, promote their transmigration across the intima, and accelerate the process of atherosclerosis by the engagement of surface receptors or the release of inflammatory factors [10]. Several reviews about platelets in atherosclerosis are available, each with a different emphasis and perspective [1,3,11,12]. Nording et al. [12] summarized the important role of platelets in atherosclerosis and atherothrombosis, and concluded that antiplatelet therapy is not suitable for primary prevention treatment due to its bleeding risk in the treatment of clinical cardiovascular disease. In this review, we try to focus on those basic studies that are related to how platelets, as inflammatory mediators, respond to atherosclerosis risk factors and regulate atherosclerotic plaque formation. Specifically, we illustrate the important roles of molecules derived from platelets in atherogenesis. Finally, we discuss whether platelet migration is involved in the process. We also raise the unsolved questions of platelets in atherogenesis as well as the highlights and perspectives in future research.

2. Platelets and Risk Factors of Atherosclerosis

2.1. Disturbed Flow Modulated Platelets in AS

Atherosclerosis preferentially develops at the curved bifurcated sites under d-flow [13], while straight blood vessels exhibit uniform laminar flow, which is essential to maintain the vascular homeostasis, and protect against AS. Endothelial cells (ECs) are located in the inner layer of the vascular wall, which is the sensor of hemodynamic shear stress. Under physiological conditions, endothelial cells undergo unidirectional laminar flow, leading to uniform cell alignment, vasodilation, anti-inflammation, and anticoagulation. In contrast, d-flow stimulates proinflammatory responses, including junction damage, leukocyte recruitment, and coagulation [13,14]. Besides, circulating platelets can also rapidly sense and respond to hemodynamic forces to regulate vascular homeostasis. When subjected to d-flow, inflamed ECs express or expose high levels of adhesion molecules (e.g., P-selectin, intercellular adhesion molecule-1 (ICAM-1), vascular cell adhesion molecule 1 (VCAM-1)) [15] and adhesion proteins (e.g., Von Willebrand factor (vWF), Fibrin) [16,17]. These molecules stimulate platelets to adhere and roll to damaged sites via platelet receptors, such as glycoprotein (GP) Ibα, glycoprotein VI (GPVI), or integrin αIIbβ3 (see Figure 1). Subsequently, the adhered platelets can capture the circulating leukocytes, which is limited to the area where P-selectin is expressed under disturbed flow [18]. Interestingly, Tersteeg et al. [19] showed that adherent and activated platelets under shear will expose long negatively charged membrane strands, called flow-induced protrusions (FLIPRs). FLIPRs can capture circulating monocytes and neutrophils in a P-selectin/PSGL-1-dependent manner, and then promote the formation and activation of platelet-leukocyte microparticle complexes, leading to the progression of inflammatory processes. In addition, FLIPR also promotes the formation of platelet microparticles (PMPs), while it is well known that PMPs play an important role in inducing foam cell formation, and promoting atherosclerosis [20]. Although FLIPR promotes platelet-leukocyte microparticle complexes and the release of platelet microparticles, to date, there is no direct evidence that FLIPR plays a role in atherosclerosis or inflammatory diseases in vivo. In addition, platelet endothelial cell adhesion molecule-1 (PECAM-1) can mediate platelet adhesion to endothelial cells under pathological flow, and a lack of PECAM-1 on either the endothelium or platelets results in reduced platelet adhesion to the endothelium [21]. PECAM-1 is also an important factor in atherosclerosis, as a lack of PECAM-1 in ApoE$^{-/-}$ mice will significantly reduce the lesion size of the aortic arch and aortic sinus [22]. Therefore, the atherogenic effect of PECAM-1 may be attributed to platelet adhesion, and the adhered platelets recruit circulating leukocytes to promote vascular inflammation and atherosclerosis. All in all, there is still no conclusive and direct evidence regarding whether and how platelets participate in the formation of early atherosclerotic plaques under d-flow conditions.

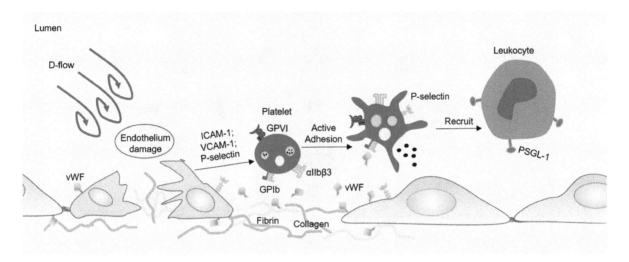

Figure 1. Disturbed flow-regulated platelets participate in the plaque formation. Disturbed flow activates endothelial cells (ECs), resulting in elevated expression of adhesion molecules and deposition of adhesion proteins. All these adhesion molecules and proteins interact with platelets via surface receptors, leading to platelet activation. Activated platelets recruit circulating leukocytes by P-selectin or other releasing inflammatory factors, therefore participating atherogenesis.

2.2. Hyperlipidemia Modulated Platelets in AS

Dyslipidemia is a major risk factor of coronary artery disease and is associated with a poor prognosis, such as the major cardiovascular adverse event (MACE) [23–25]. The effects of chronic hyperlipidemia are complex, which causes lipid deposition in atherosclerotic lesions, primary endothelial damage, and increased platelet reactivity. Thus, the mechanism leading to enhanced platelet reactivity is one of the key points in the treatment of vascular diseases. Evidence suggests that lipoprotein–platelet interaction plays an important role in atherogenesis. Platelets in hyperlipidemia show high activity and are more prone to be activated and aggregated [8]. In addition to lipid-lowering effects, statins can also effectively reduce the platelet activity [26,27]. Furthermore, platelet can also mediate lipoprotein transport to promote foam cell formation and exacerbate atherosclerosis (see Figure 2).

It is well known that platelets, through specific binding receptors, affect low-density lipoprotein (LDL) per se triggers platelet activation, and enhances platelet aggregation and secretion, whereas HDL desensitizes platelets, underlining the anti-atherosclerotic properties of high-density lipoprotein (HDL) [28,29]. Omics analysis showed that resting human platelets contained 1500 LDL-binding sites and 3200 HDL-binding sites [30]. Human platelets express LDL receptor-related protein 8 (LRP8) [31]. LDL binding to LDL receptors on platelets promotes lipid exchange between LDL particles and platelet plasma membrane, initiates phosphorylation of focal adhesion kinase (FAK), enhances the binding of fibrinogen and integrin $\alpha IIb\beta 3$, and induces an increase in intracellular Ca^{2+}. The changes of the signal transduction cascade in platelets result in increased sensitivity of platelet-activating agents [32]. Native HDL regulates platelet signaling pathways by binding to platelet HDL receptors (such as SR-BI and apoER2′), as well as by balancing the cholesterol content in platelets to prevent platelet hyperresponsiveness. [33].

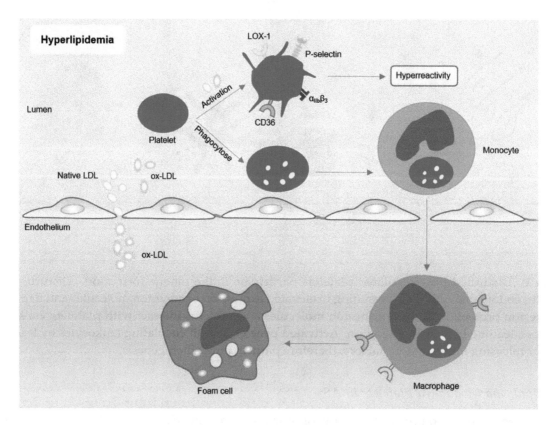

Figure 2. Platelets participate in atherosclerosis under hyperlipidemic conditions. Lipoproteins, such as low-density lipoproteins in plasma, trigger platelet activation by binding sites. Or monocytes engulf low-density lipoprotein (LDL)-containing apoptotic platelets and migrate under the inner membrane to differentiate into macrophages and foam cells. Subendothelial oxidized LDL further participates in atherosclerotic plaque formation by binding to scavenger receptor CD36 and LOX-1.

The increased lipid in the plasma of patients with hyperlipidemia invades the intimal endothelium in the form of LDL through their receptor, and is oxidized to oxidized low-density lipoprotein (oxLDL) [34]. OxLDL loses its ability to bind to natural LDL receptors, and can be recognized by scavenger receptors (CD36, LOX-1) on platelets to exert additional pro-atherosclerotic effects [8]. OxLDL can enhance the adhesion of platelets to collagen and activated ECs and the formation of platelet-monocyte aggregates [35]. OxLDL binding to CD36 actives platelet and increases exposure of platelet P-selectin and activates integrin αIIbβ3, which may involve the signal pathway including Src family kinases, Syk, and phospholipase C-γ [36,37]. Furthermore, activated platelets internalize oxLDL, while platelets loaded with oxLDL further activate the endothelium, release chemokines to recruit monocytes, and promote foam cell development [38]. CD36 deficiency in ApoE$^{-/-}$ mice can inhibit neointimal hyperplasia and vascular smooth muscle cells (VSMCs) proliferation, which may prevent atherosclerosis and restenosis [39]. Lectin-like oxidized LDL receptor 1 (LOX-1) was identified as another major receptor of oxLDL in human platelets [40]. Activated LOX-1 stimulates adhesion molecules, pro-inflammatory factors, and angiogenic factors in vascular ECs and macrophages [41]. LOX-1 activation can also indicate the occurrence of acute cardiovascular disease after plaque rupture [42]. These studies have shown that oxLDL and its receptors (CD36 and LOX-1) are involved in the regulation of atherosclerotic process. However, there is no direct evidence that specific knockout of CD36 or LOX-1 on platelets in atherosclerosis-prone mice affects atherosclerotic plaque formation.

2.3. Hyperglycemia-Modulated Platelets in AS

It is believed that hyperglycemia accelerates the progression of atherosclerosis [43]. Hyperglycemia from non-diabetic patients is also related to the increase in mortality and morbidity of patients with acute stroke [44]. Diabetes can alter the functional properties of many cell types, including ECs and platelets. Many earlier studies have shown that in patients with diabetes mellitus (DM), especially type 2 diabetes mellitus (T2DM), platelet degranulation and cytoplasmic calcification and thromboxane A2 content increase [45]. Hyperglycemia will also promote the binding of platelets and fibrinogen, and enhance p-selectin exposure [46]. Furthermore, platelets from DM patients are less sensitive to natural anticoagulants, such as prostacyclin (PGI2) [47]. These may be the key triggers leading to platelet hyperreactivity and a hypercoagulable state in blood.

Several mechanisms have been proposed to influence platelet activation and platelet hyperreactivity induced by hyperglycemia. Hyperglycemia can cause an increase in non-enzymatic glycosylated LDL (glycLDL), which may lead to changes in protein structure and conformation, as well as changes in membrane lipid dynamics [48]. GlycLDL may increase the expression of platelet key ligand receptors, such as P-selectin and GPIIb/IIIa, by elevating intracellular Ca^{2+} concentration and platelet NO production, and inhibiting changes in platelet membrane dynamics, leading to platelet dysfunction [49]. Recent research showed that chronic hyperglycemia leads to enhanced activation of biomechanical αIIbβ3, which leads to increased shear and erythrocyte dependence of discoid platelet adhesion and aggregation [50]. Moreover, the content of sorbitol in platelets is increased after prolonged high glucose treatment, and the accumulation of sorbitol is closely related to cell swelling. Addition of sorbitol can increase the mean platelet volume (MPV) by regulating platelet microtubule polymerization, and accelerate the production of platelet-related thrombin [51].

In further, circulating platelet-leukocyte aggregates are significantly increased in diabetes patients [52]. Elevated monocyte-platelet aggregates are normally used as an early marker of T2DM [53]. Platelet–leukocyte cross-talk is generally considered to be related to platelet hyper-responsiveness, which may contribute to excess microvascular risk in DM patients. Kraakman et al.'s research found that hyperglycemia triggers the release of S100 calcium-binding protein A8/A9. These proteins then bind to their receptors on Kupffer cells for advanced glycation end products, triggering the production of IL-6, and causing hepatocytes to secrete TPO, which further leads to increased megakaryocyte proliferation and reticulated platelet production [54,55]. Another study reported that hyperglycemia can enhance sodium arsenite-induced megakaryocyte adhesion, platelet P-selectin expression, and leukocyte-platelet aggregation [56]. Megakaryocyte adhesion is often considered one of the markers of atherothrombosis risk [57]. In summary, hyperglycemia can regulate the atherosclerotic process by regulating platelet signaling and the state of platelet receptors.

3. Platelet Receptors in Atherogenesis

There are abundant receptors on the surface that bind to extracellular matrix and adhesion proteins to cause platelet adhesion and activation. Major platelet receptors include integrins (αIIbβ3, αVβ3), immunoglobulin superfamily adhesion receptors (GPVI, FcγRIIa), leucine-rich adhesive receptors (GPIb-IX-V complex, toll-like receptors), G-protein-coupled receptors (PAR1, PAR4, $P2Y_{12}$), and C-type lectin receptors (P-selectin) etc. [58,59]. These receptors interact with various adhesion matrices and cells (endothelial, monocytes, smooth muscle cells, etc.) to participate in inflammatory reactions (Figure 3).

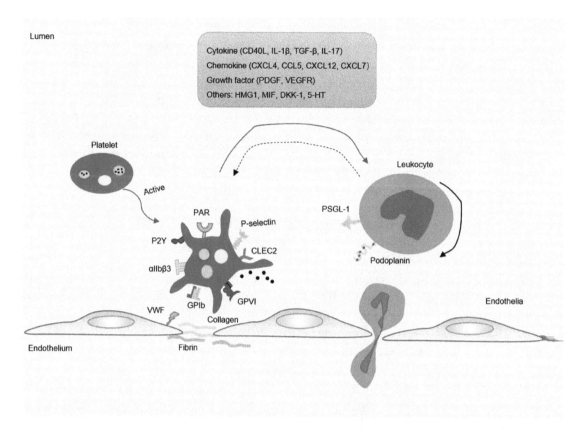

Figure 3. As an inflammatory mediator, platelets interact with ECs and leukocytes (mainly monocytes) to participate in the formation of atherosclerotic lesions. Pro-atherosclerosis factors can easily lead to platelet activation. The activated platelets express a variety of adhesion receptors. These receptors bind their matrix proteins (GPIb-vWF, GPVI-collagen, and GPIIb-IIIa-fibrinogen) to mediate platelet adhesion on ECs or leukocytes (P-selectin-PSGL-1 and Clec2-PDPN). Moreover, platelet activation releases a variety of inflammatory factors (cytokines, chemokines, growth factors, and others). These inflammatory mediators can also be induced and expressed in neighboring cells, such as monocytes/macrophages, neutrophils, and ECs, which in turn affected platelets. Blue arrow: the factor released by platelets interact with leukocytes; Black solid arrow: the rolling of leukocytes; Blue dotted arrow: activated leukocytes in turn affect platelets.

3.1. Integrin αIIbβ3

The platelet cascade activation is inseparable from the expression of αIIbβ3. The αIIbβ3 on resting platelets is in an inactive state, but when the signal transduction inside the platelets is activated, αIIbβ3 receptor activation and fibrinogen binding further promote platelet aggregation [60]. Numerous clinical trials have shown that the inhibitors of platelet αIIbβ3 receptors can effectively prevent and treat unstable angina pectoris or myocardial infarction caused by acute ischemic events [61]. However, whether platelet αIIbβ3 promotes the development of atherosclerotic lesions is currently controversial. It is reported that the absence of integrin β3 in atherosclerosis-prone mice (ApoE-null and LDLR-null mice) enhances the susceptibility of inflammation and atherosclerosis lesions caused by a high-fat diet [62]. Further research found that global β3 deletion or transplantation of $\beta3^{-/-}$ bone marrow caused atherosclerotic lesions to aggravate due to the increase in the number of smooth muscle cells (SMCs) recruited into the plaque. The authors believe that macrophage β3 deletion plays a leading role in this progress [63]. However, there are reports contrary to the above studies. The adhesion of platelets to ECs depends on the interaction of soluble fibrinogen and αIIbβ3. Platelets lacking αIIbβ3 cannot firmly adhere to activated ECs [64]. In a study of primary stroke, it was shown that the area of cerebral infarction in mice lacking GPIIb compared to wild-type mice significantly decreased. Similarly, the atherosclerotic lesions in the carotid artery and aortic arch in $ApoE^{-/-}$ mice lacking GPIIb were significantly reduced or even absent. The authors suggest that this may be due to the decrease in the number of recruited platelets adhering to active ECs [65]. The degree of atherosclerotic lesions in GPIIb or GPIIIa deficiency in atherosclerosis-prone mice may be related to the vitronectin receptor $\alpha V\beta 3$. After all, $\alpha IIb\beta 3$ is only expressed by megakaryocytes and platelets, while $\alpha V\beta 3$ is expressed on both vascular cells and monocytes. $\alpha v\beta 3$ also plays a vital role in promoting platelet adhesion. Inhibiting $\alpha v\beta 3$ can suppress inflammation and smooth muscle recruitment, thereby weakening atherosclerosis [66]. In order to clarify the specific role of $\alpha IIb\beta 3$ in AS, it is necessary to use platelet-specific knockout $\beta 3$ for in-depth research.

3.2. GPIb-V-IX Complex

One of the important adhesion receptors on platelets is glycoprotein (GP) Ib. After vascular injury, collagen fibers are exposed, and the GPIb-V-IX complex binds to vWF and is fixed on the collagen fibers. This process promotes platelet actin aggregation and skeletal reorganization on the platelet surface, and mediates platelet activation and adhesion to ECs [67]. The number of platelets was significantly decreased, and plaque formation was dramatically limited in ApoE$^{-/-}$ mice after GPIb antibody treatment [68]. Consistent with this, atherosclerotic lesions were reduced after GPIbα-specific knockout of bone marrow cells in Ldlr$^{-/-}$ mice. However, only removing the extracellular domain of GPIbα that interacts with various ligands (vWF, P-selectin, Mac-1) can reverse this phenotype [69]. This result seems to indicate that the interaction of the extracellular domain of GPIbα on platelets with leukocytes or ECs may be redundant during plaque formation. However, this is contrary to previous research, which shows that vWF or P-selectin deficiency can reduce atherosclerotic lesions [70,71], suggesting that VWF and P-selectin may also affect atherosclerosis by binding to other receptors instead of GPIb. Low-fat feeding on GPIb$^{-/-}$/ApoE$^{-/-}$ mice showed no decrease in atherosclerotic plaque size and composition, and even an increasing trend [72]. This is contrary to the above GPIbα study, which may be caused by the different feed formula, the changes in the number and the state of platelets in mice after gene deletion, the release of platelet particles, and the number of inflammatory cells (SMCs, monocytes).

3.3. GPVI

The platelet-specific immunoglobulin superfamily receptor GPVI can induce platelet activation, adhesion, and aggregation, when activated by collagen or fibrinogen [73,74]. Platelet aggregation may have certain effects on atherosclerotic vessel wall homeostasis and atherosclerotic plaque rupture. Previous studies have found GPVI expression in the core region of human plaques [75]. Clinical studies have found that in patients with acute coronary syndrome (ACS) and unclear electrocardiogram, soluble dimeric GPVI (sGPVI) levels in coronary atherosclerotic heart disease (CAD) patients are generally elevated [76,77]. The sGPVI receptor has high affinity with immobilized collagen within atherosclerotic plaques [78]. In vitro animal experiments found that inhibition of GPVI by soluble GPVI-Fc or anti-GPVI antibodies protects atherosclerosis in cholesterol-fed rabbits and ApoE$^{-/-}$ mice [79]. This may be due to GPVI blocking partially inhibiting the adhesion of platelet and fibronectin to activated ECs. Another report showed that cross-linking GPVI-Fc enhances the inhibition of human plaque- and collagen-induced platelet aggregation, further supporting this [80]. Moreover, the use of microbubble-targeted contrast-enhanced ultrasound (CEU) combined with soluble GPVI can effectively localize and diagnose atherosclerotic lesions in ApoE$^{-/-}$ mice [81]. Subsequent studies also showed that GPIb-Fc had a stronger antithrombotic effect on the rupture site of high-risk lesions of atherosclerosis [82]. Thus, GPVI-FC may be a potential therapeutic target for plaque rupture or endothelial injury. The current research on platelet GPVI mainly focus on the damage of blood vessel integrity and thrombosis caused by platelet activation or platelet and endothelial adhesion. Although clinical studies have also shown that GPVI can be used as a marker of atherosclerotic plaque, the relative contributions of platelet GPVI in vivo contributing to atherosclerosis are still incompletely understood. The knowledge of its molecular mechanism is very limited.

3.4. P-Selectin

P-selectin is encoded by the selp gene, stored in α-granules of platelet and Weibel Palace bodies of endothelial cells [83]. P-selectin mediates the rolling of leukocytes on activated endothelium, the first step in the cell adhesion cascade [84,85]. P-selectin is not only a marker of platelet activation but also an important signaling molecule and mediator of cell–cell interactions, which seems to be very important for platelet-induced inflammation models and subsequent atherosclerosis. Destruction of the mouse p-selectin gene can significantly inhibit leukocyte rolling and delay the recruitment of monocytes to sites of inflammation [86]. Similarly, in Ldl-r$^{-/-}$ mice or ApoE$^{-/-}$ mice, the lack of P-selectin significantly reduced the fatty streak lesion size and macrophage infiltration [87,88]. Further studies have shown that both endothelial P-selectin deficiency and platelet P-selectin deficiency can reduce atherosclerosis lesions and macrophage infiltration in ApoE$^{-/-}$ mice with high-fat feeding. The latest research also reports that endothelial cell-derived P-selectin binds to p-selectin glycoprotein ligand 1 (PSGL-1) on dendritic cells (DCs), promotes an inflammatory response through the TLR4 signaling pathway, and participates in the progression of atherosclerosis [89]. In addition, platelet P-selectin can induce platelet adhesion to monocytes via the P-selectin-PSGL-1 axis, which further evokes the expression of some inflammatory factors (TNF-α, MCP-1) [90,91]. Increased binding of platelet-monocytes is also considered as a marker of acute coronary syndrome [92]. The expression of inflammatory factors accelerates the transformation of monocytes to macrophages and promotes atherosclerosis. Furthermore, Zhang et al. used mice expressing human SELP transgenes to further verify the atherosclerotic effect of P-selectin [93]. These combined data support an important role for P-selectin in murine or human atherogenesis. Treatment targeting the pathological expression or function of human p-selectin may effectively improve the prevention of atherosclerosis-related cardiovascular disease.

3.5. Thrombin Receptors

Thrombin is a multifunctional serine protease produced at the site of vascular injury, which converts fibrinogen to fibrin, activates platelets, and causes multiple actions of various cell types. The cellular effects of thrombin are mediated in part by the G protein-coupled receptor family protease-activated receptors (PARs, include PAR1~4) [94]. The role of PARs in the progression of atherosclerosis has been confirmed [95–99], but the link between platelet-derived PARs and the actual pathogenesis of AS is less clear. Interestingly, while human platelets utilize two thrombin receptors, PAR-1 and PAR-4, mouse platelets utilize PAR-3 and PAR-4 [100]. PAR1 and PAR3 mediate the activation of platelets at low thrombin concentrations and PAR4 can mediate platelet activation but only at high thrombin concentrations [100]. This may also be the reason why PAR1-inhibited human platelets are analogous to PAR3-deficient mouse platelets, as both rely on PAR4 for thrombin signaling [101,102]. However, PAR3 is rarely studied mainly because of the extremely low expression in human platelets [101]. The expression of PAR1 is abnormally elevated in human atherosclerotic arteries [103]. Application of PAR1 pepducin PZ-128 can inhibit macrophage infiltration of atherosclerotic lesions in mice [95,104]. The latest research report further confirms the role of PAR1 in the development of diet-mediated atherosclerosis, as one of the articles believes that PAR1 can promote AS in ApoE$^{-/-}$ mice by inhibiting the efflux of cholesterol in macrophages and smooth muscle cells and the recruitment of leukocytes [96]. Another article reported that thrombin can trigger the formation of foam cells by inducing the expression of CD36, and this process relies on the activation of the PKCθ signaling pathway mediated by PAR1 [105]. PAR4 has evolved a unique strategy for interacting with thrombin in human and mouse platelets. A study with PAR4 deficiency in ApoE$^{-/-}$ mice showed no significant difference in the plaque area compared with PAR4$^{+/+}$/ApoE$^{-/-}$ mice [106]. This indicates that PAR-4 is not required for the development of early atherosclerotic lesions. More recently, long-term administration of the thrombin inhibitor dabigatran in diabetic rats can cause upregulation of vascular PAR4, leading to increased platelet aggregation and coronary lipid deposition [107]. Therefore, the role of PAR4 in atherogenesis is still controversial, and platelet-derived PAR4 needs further study through platelet-specific knockout mice.

3.6. ADP Receptors

Along with thrombin, ADP has been recognized an important primary platelet agonist. ADP can be actively secreted by platelet-dense granules. Human platelets include three different ADP receptors: P2Y1, P2Y$_{12}$, and P2X1. P2X1 is a ligand-gated ion channel, and P2Y1 and P2Y$_{12}$ are receptors linked to two different G proteins. In platelets, the P2X1 receptor triggers transient shape change and participates in collagen- and shear-induced platelet aggregation, and may contribute to thrombus formation in the context of inflammation [108,109]. P2X1$^{-/-}$ mice displayed resistance to the systemic thromboembolism induced by injection of a mixture of collagen and adrenaline and also to the thrombosis triggered by a laser [108]. Overall, combined with current research, it is believed that P2X1 receptors are closely related to thrombosis and do not play a role in early atherosclerosis. Platelet P2Y1-related research mostly focuses on thrombosis and vascular inflammation. Activation of P2Y1 initiates shape change in platelet and leads to ADP-induced platelet aggregation [110,111]. The P2Y1 receptor antagonist MRS2500 can effectively inhibit experimental thrombosis in vivo [112]. In addition, the P2Y1 receptor can also facilitate the interaction between platelets and leukocytes resulting in leukocyte activation [113], which may be related to the platelet-dependent recruitment of leukocytes to lung tissue in the case of allergic airway inflammation [114]. However, this does not exclude the role of P2Y1 derived from endothelial cells or leukocytes. Indeed, the endothelial cell P2Y1 receptor strongly contributes to leukocyte recruitment and exposure of adhesion molecules (P-selectin, ICAM-1, and VCAM-1) during inflammation [115], and P2Y1$^{-/-}$/ApoE$^{-/-}$ mice showed reduced macrophage infiltration and atherosclerosis lesions [116]. The reason why platelet P2Y1 has a weak role in atherosclerosis or inflammation may be related to its expression on platelets. After all, approximately 150 copy numbers of P2Y1 receptors are expressed on each platelet, which is very low [117]. P2Y$_{12}$ is currently a clinically determined antiplatelet drug target, and P2Y$_{12}$ antagonists, such as clopidogrel, prasugrel, or ticagrelor, are clinically used in patients with coronary heart disease to inhibit platelet aggregation [118]. Moreover, animal studies have also shown that the P2Y$_{12}$ receptor may participate in atherogenesis by promoting the proliferation and migration of VSMCs, and endothelial dysfunction [119–121]. Deletion of the P2Y$_{12}$ gene in ApoE$^{-/-}$ mice or LDL$^{-/-}$ mice resulted in shrinking of the lesion area, decreased monocyte/macrophage infiltration, and increased fiber in plaque after a high-fat diet for 12 weeks [119,122]. Bone marrow transplantation experiments further demonstrate that platelet-expressed P2Y$_{12}$ is a key factor leading to atherosclerosis, but the role of smooth muscle cell P2Y12 is not excluded [119]. Subsequently, a study by West et al. [120] showed that the lack of P2Y$_{12}$ derived from the blood vessel wall rather than platelet can reduce the lesion size of atherosclerotic plaques in ApoE$^{-/-}$ mice. In summary, these results indicate that the early occurrence of atherosclerosis is mainly related to the expression of P2Y$_{12}$ in the vessel wall not in the platelet.

4. Platelet-Derived Proinflammatory Mediators in Atherogenesis

After platelet activation, a large amount of adhesive and proinflammatory substances stored in α granules and dense tubular systems are released. These substances interact with circulating leukocytes and blood vessel wall cells to induce a strong inflammatory response [1]. Proinflammatory substances released by platelets usually include various cytokines (IL1β, CD40L), chemokines (CCL5, CXCL4, CXCL7, CXCL12), growth factors (PDGF), and damage-related molecular model molecules DAMPs (HMGB, cyclophilin A) (Figure 3) [68,123]. The complex functional relationships of different platelet-derived mediators provide a mechanistic framework for the insight into the mechanisms by which platelets promote atherosclerosis.

4.1. Cytokines

IL-1β and CD40 ligand (CD40L, CD154) are important proinflammatory cytokines. IL-1β is synthesized and released after platelet activation and has become a target for coronary heart disease treatment. Activated platelet-synthesized interleukin (IL)-1β can induce the inflammatory response of ECs and promote the adhesion of platelets to leukocytes under the synergistic effect of e-selectin, ICAM-1, and chemokines [123]. In patients prone to development of atherosclerosis, polymorphism of the IL-1β gene cluster is associated with the extent of coronary arteries lesions, especially IL1B: −511 and −31 C/T polymorphism [124,125]. CD40L is stored in the cytoplasm of resting platelets, and is rapidly released to the membrane surface after platelet activation, and then it is cleaved to form a soluble functional fragment, sCD40L [1]. Platelets are the main source of circulating sCD40L, and elevated levels of circulating sCD40L have been reported in patients with hypercholesterolemia and diabetes [126–128]. This suggests that platelet-derived sCD40L can be an indicator for predicting postoperative risk of cardiovascular disease. IL-1β and CD40L on platelets induces ECs to express adhesion molecules (ICAM-1/VCAM-1) and secrete inflammatory factors (IL-8 and MCP-1), and promote the recruitment and extravasation of leukocytes at the site of injury, directly triggering an inflammatory response in the vessel wall [129]. Interrupting CD40 signal transduction with CD40L antibodies or CD40L deficiency in ApoE$^{-/-}$ mice can improve atherosclerotic lesions, reducing the infiltration of intermediate macrophages and T lymphocytes [130,131]. In clinical studies, the upregulation of platelet CD40L indicates a poor prognosis in stroke patients and is associated with increased platelet-mononuclear aggregate formation [132]. These results indicate that CD40L plays an important role in AS. However, Bavendiek et al. [133] showed that a CD40L deficiency on bone marrow-derived cells does not alter diet-induced atherosclerosis in hypercholesterolemia mice. This suggests that CD40L mainly regulates the occurrence of atherosclerosis through its expression on non-hematopoietic cell types, and platelet CD40L may not participate in AS. Moreover, the lack of CD40L will affect the stability of arterial thrombosis and delay arterial occlusion in vivo [134]. Therefore, simply blocking CD40L may not be feasible in the clinical treatment of atherosclerosis and other cardiovascular diseases, because long-term inhibition will increase the risk of thromboembolic events. Conceivably, more targeted intervention strategies in CD40 signaling will have less deleterious side effects.

Meanwhile, platelets also express substantial levels of CD40, which is the alleged counter receptor for CD40L [135]. CD40 is different from CD40L, and the role of the receptor CD40 in the development of atherosclerosis remains disputable. Zirlik [136] reported that CD40 deficiency in Ldlr$^{-/-}$ mice does not ameliorate atherosclerosis, although the endothelial CD40-TNF receptor-related factor (TRAF) signaling pathways have been proven to promote atherosclerosis. Lutgens [137] also reported that deficiency in hematopoietic CD40 in Ldlr$^{-/-}$ mice or genetic interruption of CD40-TRAF6 signaling in ApoE$^{-/-}$ mice reduces atherosclerosis and increases plaque fibrosis. Gerdes [138] further reported that platelet CD40 promotes atherogenesis by stimulating endothelial cell activation and recruiting leukocytes. In summary, the current findings suggest that platelet CD40 and CD40L can serve as a key interface between inflammation, thrombosis, and atherosclerosis and are attractive potential therapeutic targets for cardiovascular disease.

4.2. Chemokines

4.2.1. CXCL4

Platelet factor 4 (PF-4 or CXCL4), a member of the C-X-C subfamily of chemokines, is stored in the α-particles of platelet, and is extremely abundant in platelets. It is quickly mobilized and released into plasma when platelets are activated, and is the first type of medium for early thrombosis or plaque formation [139]. The presence of PF4 in atherosclerotic lesions correlates with clinical parameters in patients with atherosclerosis [140]. Additionally, co-localization of PF4 and ox-LDL can be observed in human atherosclerotic lesions, especially in macrophage-derived foam cells [139,141]. In vitro experiments found that PF4 not only induces the differentiation of monocytes into macrophages, named "M4" [142,143], but also promoted the binding of ox-LDL to vascular cells and macrophages and the accumulation of cholesterol esters [140]. These observations suggest that platelet activation may promote the accumulation of harmful lipoproteins and thus promote atherosclerosis. The more direct evidence is that PF4$^{-/-}$; ApoE$^{-/-}$ mice have a strong decrease in atherosclerotic lesion formation compared to ApoE$^{-/-}$ mice [144]. The reason for the reduction in plaque is most likely that PF4 inhibits the expression of the hemoglobin scavenger receptor (CD163) in proinflammatory macrophages, and CD163 has anti-lipid peroxidation and anti-inflammatory effects [145]. Normally, PF4 is more likely to form heterodimers, dimers, and oligomers with CCL5, inducing the binding of monocytes to ECs, thereby promoting the transmigration of monocyte into the subendothelial space.

4.2.2. CCL5

CCL5 (RANTES) is the most expressed chemokine during platelet transcription, and mainly activates CCR5 and CCR1 receptors. The microparticles released after platelet activation promotes the delivery of RANTES to the surface of monocytes in atherosclerotic arteries [146]. RANTES deposition enhances the recruitment of monocytes by inflammatory microvascular or aortic ECs, a process that depends on P-selectin expression [147,148]. Treatment with the RANTES antagonist Met-RANTES in Ldlr$^{-/-}$ mice reduces leukocyte infiltration and diet-induced atherosclerosis [149,150]. Clinical studies in patients with acute myocardial infarction and stable angina pectoris indicate that RANTES is more likely to be a biomarker for the presence of chronic coronary artery disease and is critical for the initial stage of atherosclerotic plaque formation [151]. Although RANTEs can be used as an indicator of AS inflammation, the specific role of platelet-derived RANTEs in AS needs more evidence. In fact, platelet-derived RANTES, in most cases, together with other mediators, induce monocyte inflammatory factor secretion (McP-1, McP-4, and IL-8) and accelerate AS [3]. One of the most common combinations is that CXCL4 and CCL5 interact to form heterodimers, then synergistically recruit monocytes to inflammatory vascular ECs [146] and induce the release of neutrophil extracellular traps (NETs) [152]. Disrupting the synergistic effect of CXCL4/CCL5 with peptide inhibitors MKEY will reduce leukocyte recruitment, NETosis formation, and ultimately reduce infarction size [153–155]. In conclusion, compared with CCL5 deficiency [156], blocking chemokine heterodimers can reduce inflammatory side effects and maintain normal immune defense.

4.2.3. CXCL7

CXCL7 is abundant in platelets; it is divided into several variants by pre-platelet basic protein (pre-PBP), including platelet basic protein (PBP), connective tissue-activating peptide III (CTAP-III), β thrombin (β-TG), and neutrophil-activating peptide 2 (NAP-2) [157]. NAP-2 is considered to be the only variant with chemotactic activity. Platelet-derived NAP-2 (CXCL7) deficiency or blockade of its receptor CXCR1/2 can significantly reduce thrombosis-induced neutrophil migration [158]. Patients with acute myocardial infarction were treated with PCI and found that plasma CXCL7 levels were negatively correlated with myocardial dysfunction [159]. However, there is no more relevant research reported in cardiovascular, especially atherosclerosis, patients. To the best of our knowledge, there are few studies on CXCL7 in the progress of AS. Additionally, there are few reports related to mononuclear/macrophages either. Further research is still needed on the role of platelet-derived CXCL7 in atherosclerosis.

4.2.4. CXCL12

The chemokine CXCL12, also known as stromal cell-derived factor-1 (SDF-1), is stored in platelet α granules. Early research found that high expression of CXCL12 was detected in SMCs, ECs, and macrophages of human atherosclerotic plaques from human carotid arteries [160]. However, recent studies by Merckelbach et al. [161] on human carotid atherosclerotic plaques have shown that CXCL12 is expressed only on the macrodissected areas of macrophages. The CXCR12 receptor CXCR4 is expressed on plaque macrophages, SMCs, and leukocytes. The reason for this difference may be related to the disease status and complications of patients with different plaque samples. In addition, the lower sensitivity of IHC staining and the shorter half-life of CXCL12 may also lead to poor observation of CXCL12 staining. In vitro experimental studies have found that platelet-derived CXCL12 can participate in the regulation of monocyte function, and induce the differentiation of monocytes into macrophages and foam cells through the receptors CXCR4-CXCR7 [162]. Therefore, CXCL12 may participate in AS through mononuclear differentiation. Animal studies further found that systemic treatment of CXCL12 in ApoE$^{-/-}$ mice promoted the mobilization and accumulation of smooth muscle progenitor cells at the site of vascular injury, thereby increasing plaque stability [163]. However, there is no evidence to show whether platelet-derived CXCL12 is playing a role here, thus further studies are necessary to elucidate the exact role of the platelet-derived CXCL12 in atherosclerotic plaques and potential impact on plaque vulnerability.

4.3. Other Platelet-Derived Inflammatory Mediators

The number of inflammatory mediators released from activated platelets is rapidly increasing. Platelet-derived growth factor (PDGF) is stored and released by α granules from activated platelets but can be widely secreted by macrophages, VSMCs, and endothelial cells [164]. The presence of PDGF was detected in the atherosclerotic vessel wall, especially PDGF-A and PDGF-B [165]. Simultaneously, PDGF receptors (PDGFR), PDGFR-α and PDGFR-β, expressed by macrophages and SMCs, are also significantly upregulated [166]. Multiple studies have shown that PDGF and PDGFR mainly regulate the development of atherosclerotic lesions by inducing the migration and proliferation of SMCs [167–169]. In ApoE$^{-/-}$ mice, blocking the PDGF-PDGFR-β pathway by neutralizing antibodies or chemical inhibitors prevented vascular smooth muscle cell accumulation and delayed fibrous cap formation [170,171]. In addition, enhancement of PDGF signaling led to severer inflammation, and promoted the progression of atherosclerosis in ApoE$^{-/-}$ mice [172]. However, at present, all studies have not pointed out how PDGF derived from platelets affects the expression of PDGFR in ECs, VSMCs, and infiltrating macrophages participating in vascular inflammation and remodeling.

Amphoterin (HMG1) is an endogenous protein in human platelets, which is exposed on the surface during platelet activation [173]. HMGB1 expression in human atherosclerotic plaques and coronary artery thrombi was identified. Therapeutic blockade of HMGB1 reduced the development of diet-induced atherosclerosis in ApoE$^{-/-}$ mice [174]. Furthermore, platelet-derived HMGB1 induces NETs formation and thrombosis [175,176]. This suggests that platelet-derived HMGB1 may be involved in the progression of both atherosclerosis and atherosclerotic thrombosis. Cyclophilin A (CyPA), a protein released when platelets are activated, is found in atherosclerotic plaques [177]. CyPA stimulates migration and proliferation of VSMCs, expression of adhesion molecules in endothelial cells, and inflammatory cell chemotaxis, and promotes atherosclerosis in ApoE$^{-/-}$ mice [178,179]. In addition, platelets also release several other proteins that may be related to atherosclerosis, such as granule protein III, histamine, etc. At present, we have less research on these "new" platelet-derived mediators, and future research should be an attempt to determine the role of these inflammatory factors in the formation of plaque.

5. Platelet Migration in Atherogenesis

Platelets guard blood vessels as a "patrol" to maintain vascular homeostasis in the physiological environment. Upon encountering endothelial injury or inflammation, the circulating platelets are recruited to the damaged sites of inflammation by various inflammatory factors and chemokines. Meanwhile, the platelets activated in the circulation can also release inflammatory factors and chemokines to promote the combination of platelets and immune cells. The interaction between these molecules and cells has been widely reported in atherosclerosis. However, the direct interaction of platelets with different subpopulations of leukocytes in atherosclerotic plaques remains unclear. Barrett et al. [180] found PF4 expression in a subset of plaque macrophages based on their single-cell

RNA sequencing in hypercholesterolemic mice, thus they suggested increased macrophage-platelet aggregates accumulate in atherosclerotic plaques. However, PF4 can also be expressed by a small number of macrophages [140,181], so whether platelets are present in atherosclerotic plaques needs further evidence for this to be confirmed. This may be proved by directly observing platelet markers (e.g., CD41, CD42d) at different stages of plaque formation by immunofluorescence staining. The study published by Gaertner et al. [182] identified that platelets have the capacity for locomotion at the level of cell biology for the first time, and they can migrate autonomously at the site of vascular injury. Platelets that migrate at the site of infection can help trap bacteria and promote the activation of NETs. In addition, platelets can penetrate into the lung tissue of allergic asthma through the reaction to allergens [183]. All these data indicate that the migrated platelets may promote tissue damage as inflammatory cells. In the process of atherosclerosis, whether platelets can actively migrate into the plaque, and how the migrated platelets act on the plaque formation needs in-depth study. Kraemer et al. [184] used transwell experiments in vitro found that CXCL12 can stimulate the migration of platelets on the surface of fibrinogen and collagen. The migration of platelets did not depend on either GPVI or GPIb/GPIIbIIIa. Receptors on the platelet surface recognizing and participating in the process of platelet migration need further exploration. Interestingly, Witte et al. [185] used platelet CXCR4-specific knockout mice, and for the first time showed that platelet-derived CXCL14 could induce monocyte migration through CXCR4 and enhance monocyte phagocytosis [186]. Controversially, some early in vitro flow chamber experiments believed that the platelets were still retained on the top of endothelial surface after they promoted monocyte transmigration [187,188]. Conclusively, whether platelets autonomously transmigrate, or could be carried by leukocytes into the subendothelium and play a role in atherogenesis still requires further proof. This could be addressed in in vitro transmigration models using cultured endothelial cells, or an in vivo animal model, combined with a pro-atherosclerotic factor, such as pathological blood flow.

6. Concluding Remarks and Future Perspectives

Platelets are important blood cells in the body. The initial physiological functions of platelets are mainly to stop the bleeding and keep the vascular endothelium intact. However, now, accumulating evidence indicates that platelets, as a novel immune and inflammatory cell, can modulate the inflammatory response of neighboring cells, such as leukocytes, ECs, and vascular SMCs. Simultaneously, platelets also receive the inflammatory signals produced by their neighboring cells. This double effect between platelets and neighboring cells plays roles in both the early and late stage during atherosclerosis. Although a variety of antiplatelet drugs have been widely used in patients with atherosclerotic diseases, platelet-mediated inflammation (complications due to side effects of the drug) appears to be operating. Therefore, the latest advances in understanding how platelets participate in the formation of atherosclerotic plaques will provide important clues for antiplatelet drugs in the prevention and treatment of cardiovascular diseases, especially atherosclerosis. Several issues need to be addressed in future studies: (1) whether and how platelets regulate atherosclerotic plaque formation under disturbance flow; (2) how platelets foster monocyte recruitment to atherosclerotic lesions and how they reprogram macrophages; (3) the association of platelet-derived inflammation mediators with atherogenesis should be explored in detail, such as using platelet-specific knockout mice; (4) further study is required to confirm whether platelet heterogeneity has been involved by using single-cell sequencing technology; and (5) whether platelets actively migrate to the subintima to participate in atherogenesis.

Author Contributions: Both authors contributed to writing, reviewing and editing of this work and consented to the final version. Both authors have read and agreed to the published version of the manuscript.

Abbreviations

AS	Atherosclerosis
D-flow	Disturbed flow
ECs	Endothelial cells
ICAM-1	Intercellular adhesion molecule-1
VCAM-1	Vascular cell adhesion molecule 1
vWF	Von Willebrand factor
GPIbα	Glycoprotein (GP) Ibα
GPVI	Glycoprotein VI
αIIbβ3	Integrin αIIbβ3
FLIPRs	Flow-induced protrusions
PMPs	Platelet microparticles
PECAM-1	Platelet endothelial cell adhesion molecule-1
MACE	Major cardiovascular adverse event
LDL	Low-density lipoprotein
HDL	High-density lipoprotein
LRP	LDL receptor-related protein
FAK	Focal adhesion kinase
oxLDL	Oxidized low-density lipoprotein
VSMCs	Vascular smooth muscle cells
SMCs	Smooth muscle cells
LOX-1	Lectin-like oxidized LDL receptor 1
DM	Diabetes mellitus
T2DM	Type 2 diabetes mellitus
PGI2	Prostacyclin
glycLDL	Glycosylated LDL
MPV	Mean platelet volume
sGPVI	Soluble dimeric GPVI
CAD	Coronary atherosclerotic heart disease
CEU	Contrast-enhanced ultrasound
PSGL-1	P-selectin glycoprotein ligand 1
DCs	Dendritic cells
PARs	Protease-activated receptors
IL-1β	Interleukin (IL)-1β
TRAF	TNF receptor-related factor
PF-4	Platelet factor 4
NETs	Neutrophil extracellular traps
PBP	Platelet basic protein
CTAP-III	Connective tissue-activating peptide III
β-TG	β thrombin
NAP-2	Neutrophil-activating peptide 2
SDF-1	Stromal cell-derived factor-1
PDGF	Platelet-derived growth factor
PDGFR	Platelet-derived growth factor receptors
CyPA	Cyclophilin A
HMG1	Amphoterin

References

1. Huo, Y.; Ley, K.F. Role of platelets in the development of atherosclerosis. *Trends Cardiovasc. Med.* **2004**, *14*, 18–22. [CrossRef] [PubMed]
2. Lievens, D.; von Hundelshausen, P. Platelets in atherosclerosis. *Thromb. Haemost.* **2011**, *106*, 827–838.
3. Aukrust, P.; Halvorsen, B.; Ueland, T.; Michelsen, A.E.; Skjelland, M.; Gullestad, L.; Yndestad, A.; Otterdal, K. Activated platelets and atherosclerosis. *Expert Rev. Cardiovasc. Ther.* **2010**, *8*, 1297–1307. [CrossRef] [PubMed]

4.   Kobiyama, K.; Ley, K. Atherosclerosis. *Circ. Res.* **2018**, *123*, 1118–1120. [CrossRef] [PubMed]

5.   Zhao, Y.; Yang, Y.; Xing, R.; Cui, X.; Xiao, Y.; Xie, L.; You, P.; Wang, T.; Zeng, L.; Peng, W.; et al. Hyperlipidemia induces typical atherosclerosis development in Ldlr and Apoe deficient rats. *Atherosclerosis* **2018**, *271*, 26–35. [CrossRef] [PubMed]

6.   Aronson, D.; Rayfield, E.J. How hyperglycemia promotes atherosclerosis: Molecular mechanisms. *Cardiovasc. Diabetol.* **2002**, *1*, 1–10. [CrossRef] [PubMed]

7.   Von Hundelshausen, P.; Weber, C. Platelets as Immune Cells Bridging Inflammation and Cardiovascular Disease. *Circ. Res.* **2007**, *100*, 27–40. [CrossRef]

8.   Siegel-Axel, D.; Daub, K.; Seizer, P.; Lindemann, S.; Gawaz, M. Platelet lipoprotein interplay: Trigger of foam cell formation and driver of atherosclerosis. *Cardiovasc. Res.* **2008**, *78*, 8–17. [CrossRef]

9.   Hartwig, J.H. The Platelet: Form and Function. *Semin. Hematol.* **2006**, *43*, S94–S100. [CrossRef]

10. Li, Z.; Yang, F.; Dunn, S.; Gross, A.K.; Smyth, S.S. Platelets as immune mediators: Their role in host defense responses and sepsis. *Thromb. Res.* **2011**, *127*, 184–188. [CrossRef]

11. Von Hundelshausen, P.; Duchene, J. Platelet-derived chemokines in atherosclerosis. *Hämostaseologie* **2017**, *35*, 137–141. [CrossRef] [PubMed]

12. Nording, H.; Baron, L.; Langer, H.F. Platelets as therapeutic Targets to prevent Atherosclerosis. *Atherosclerosis* **2020**, *307*, 97–108. [CrossRef] [PubMed]

13. Nam, D.; Ni, C.W.; Rezvan, A.; Suo, J.; Budzyn, K.; Llanos, A.; Harrison, D.; Giddens, D.; Jo, H. Partial carotid ligation is a model of acutely induced disturbed flow, leading to rapid endothelial dysfunction and atherosclerosis. *Am. J. Physiol. Heart Circ. Physiol.* **2009**, *297*, H1535–H1543. [CrossRef] [PubMed]

14. Berk, B.C. Atheroprotective signaling mechanisms activated by steady laminar flow in endothelial cells. *Circulation* **2008**, *117*, 1082–1089. [CrossRef]

15. Chiu, J.J.; Chen, C.N.; Lee, P.L.; Yang, C.T.; Chuang, H.S.; Chien, S.; Usami, S. Analysis of the effect of disturbed flow on monocytic adhesion to endothelial cells. *J. Biomech.* **2003**, *36*, 1883–1895. [CrossRef]

16. Coenen, D.M.; Mastenbroek, T.G.; Cosemans, J.M.E.M. Platelet interaction with activated endothelium: Mechanistic insights from microfluidics. *Blood* **2017**, *130*, 2819–2828. [CrossRef]

17. Glise, L.; Larsson, P.; Jern, S.; Borén, J.; Levin, M.; Ny, T.; Fogelstrand, P.; Bergh, N. Disturbed Laminar Blood Flow Causes Impaired Fibrinolysis and Endothelial Fibrin Deposition In Vivo. *Thromb. Haemost.* **2019**, *119*, 223–233. [CrossRef]

18. Skilbeck, C.A.; Walker, P.G.; David, T.; Nash, G.B. Disturbed flow promotes deposition of leucocytes from flowing whole blood in a model of a damaged vessel wall. *Br. J. Haematol.* **2004**, *126*, 418–427. [CrossRef]

19. Tersteeg, C.; Heijnen, H.F.G.; Eckly, A.; Pasterkamp, G.; Urbanus, R.T.; Maas, C.; Hoefer, I.E.; Nieuwland, R.; Farndale, R.W.; Gachet, C. FLow-Induced PRotrusions (FLIPRs): A Platelet-Derived Platform for the Retrieval of Microparticles by Monocytes and Neutrophils. *Circ. Res.* **2014**, *114*, 780–791. [CrossRef]

20. Wang, Z.; Wang, Z.; Hu, Y. Possible roles of platelet-derived microparticles in atherosclerosis. *Atherosclerosis* **2016**, *248*, 10–16. [CrossRef]

21. Meza, D.; Shanmugavelayudam, S.K.; Mendoza, A.; Sanchez, C.; Rubenstein, D.A.; Yin, W. Platelets modulate endothelial cell response to dynamic shear stress through PECAM-1. *Thromb Res.* **2017**, *150*, 44–50. [CrossRef] [PubMed]

22. Stevens, H.Y.; Melchior, B.; Bell, K.S.; Yun, S.J.; Yeh, J.C.; Frangos, J.A. PECAM-1 is a critical mediator of atherosclerosis. *Dis. Model Mech.* **2008**, *1*, 175–181. [CrossRef] [PubMed]

23. Libby, P.; Ridker, P.M.; Maseri, A. Inflammation and Atherosclerosis. *Circulation* **2002**, *105*, 1135–1143. [CrossRef] [PubMed]

24. Halcox, J.P.; Banegas, J.R.; Roy, C.; Dallongeville, J.; De Backer, G.; Guallar, E.; Perk, J.; Hajage, D.; Henriksson, K.M.; Borghi, C. Prevalence and treatment of atherogenic dyslipidemia in the primary prevention of cardiovascular disease in Europe: EURIKA, a cross-sectional observational study. *BMC Cardiovasc. Disord.* **2017**, *17*, 160. [CrossRef]

25. Wang, X.; Cai, G.; Wang, Y.; Liu, R.; Xi, Z.; Li, G.; Wen, W.; Wu, Y.; Wang, C.; Ji, Q.; et al. Comparison of long-term outcomes of young patients after a coronary event associated with familial hypercholesterolemia. *Lipids Health Dis.* **2019**, *18*, 131. [CrossRef]

26. Barale, C.; Frascaroli, C.; Senkeev, R.; Cavalot, F.; Russo, I. Simvastatin Effects on Inflammation and Platelet Activation Markers in Hypercholesterolemia. *BioMed Res. Int.* **2018**, *2018*, 6508709. [CrossRef]

27. Hamilton, P.K.; Hughes, S.M.T.; Plumb, R.D.; Devine, A.; Mcveigh, G.E. Statins have beneficial effects on platelet free radical activity and intracellular distribution of GTPases in hyperlipidaemia. *Clin. Sci.* **2010**, *118*, 359–366. [CrossRef]

28. Surya, I.I.; Akkerman, J.N. The influence of lipoproteins on blood platelets. *Am. Heart J.* **1993**, *125*, 272–275. [CrossRef]

29. Sener, A.; Enc, E.; Ozsavci, D.; Vanizor-Kural, B.; Demir, M. Exogenous L-Arginine and HDL Can Alter LDL and ox-LDL-Mediated Platelet Activation: Using Platelet P-Selectin Receptor Numbers. *Clin. Appl. Thromb./Hemost.* **2010**, *17*, E79–E86. [CrossRef]

30. Koller, E.; Koller, F.; Doleschel, W. Specific Binding Sites on Human Blood Platelets for Plasma Lipoproteins. *Biol. Chem.* **1982**, *363*, 395–406. [CrossRef]

31. Riddell, D.R.; Vinogradov, D.V.; Stannard, A.K.; Chadwick, N.; Owen, J.S. Identification and characterization of LRP8 (apoER2) in human blood platelets. *J. Lipid Res.* **1999**, *40*, 1925–1930. [PubMed]

32. Relou, I.A.M.; Hackeng, C.M.; Akkerman, J.N.; Malle, E. Low-density lipoprotein and its effect on human blood platelets. *Cell. Mol. Life Sci.* **2003**, *60*, 961–971. [CrossRef] [PubMed]

33. van der Stoep, M.; Korporaal, S.J.; Van Eck, M. High-density lipoprotein as a modulator of platelet and coagulation responses. *Cardiovasc. Res.* **2014**, *103*, 362–371. [CrossRef] [PubMed]

34. Podrez, E.A.; Byzova, T.V.; Febbraio, M.; Salomon, R.G.; Ma, Y.; Valiyaveettil, M.; Poliakov, E.; Sun, M.; Finton, P.J.; Curtis, B.R. Platelet CD36 links hyperlipidemia, oxidant stress and a prothrombotic phenotype. *Nat. Med.* **2007**, *13*, 1086–1095. [CrossRef] [PubMed]

35. Stellos, K.; Sauter, R.; Fahrleitner, M.; Grimm, J.; Stakos, D.; Emschermann, F.; Panagiota, V.; Gnerlich, S.; Perk, A.; Schonberger, T. Binding of Oxidized Low-Density Lipoprotein on Circulating Platelets Is increased in Patients With Acute Coronary Syndromes and Induces Platelet Adhesion to Vascular Wall In Vivo—Brief Report. *Arterioscler. Thromb. Vasc. Biol.* **2012**, *32*, 2017–2020. [CrossRef]

36. Magwenzi, S.; Woodward, C.; Wraith, K.S.; Aburima, A.; Raslan, Z.; Jones, H.S.; Mcneil, C.; Wheatcroft, S.B.; Yuldasheva, N.; Febbraio, M. Oxidized LDL activates blood platelets through CD36/NOX2–mediated inhibition of the cGMP/protein kinase G signaling cascade. *Blood* **2015**, *125*, 2693–2703. [CrossRef]

37. Zimman, A.; Titz, B.; Komisopoulou, E.; Biswas, S.; Graeber, T.G.; Podrez, E.A. Phosphoproteomic analysis of platelets activated by pro-thrombotic oxidized phospholipids and thrombin. *PLoS ONE* **2014**, *9*, e84488. [CrossRef]

38. Daub, K.; Seizer, P.; Stellos, K.; Kramer, B.F.; Bigalke, B.; Schaller, M.; Fatehmoghadam, S.; Gawaz, M.; Lindemann, S. Oxidized LDL-Activated Platelets Induce Vascular Inflammation. *Semin. Thromb. Hemost.* **2010**, *36*, 146–156. [CrossRef]

39. Yue, H.; Febbraio, M.; Klenotic, P.A.; Kennedy, D.J.; Wu, Y.; Chen, S.; Gohara, A.F.; Li, O.; Belcher, A.; Kuang, B. CD36 Enhances Vascular Smooth Muscle Cell Proliferation and Development of Neointimal Hyperplasia. *Arterioscler. Thromb. Vasc. Biol.* **2019**, *39*, 263–275. [CrossRef]

40. Chen, M.; Kakutani, M.; Naruko, T.; Ueda, M.; Narumiya, S.; Masaki, T.; Sawamura, T. Activation-Dependent Surface Expression of LOX-1 in Human Platelets. *Biochem. Biophys. Res. Commun.* **2001**, *282*, 153–158. [CrossRef]

41. Balzan, S.; Lubrano, V. LOX-1 receptor: A potential link in atherosclerosis and cancer. *Life Sci.* **2018**, *198*, 79–86. [CrossRef] [PubMed]

42. Tian, K.; Ogura, S.; Little, P.J.; Xu, S.; Sawamura, T. Targeting LOX-1 in atherosclerosis and vasculopathy: Current knowledge and future perspectives. *Ann. N. Y. Acad. Sci.* **2019**, *1443*, 34–53. [CrossRef] [PubMed]

43. Katakami, N. Mechanism of Development of Atherosclerosis and Cardiovascular Disease in Diabetes Mellitus. *J. Atheroscler. Thromb.* **2018**, *25*, 27–39. [CrossRef] [PubMed]

44. Capes, S.E.; Hunt, D.L.; Malmberg, K.; Pathak, P.; Gerstein, H.C. Stress hyperglycemia and prognosis of stroke in nondiabetic and diabetic patients: A systematic overview. *Stroke* **2001**, *32*, 2426–2432. [CrossRef] [PubMed]

45. Li, Y.; Woo, V.; Bose, R. Platelet hyperactivity and abnormal Ca2+ homeostasis in diabetes mellitus. *Am. J. Physiol.-Heart Circ. Physiol.* **2001**, *280*, H1480–H1489. [CrossRef] [PubMed]

46. Keating, F.K.; Sobel, B.E.; Schneider, D.J. Effects of Increased Concentrations of Glucose on Platelet Reactivity in Healthy Subjects and in Patients With and Without Diabetes Mellitus. *Am. J. Cardiol.* **2003**, *92*, 1362–1365. [CrossRef]

47. Ferroni, P.; Basili, S.; Falco, A.; Davi, G. Platelet activation in type 2 diabetes mellitus. *J. Thromb. Haemost.* **2004**, *2*, 1282–1291. [CrossRef]

48. Winocour, P.D. Platelet Abnormalities in Diabetes Mellitus. *Diabetes* **1992**, *41*, 26–31. [CrossRef]

49. Ferretti, G.; Rabini, R.A.; Bacchetti, T.; Vignini, A.; Salvolini, E.; Ravaglia, F.; Curatola, G.; Mazzanti, L. Glycated Low Density Lipoproteins Modify Platelet Properties: A Compositional and Functional Study. *J. Clin. Endocrinol. Metab.* **2002**, *87*, 2180–2184. [CrossRef]

50. Ju, L.; McFadyen, J.D.; Al-Daher, S.; Alwis, I.; Chen, Y.; Tønnesen, L.L.; Maiocchi, S.; Coulter, B.; Calkin, A.C.; Felner, E.I.; et al. Compression force sensing regulates integrin αIIbβ3 adhesive function on diabetic platelets. *Nat. Commun.* **2018**, *9*, 1087. [CrossRef]

51. Rusak, T.; Misztal, T.; Rusak, M.; Branskajanuszewska, J.; Tomasiak, M. Involvement of hyperglycemia in the development of platelet procoagulant response: The role of aldose reductase and platelet swelling. *Blood Coagul. Fibrinolysis* **2017**, *28*, 443–451. [CrossRef] [PubMed]

52. Hu, H.; Li, N.; Yngen, M.; Ostenson, C.; Wallen, N.H.; Hjemdahl, P. Enhanced leukocyte–platelet cross-talk in Type 1 diabetes mellitus: Relationship to microangiopathy. *J. Thromb. Haemost.* **2004**, *2*, 58–64. [CrossRef] [PubMed]

53. Patko, Z.; Csaszar, A.; Acsady, G.; Őry, I.; Takacs, E.; Fűresz, J. Elevation of monocyte-platelet aggregates is an early marker of type 2 diabetes. *Interv. Med. Appl. Sci.* **2012**, *4*, 181–185. [CrossRef] [PubMed]

54. Kraakman, M.J.; Lee, M.K.S.; Alsharea, A.; Dragoljevic, D.; Barrett, T.J.; Montenont, E.; Basu, D.; Heywood, S.E.; Kammoun, H.L.; Flynn, M.C. Neutrophil-derived S100 calcium-binding proteins A8/A9 promote reticulated thrombocytosis and atherogenesis in diabetes. *J. Clin. Investig.* **2017**, *127*, 2133–2147. [CrossRef] [PubMed]

55. Lee, R.H.; Bergmeier, W. Sugar makes neutrophils RAGE: Linking diabetes-associated hyperglycemia to thrombocytosis and platelet reactivity. *J. Clin. Investig.* **2017**, *127*, 2040–2043. [CrossRef] [PubMed]

56. Newman, J.D.; Echagarruga, C.; Ogando, Y.; Montenont, E.; Chen, Y.; Fisher, E.A.; Berger, J.S. Hyperglycemia enhances arsenic-induced platelet and megakaryocyte activation. *J. Transl. Med.* **2017**, *15*, 55. [CrossRef]

57. Beaulieu, L.M.; Lin, E.; Mick, E.; Koupenova, M.; Weinberg, E.O.; Kramer, C.D.; Genco, C.A.; Tanriverdi, K.; Larson, M.G.; Benjamin, E.J. Interleukin 1 Receptor 1 and Interleukin 1β Regulate Megakaryocyte Maturation, Platelet Activation, and Transcript Profile During Inflammation in Mice and Humans. *Arterioscler. Thromb. Vasc. Biol.* **2014**, *34*, 552–564. [CrossRef]

58. Pretorius, L.; Thomson, G.J.A.; Adams, R.C.M.; Nell, T.A.; Laubscher, W.A.; Pretorius, E. Platelet activity and hypercoagulation in type 2 diabetes. *Cardiovasc. Diabetol.* **2018**, *17*, 141. [CrossRef]

59. Ibrahim, H.; Kleiman, N.S. Platelet pathophysiology, pharmacology, and function in coronary artery disease. *Coron. Artery Dis.* **2017**, *28*, 614–623. [CrossRef]

60. Shattil, S.J. Signaling through platelet integrin αIIbβ3: Inside-out, outside-in, and sideways. *Thromb. Haemost.* **1999**, *82*, 318–325. [CrossRef]

61. Shpilberg, O.; Rabi, I.; Schiller, K.; Walden, R.; Harats, D.; Tyrrell, K.S.; Coller, B.; Seligsohn, U. Patients With Glanzmann Thrombasthenia Lacking Platelet Glycoprotein αIIbβ3 (GPIIb/IIIa) and αvβ3 Receptors Are Not Protected From Atherosclerosis. *Circulation* **2002**, *105*, 1044–1048. [CrossRef] [PubMed]

62. Weng, S.; Zemany, L.; Standley, K.N.; Novack, D.V.; La Regina, M.; Bernalmizrachi, C.; Coleman, T.; Semenkovich, C.F. β3 integrin deficiency promotes atherosclerosis and pulmonary inflammation in high-fat-fed, hyperlipidemic mice. *Proc. Natl. Acad. Sci. USA* **2003**, *100*, 6730–6735. [CrossRef] [PubMed]

63. Misra, A.; Feng, Z.; Chandran, R.R.; Kabir, I.; Rotllan, N.; Aryal, B.; Sheikh, A.Q.; Ding, L.; Qin, L.; Fernandezhernando, C. Integrin beta3 regulates clonality and fate of smooth muscle-derived atherosclerotic plaque cells. *Nat. Commun.* **2018**, *9*, 2073. [CrossRef] [PubMed]

64. Massberg, S.; Enders, G.; Matos, F.C.; Tomic, L.I.; Leiderer, R.; Eisenmenger, K.; Krombach, F. Fibrinogen Deposition at the Postischemic Vessel Wall Promotes Platelet Adhesion During Ischemia-Reperfusion In Vivo. *Blood* **1999**, *94*, 3829–3838. [CrossRef]

65. Massberg, S.; Schurzinger, K.; Lorenz, M.; Konrad, I.; Schulz, C.; Plesnila, N.; Kennerknecht, E.; Rudelius, M.; Sauer, S.; Braun, S. Platelet Adhesion Via Glycoprotein IIb Integrin Is Critical for Atheroprogression and Focal Cerebral Ischemia An In Vivo Study in Mice Lacking Glycoprotein IIb. *Circulation* **2005**, *112*, 1180–1188. [CrossRef] [PubMed]

66. Maile, L.A.; Busby, W.H.; Xi, G.; Gollahan, K.P.; Flowers, W.L.; Gafbacik, N.; Gafbacik, S.; Stewart, K.; Merricks, E.P.; Nichols, T.C. An anti-αVβ3 antibody inhibits coronary artery atherosclerosis in diabetic pigs. *Atherosclerosis* **2017**, *258*, 40–50. [CrossRef]

67. Lopez, J.A. The platelet glycoprotein Ib-IX complex. *Blood Coagul. Fibrinolysis* **2017**, *5*, 97–120. [CrossRef]

68. Massberg, S.; Brand, K.; Gruner, S.; Page, S.; Muller, E.; Muller, I.; Bergmeier, W.; Richter, T.; Lorenz, M.; Konrad, I.; et al. A critical role of platelet adhesion in the initiation of atherosclerotic lesion formation. *J. Exp. Med.* **2002**, *196*, 887–896. [CrossRef]

69. Koltsova, E.K.; Sundd, P.; Zarpellon, A.; Ouyang, H.; Mikulski, Z.; Zampolli, A.; Ruggeri, Z.M.; Ley, K. Genetic deletion of platelet glycoprotein Ib alpha but not its extracellular domain protects from atherosclerosis. *Thromb. Haemost.* **2014**, *112*, 1252–1263. [CrossRef]

70. Methia, N.; Andre, P.; Denis, C.V.; Economopoulos, M.; Wagner, D.D. Localized reduction of atherosclerosis in von Willebrand factor–deficient mice. *Blood* **2001**, *98*, 1424–1428. [CrossRef]

71. Manka, D.; Forlow, S.B.; Sanders, J.M.; Hurwitz, D.; Bennett, D.K.; Green, S.A.; Ley, K.; Sarembock, I.J. Critical Role of Platelet P-Selectin in the Response to Arterial Injury in Apolipoprotein-E–Deficient Mice. *Arterioscler. Thromb. Vasc. Biol.* **2004**, *24*, 1124–1129. [CrossRef]

72. Strassel, C.; Hechler, B.; Bull, A.; Gachet, C.; Lanza, F. Studies of mice lacking the GPIb-V-IX complex question the role of this receptor in atherosclerosis. *J. Thromb. Haemost.* **2009**, *7*, 1935–1938. [CrossRef] [PubMed]

73. Mangin, P.H.; Onselaer, M.; Receveur, N.; Lay, N.L.; Hardy, A.T.; Wilson, C.; Sanchez, X.; Loyau, S.; Dupuis, A.; Babar, A.K. Immobilized fibrinogen activates human platelets through glycoprotein VI. *Haematologica* **2018**, *103*, 898–907. [CrossRef] [PubMed]

74. Alshehri, O.; Hughes, C.E.; Montague, S.J.; Watson, S.; Frampton, J.; Bender, M.; Watson, S.P. Fibrin activates GPVI in human and mouse platelets. *Blood* **2015**, *126*, 1601–1608. [CrossRef] [PubMed]

75. Schonberger, T.; Siegel-Axel, D.; Bussl, R.; Richter, S.; Judenhofer, M.S.; Haubner, R.; Reischl, G.; Klingel, K.; Munch, G.; Seizer, P.; et al. The immunoadhesin glycoprotein VI-Fc regulates arterial remodelling after mechanical injury in ApoE-/- mice. *Cardiovasc. Res.* **2008**, *80*, 131–137. [CrossRef] [PubMed]

76. Gawaz, M.; Vogel, S.; Pfannenberg, C.; Pichler, B.J.; Langer, H.F.; Bigalke, B. Implications of glycoprotein VI for theranostics. *Thromb. Haemost.* **2014**, *112*, 26–31.

77. Villmann, J.M.; Burkhardt, R.; Teren, A.; Villmann, T.; Thiery, J.; Drogies, T. Atherosclerosis, myocardial infarction and primary hemostasis: Impact of platelets, von Willebrand factor and soluble glycoprotein VI. *Thromb. Res.* **2019**, *180*, 98–104. [CrossRef]

78. Massberg, S.; Konrad, I.; Bultmann, A.; Schulz, C.; Munch, G.; Peluso, M.; Lorenz, M.; Schneider, S.; Besta, F.; Muller, I. Soluble glycoprotein VI dimer inhibits platelet adhesion and aggregation to the injured vessel wall in vivo. *FASEB J.* **2003**, *18*, 397–399. [CrossRef]

79. Bultmann, A.; Li, Z.; Wagner, S.; Peluso, M.; Schonberger, T.; Weis, C.; Konrad, I.; Stellos, K.; Massberg, S.; Nieswandt, B.; et al. Impact of glycoprotein VI and platelet adhesion on atherosclerosis—A possible role of fibronectin. *J. Mol. Cell Cardiol.* **2010**, *49*, 532–542. [CrossRef]

80. Jamasbi, J.; Megens, R.T.A.; Bianchini, M.; Uhland, K.; Munch, G.; Ungerer, M.; Sherman, S.; Faussner, A.; Brandl, R.; John, C. Cross-Linking GPVI-Fc by Anti-Fc Antibodies Potentiates Its Inhibition of Atherosclerotic Plaque- and Collagen-Induced Platelet Activation. *JACC Basic Transl. Sci.* **2016**, *1*, 131–142. [CrossRef]

81. Metzger, K.; Vogel, S.; Chatterjee, M.; Borst, O.; Seizer, P.; Schonberger, T.; Geisler, T.; Lang, F.; Langer, H.F.; Rheinlaender, J. High-frequency ultrasound-guided disruption of glycoprotein VI-targeted microbubbles targets atheroprogressison in mice. *Biomaterials* **2015**, *36*, 80–89. [CrossRef] [PubMed]

82. Jamasbi, J.; Megens, R.T.A.; Bianchini, M.; Munch, G.; Ungerer, M.; Faussner, A.; Sherman, S.; Walker, A.; Goyal, P.; Jung, S.M. Differential Inhibition of Human Atherosclerotic Plaque-Induced Platelet Activation by Dimeric GPVI-Fc and Anti-GPVI Antibodies Functional and Imaging Studies. *J. Am. Coll. Cardiol.* **2015**, *65*, 2404–2415. [CrossRef] [PubMed]

83. Vestweber, D.; Blanks, J.E. Mechanisms that regulate the function of the selectins and their ligands. *Physiol. Rev.* **1999**, *79*, 181–213. [CrossRef] [PubMed]

84. Ramos, C.L.; Huo, Y.; Jung, U.; Ghosh, S.; Manka, D.; Sarembock, I.J.; Ley, K. Direct Demonstration of P-Selectin– and VCAM-1–Dependent Mononuclear Cell Rolling in Early Atherosclerotic Lesions of Apolipoprotein E–Deficient Mice. *Circ. Res.* **1999**, *84*, 1237–1244. [CrossRef] [PubMed]

85. Burger, P.C.; Wagner, D.D. Platelet P-selectin facilitates atherosclerotic lesion development. *Blood* **2003**, *101*, 2661–2666. [CrossRef] [PubMed]

86. Subramaniam, M.; Saffaripour, S.; Watson, S.R.; Mayadas, T.N.; Hynes, R.O.; Wagner, D.D. Reduced recruitment of inflammatory cells in a contact hypersensitivity response in P-selectin-deficient mice. *J. Exp. Med.* **1995**, *181*, 2277–2282. [CrossRef]

87.	Johnson, R.C.; Schaefer, E.J.; Wagner, D.D. Absence of P-selectin delays fatty streak formation in mice. *J. Clin. Investig.* **1997**, *99*, 1037–1043. [CrossRef]
88.	Dong, Z.M.; Brown, A.A.; Wagner, D.D. Prominent Role of P-Selectin in the Development of Advanced Atherosclerosis in ApoE-Deficient Mice. *Circulation* **2000**, *101*, 2290–2295. [CrossRef]
89.	Ye, Z.; Zhong, L.; Zhu, S.; Wang, Y.; Zheng, J.; Wang, S.; Zhang, J.; Huang, R. The P-selectin and PSGL-1 axis accelerates atherosclerosis via activation of dendritic cells by the TLR4 signaling pathway. *Cell Death Dis.* **2019**, *10*, 507. [CrossRef]
90.	Sarma, J.; Laan, C.A.; Alam, S.; Jha, A.; Fox, K.A.A.; Dransfield, I. Increased Platelet Binding to Circulating Monocytes in Acute Coronary Syndromes. *Circulation* **2002**, *105*, 2166–2171. [CrossRef]
91.	Weyrich, A.S.; Mcintyre, T.M.; Mcever, R.P.; Prescott, S.M.; Zimmerman, G.A. Monocyte tethering by P-selectin regulates monocyte chemotactic protein-1 and tumor necrosis factor-alpha secretion. Signal integration and NF-kappa B translocation. *J. Clin. Investig.* **1995**, *95*, 2297–2303. [CrossRef] [PubMed]
92.	Gremmel, T.; Ay, C.; Riedl, J.; Kopp, C.W.; Eichelberger, B.; Koppensteiner, R.; Panzer, S. Platelet-specific markers are associated with monocyte-platelet aggregate formation and thrombin generation potential in advanced atherosclerosis. *Thromb. Haemost.* **2015**, *115*, 615–621. [PubMed]
93.	Zhang, N.; Liu, Z.; Yao, L.; Mehtadsouza, P.; Mcever, R.P. P-Selectin Expressed by a Human SELP Transgene Is Atherogenic in Apolipoprotein E–Deficient Mice. *Arterioscler. Thromb. Vasc. Biol.* **2016**, *36*, 1114–1121. [CrossRef] [PubMed]
94.	Martorell, L.; Martinez-Gonzalez, J.; Rodriguez, C.; Gentile, M.; Calvayrac, O.; Badimon, L. Thrombin and protease-activated receptors (PARs) in atherothrombosis. *Thromb. Haemost.* **2008**, *99*, 305–315. [CrossRef] [PubMed]
95.	Rana, R.; Huang, T.; Koukos, G.; Fletcher, E.K.; Turner, S.E.; Shearer, A.M.; Gurbel, P.A.; Rade, J.J.; Kimmelstiel, C.; Bliden, K.P. Noncanonical Matrix Metalloprotease 1–Protease-Activated Receptor 1 Signaling Drives Progression of Atherosclerosis. *Arterioscler. Thromb. Vasc. Biol.* **2018**, *38*, 1368–1380. [CrossRef] [PubMed]
96.	Raghavan, S.; Singh, N.K.; Mani, A.M.; Rao, G.N. Protease-activated receptor 1 inhibits cholesterol efflux and promotes atherogenesis via cullin 3–mediated degradation of the ABCA1 transporter. *J. Biol. Chem.* **2018**, *293*, 10574–10589. [CrossRef] [PubMed]
97.	Jones, S.M.; Mann, A.; Conrad, K.; Saum, K.; Hall, D.; Mckinney, L.M.; Robbins, N.; Thompson, J.C.; Peairs, A.; Camerer, E. PAR2 (Protease-Activated Receptor 2) Deficiency Attenuates Atherosclerosis in Mice. *Arterioscler. Thromb. Vasc. Biol.* **2018**, *38*, 1271–1282. [CrossRef]
98.	Hara, T.; Phuong, P.T.; Fukuda, D.; Yamaguchi, K.; Murata, C.; Nishimoto, S.; Yagi, S.; Kusunose, K.; Yamada, H.; Soeki, T. Protease-Activated Receptor-2 Plays a Critical Role in Vascular Inflammation and Atherosclerosis in Apolipoprotein E–Deficient Mice. *Circulation* **2018**, *138*, 1706–1719. [CrossRef]
99.	Hikita, T.; Mirzapourshafiyi, F.; Barbacena, P.; Riddell, M.; Pasha, A.; Li, M.; Kawamura, T.; Brandes, R.P.; Hirose, T.; Ohno, S. PAR-3 controls endothelial planar polarity and vascular inflammation under laminar flow. *EMBO Rep.* **2018**, *19*, e45253. [CrossRef]
100.	Coughlin, S.R. Thrombin signalling and protease-activated receptors. *Nature* **2000**, *407*, 258–264. [CrossRef]
101.	Nakanishimatsui, M.; Zheng, Y.; Sulciner, D.; Weiss, E.J.; Ludeman, M.J.; Coughlin, S.R. PAR3 is a cofactor for PAR4 activation by thrombin. *Nature* **2000**, *404*, 609–613. [CrossRef] [PubMed]
102.	Leger, A.J.; Covic, L.; Kuliopulos, A. Protease-Activated Receptors in Cardiovascular Diseases. *Circulation* **2006**, *114*, 1070–1077. [CrossRef] [PubMed]
103.	Nelken, N.A.; Soifer, S.J.; Okeefe, J.; Vu, T.H.; Charo, I.F.; Coughlin, S.R. Thrombin receptor expression in normal and atherosclerotic human arteries. *J. Clin. Investig.* **1992**, *90*, 1614–1621. [CrossRef]
104.	Ruf, W. Proteases, Protease-Activated Receptors, and Atherosclerosis. *Arterioscler. Thromb. Vasc. Biol.* **2018**, *38*, 1252–1254. [CrossRef] [PubMed]
105.	Raghavan, S.; Singh, N.K.; Gali, S.; Mani, A.M.; Rao, G.N. Protein Kinase Cθ Via Activating Transcription Factor 2-Mediated CD36 Expression and Foam Cell Formation of Ly6Chi Cells Contributes to Atherosclerosis. *Circulation* **2018**, *138*, 2395–2412. [CrossRef]
106.	Hamilton, J.R.; Cornelissen, I.; Mountford, J.K.; Coughlin, S.R. Atherosclerosis proceeds independently of thrombin-induced platelet activation in ApoE-/- mice. *Atherosclerosis* **2009**, *205*, 427–432. [CrossRef]

107. Scridon, A.; Mărginean, A.; Huțanu, A.; Chinezu, L.; Gheban, D.; Perian, M.; Vântu, A.; Gherțescu, D.; Fișcă, P.C.; Șerban, R.C. Vascular protease-activated receptor 4 upregulation, increased platelet aggregation, and coronary lipid deposits induced by long-term dabigatran administration—results from a diabetes animal model. *J. Thromb. Haemost.* **2019**, *17*, 538–550. [CrossRef]

108. Hechler, B.; Lenain, N.; Marchese, P.; Vial, C.; Heim, V.; Freund, M.; Cazenave, J.; Cattaneo, M.; Ruggeri, Z.M.; Evans, R.J. A role of the fast ATP-gated P2X1 cation channel in thrombosis of small arteries in vivo. *J. Exp. Med.* **2003**, *198*, 661–667. [CrossRef]

109. Hechler, B.; Gachet, C. Purinergic Receptors in Thrombosis and Inflammation. *Arterioscler. Thromb. Vasc. Biol.* **2015**, *35*, 2307–2315. [CrossRef]

110. Hechler, B.; Leon, C.; Vial, C.; Vigne, P.; Frelin, C.; Cazenave, J.; Gachet, C. The P2Y1 receptor is necessary for adenosine 5′-diphosphate-induced platelet aggregation. *Blood* **1998**, *92*, 152–159. [CrossRef]

111. Burnstock, G. Purinergic Signaling in the Cardiovascular System. *Circ. Res.* **2017**, *120*, 207–228. [CrossRef] [PubMed]

112. Hechler, B.; Nonne, C.; Roh, E.J.; Cattaneo, M.; Cazenave, J.; Lanza, F.; Jacobson, K.A.; Gachet, C. MRS2500 [2-Iodo-N6-methyl-(N)-methanocarba-2′-deoxyadenosine-3′,5′-bisphosphate], a Potent, Selective, and Stable Antagonist of the Platelet P2Y1 Receptor with Strong Antithrombotic Activity in Mice. *J. Pharmacol. Exp. Ther.* **2006**, *316*, 556–563. [CrossRef] [PubMed]

113. Leon, C.; Ravanat, C.; Freund, M.; Cazenave, J.; Gachet, C. Differential Involvement of the P2Y1 and P2Y12 Receptors in Platelet Procoagulant Activity. *Arterioscler. Thromb. Vasc. Biol.* **2003**, *23*, 1941–1947. [CrossRef] [PubMed]

114. Amison, R.T.; Momi, S.; Morris, A.; Manni, G.; Keir, S.; Gresele, P.; Page, C.P.; Pitchford, S.C. RhoA signaling through platelet P2Y1 receptor controls leukocyte recruitment in allergic mice. *J. Allergy Clin. Immunol.* **2015**, *135*, 528–538. [CrossRef]

115. Zerr, M.; Hechler, B.; Freund, M.; Magnenat, S.; Lanois, I.; Cazenave, J.; Leon, C.; Gachet, C. Major Contribution of the P2Y1 Receptor in Purinergic Regulation of TNFα-Induced Vascular Inflammation. *Circulation* **2011**, *123*, 2404–2413. [CrossRef]

116. Hechler, B.; Freund, M.; Ravanat, C.; Magnenat, S.; Cazenave, J.P.; Gachet, C. Reduced atherosclerotic lesions in P2Y1/apolipoprotein E double-knockout mice: The contribution of non-hematopoietic-derived P2Y1 receptors. *Circulation* **2008**, *118*, 754–763. [CrossRef]

117. Gachet, C. Regulation of platelet functions by p2 receptors. *Annu. Rev. Pharmacol. Toxicol.* **2006**, *46*, 277–300. [CrossRef]

118. Cattaneo, M. Platelet P2 receptors: Old and new targets for antithrombotic drugs. *Expert Rev. Cardiovasc. Ther.* **2007**, *5*, 45–55. [CrossRef]

119. Li, D.; Wang, Y.; Zhang, L.; Luo, X.; Li, J.; Chen, X.; Niu, H.; Wang, K.; Sun, Y.; Wang, X. Roles of Purinergic Receptor P2Y, G Protein–Coupled 12 in the Development of Atherosclerosis in Apolipoprotein E–Deficient Mice. *Arterioscler. Thromb. Vasc. Biol.* **2012**, *32*, e81–e89. [CrossRef]

120. West, L.; Steiner, T.; Judge, H.M.; Francis, S.E.; Storey, R.F. Vessel wall, not platelet, P2Y12 potentiates early atherogenesis. *Cardiovasc. Res.* **2014**, *102*, 429–435. [CrossRef]

121. Gao, Y.; Yu, C.; Pi, S.; Mao, L.; Hu, B. The role of P2Y 12 receptor in ischemic stroke of atherosclerotic origin. *Cell. Mol. Life Sci.* **2019**, *76*, 341–354. [CrossRef] [PubMed]

122. Boulaftali, Y.; Owens, A.P.; Beale, A.; Piatt, R.; Casari, C.; Lee, R.H.; Conley, P.B.; Paul, D.S.; Mackman, N.; Bergmeier, W. CalDAG-GEFI Deficiency Reduces Atherosclerotic Lesion Development in Mice. *Arterioscler. Thromb. Vasc. Biol.* **2016**, *36*, 792–799. [CrossRef] [PubMed]

123. Lindemann, S.; Tolley, N.D.; Dixon, D.A.; Mcintyre, T.M.; Prescott, S.M.; Zimmerman, G.A.; Weyrich, A.S. Activated platelets mediate inflammatory signaling by regulated interleukin 1β synthesis. *J. Cell Biol.* **2001**, *154*, 485–490. [CrossRef] [PubMed]

124. Rechciński, T.; Grębowska, A.; Kurpesa, M.; Sztybrych, M.; Peruga, J.Z.; Trzos, E.; Rudnicka, W.; Krzemińskapakuła, M.; Chmiela, M. Interleukin-1b and interleukin-1 receptor inhibitor gene cluster polymorphisms in patients with coronary artery disease after percutaneous angioplasty or coronary artery bypass grafting. *Kardiologia Polska* **2009**, *67*, 601.

125. Goracy, I.; Kaczmarczyk, M.; Ciechanowicz, A.; Lewandowska, K.; Jakubiszyn, P.; Bodnar, O.; Kopijek, B.; Brodkiewicz, A.; Cyrylowski, L. Polymorphism of Interleukin 1B May Modulate the Risk of Ischemic Stroke in Polish Patients. *Med.-Buenos Aires* **2019**, *55*, 558. [CrossRef]

126. Garlichs, C.D.; Kozina, S.; Fatehmoghadam, S.; Tomandl, B.; Stumpf, C.; Eskafi, S.; Raaz, D.; Schmeiser, A.; Yilmaz, A.; Ludwig, J. Upregulation of CD40-CD40 Ligand (CD154) in Patients with Acute Cerebral Ischemia. *Stroke* **2003**, *34*, 1412–1418. [CrossRef]

127. Varo, N.; De Lemos, J.A.; Libby, P.; Morrow, D.A.; Murphy, S.A.; Nuzzo, R.; Gibson, C.M.; Cannon, C.P.; Braunwald, E.; Schonbeck, U. Soluble CD40L: Risk prediction after acute coronary syndromes. *Circulation* **2003**, *108*, 1049–1052. [CrossRef]

128. Sanguigni, V.; Pignatelli, P.; Lenti, L.; Ferro, D.; Bellia, A.; Carnevale, R.; Tesauro, M.; Sorge, R.; Lauro, R.; Violi, F. Short-term treatment with atorvastatin reduces platelet CD40 ligand and thrombin generation in hypercholesterolemic patients. *Circulation* **2005**, *111*, 412–419. [CrossRef]

129. Henn, V.; Slupsky, J.R.; Grafe, M.; Anagnostopoulos, I.; Forster, R.; Mullerberghaus, G.; Kroczek, R.A. CD40 ligand on activated platelets triggers an inflammatory reaction of endothelial cells. *Nature* **1998**, *391*, 591–594. [CrossRef]

130. Mach, F.; Schonbeck, U.; Sukhova, G.K.; Atkinson, E.; Libby, P. Reduction of atherosclerosis in mice by inhibition of CD40 signalling. *Nature* **1998**, *394*, 200–203. [CrossRef]

131. Lutgens, E.; Gorelik, L.; Daemen, M.J.A.P.; Ed, D.M.; Grewal, I.S.; Koteliansky, V.; Flavell, R.A. Requirement for CD154 in the progression of atherosclerosis. *Nat. Med.* **1999**, *5*, 1313–1316. [CrossRef] [PubMed]

132. Lukasik, M.; Dworacki, G.; Kufelgrabowska, J.; Watala, C.; Kozubski, W. Upregulation of CD40 ligand and enhanced monocyte-platelet aggregate formation are associated with worse clinical outcome after ischaemic stroke. *Thromb. Haemost.* **2012**, *107*, 346–355. [PubMed]

133. Bavendiek, U.; Zirlik, A.; Laclair, S.; Macfarlane, L.A.; Libby, P.; Schonbeck, U. Atherogenesis in Mice Does Not Require CD40 Ligand From Bone Marrow–Derived Cells. *Arterioscler. Thromb. Vasc. Biol.* **2005**, *25*, 1244–1249. [CrossRef] [PubMed]

134. Andre, P.; Prasad, K.; Denis, C.; Papalia, J.; Wagner, D. CD40L stabilizes arterial thrombi by a 3 integrin-dependent mechanism. *Nat. Med.* **2001**, *8*, 247–252. [CrossRef]

135. Henn, V.; Steinbach, S.; Buchner, K.; Presek, P.; Kroczek, R.A. The inflammatory action of CD40 ligand (CD154) expressed on activated human platelets is temporally limited by coexpressed CD40. *Blood* **2001**, *98*, 1047–1054. [CrossRef]

136. Zirlik, A.; Bavendiek, U.; Libby, P.; Macfarlane, L.A.; Gerdes, N.; Jagielska, J.; Ernst, S.; Aikawa, M.; Nakano, H.; Tsitsikov, E. TRAF-1, -2, -3, -5, and -6 Are Induced in Atherosclerotic Plaques and Differentially Mediate Proinflammatory Functions of CD40L in Endothelial Cells. *Arterioscler. Thromb. Vasc. Biol.* **2007**, *27*, 1101–1107. [CrossRef]

137. Lutgens, E.; Lievens, D.; Beckers, L.; Wijnands, E.; Soehnlein, O.; Zernecke, A.; Seijkens, T.; Engel, D.; Cleutjens, J.P.M.; Keller, A.M. Deficient CD40-TRAF6 signaling in leukocytes prevents atherosclerosis by skewing the immune response toward an antiinflammatory profile. *J. Exp. Med.* **2010**, *207*, 391–404. [CrossRef]

138. Gerdes, N.; Seijkens, T.; Lievens, D.; Kuijpers, M.J.; Winkels, H.; Projahn, D.; Hartwig, H.; Beckers, L.; Megens, R.T.; Boon, L.; et al. Platelet CD40 Exacerbates Atherosclerosis by Transcellular Activation of Endothelial Cells and Leukocytes. *Arterioscler. Thromb. Vasc. Biol.* **2016**, *36*, 482–490. [CrossRef]

139. Nassar, T.; Sachais, B.S.; Akkawi, S.; Kowalska, M.A.; Bdeir, K.; Leitersdorf, E.; Hiss, E.; Ziporen, L.; Aviram, M.; Cines, D.B. Platelet Factor 4 Enhances the Binding of Oxidized Low-density Lipoprotein to Vascular Wall Cells. *J. Biol. Chem.* **2003**, *278*, 6187–6193. [CrossRef]

140. Pitsilos, S.; Hunt, J.L.; Mohler, E.R.; Prabhakar, A.M.; Poncz, M.; Dawicki, J.; Khalapyan, T.Z.; Wolfe, M.L.; Fairman, R.M.; Mitchell, M.E. Platelet factor 4 localization in carotid atherosclerotic plaques: Correlation with clinical parameters. *Thromb. Haemost.* **2003**, *90*, 1112–1120. [CrossRef]

141. O'brien, J.R.; Etherington, M.D.; Pashley, M.A. Intra-Platelet Platelet Factor 4 (IP.PF4) and the Heparin-Mobilisable Pool of PF4 in Health and Atherosclerosis. *Thromb. Haemost.* **1984**, *51*, 354–357. [CrossRef] [PubMed]

142. Scheuerer, B.; Ernst, M.; Durrbaumlandmann, I.; Fleischer, J.; Gragegriebenow, E.; Brandt, E.; Flad, H.D.; Petersen, F. The CXC-chemokine platelet factor 4 promotes monocyte survival and induces monocyte differentiation into macrophages. *Blood* **2000**, *95*, 1158–1166. [CrossRef] [PubMed]

143. Erbel, C.; Tyka, M.; Helmes, C.M.; Akhavanpoor, M.; Rupp, G.; Domschke, G.; Linden, F.; Wolf, A.; Doesch, A.O.; Lasitschka, F. CXCL4-induced plaque macrophages can be specifically identified by co-expression of MMP7+S100A8+in vitro and in vivo. *Innate Immun.* **2015**, *21*, 255–265. [CrossRef] [PubMed]

144. Sachais, B.S.; Turrentine, T.; Mckenna, J.M.D.; Rux, A.H.; Rader, D.J.; Kowalska, M.A. Elimination of platelet factor 4 (PF4) from platelets reduces atherosclerosis in C57Bl/6 and apoE-/- mice. *Thromb. Haemost.* **2007**, *98*, 1108–1113. [PubMed]

145. Gleissner, C.A.; Shaked, I.; Erbel, C.; Bockler, D.; Katus, H.A.; Ley, K. CXCL4 Downregulates the Atheroprotective Hemoglobin Receptor CD163 in Human Macrophages. *Circ. Res.* **2010**, *106*, 203–211. [CrossRef] [PubMed]

146. Von Hundelshausen, P.; Koenen, R.R.; Sack, M.; Mause, S.F.; Adriaens, W.; Proudfoot, A.E.I.; Hackeng, T.M.; Weber, C. Heterophilic interactions of platelet factor 4 and RANTES promote monocyte arrest on endothelium. *Blood* **2005**, *105*, 924–930. [CrossRef] [PubMed]

147. Von Hundelshausen, P.; Weber, K.S.C.; Huo, Y.; Proudfoot, A.E.I.; Nelson, P.J.; Ley, K.; Weber, C. RANTES Deposition by Platelets Triggers Monocyte Arrest on Inflamed and Atherosclerotic Endothelium. *Circulation* **2001**, *103*, 1772–1777. [CrossRef]

148. Schober, A.; Manka, D.; Von Hundelshausen, P.; Huo, Y.; Hanrath, P.; Sarembock, I.J.; Ley, K.; Weber, C. Deposition of Platelet RANTES Triggering Monocyte Recruitment Requires P-Selectin and Is Involved in Neointima Formation After Arterial Injury. *Circulation* **2002**, *106*, 1523–1529. [CrossRef]

149. Veillard, N.R.; Kwak, B.R.; Pelli, G.; Mulhaupt, F.; James, R.W.; Proudfoot, A.E.I.; Mach, F. Antagonism of RANTES Receptors Reduces Atherosclerotic Plaque Formation in Mice. *Circ. Res.* **2004**, *94*, 253–261. [CrossRef]

150. Braunersreuther, V.; Steffens, S.; Arnaud, C.; Pelli, G.; Burger, F.; Proudfoot, A.E.I.; Mach, F. A Novel RANTES Antagonist Prevents Progression of Established Atherosclerotic Lesions in Mice. *Arterioscler. Thromb. Vasc. Biol.* **2008**, *28*, 1090–1096. [CrossRef]

151. Koperlenkiewicz, O.M.; Kaminska, J.; Lisowska, A.; Milewska, A.J.; Hirnle, T.; Dymickapiekarska, V. Factors Associated with RANTES Concentration in Cardiovascular Disease Patients. *BioMed Res. Int.* **2019**, *2019*, 3026453.

152. Rossaint, J.; Herter, J.M.; Van Aken, H.; Napirei, M.; Doring, Y.; Weber, C.; Soehnlein, O.; Zarbock, A. Synchronized integrin engagement and chemokine activation is crucial in neutrophil extracellular trap–mediated sterile inflammation. *Blood* **2014**, *123*, 2573–2584. [CrossRef] [PubMed]

153. Carlson, J.; Baxter, S.A.; Dreau, D.; Nesmelova, I.V. The heterodimerization of platelet-derived chemokines. *Biochim. Biophys. Acta* **2013**, *1834*, 158–168. [CrossRef] [PubMed]

154. Koenen, R.R.; Von Hundelshausen, P.; Nesmelova, I.V.; Zernecke, A.; Liehn, E.A.; Sarabi, A.; Kramp, B.; Piccinini, A.M.; Paludan, S.R.; Kowalska, M.A. Disrupting functional interactions between platelet chemokines inhibits atherosclerosis in hyperlipidemic mice. *Nat. Med.* **2009**, *15*, 97–103. [CrossRef] [PubMed]

155. Vajen, T.; Koenen, R.R.; Werner, I.; Staudt, M.; Projahn, D.; Curaj, A.; Sonmez, T.T.; Simsekyilmaz, S.; Schumacher, D.; Mollmann, J. Blocking CCL5-CXCL4 heteromerization preserves heart function after myocardial infarction by attenuating leukocyte recruitment and NETosis. *Sci. Rep.* **2018**, *8*, 10647. [CrossRef] [PubMed]

156. Tyner, J.W.; Uchida, O.; Kajiwara, N.; Kim, E.Y.; Patel, A.C.; Osullivan, M.P.; Walter, M.J.; Schwendener, R.A.; Cook, D.N.; Danoff, T.M. CCL5-CCR5 interaction provides antiapoptotic signals for macrophage survival during viral infection. *Nat. Med.* **2005**, *11*, 1180–1187. [CrossRef] [PubMed]

157. Gleissner, C.A.; Von Hundelshausen, P.; Ley, K. Platelet Chemokines in Vascular Disease. *Arterioscler. Thromb. Vasc. Biol.* **2008**, *28*, 1920–1927. [CrossRef]

158. Ghasemzadeh, M.; Kaplan, Z.S.; Alwis, I.; Schoenwaelder, S.M.; Ashworth, K.J.; Westein, E.; Hosseini, E.; Salem, H.H.; Slattery, R.; McColl, S.R.; et al. The CXCR1/2 ligand NAP-2 promotes directed intravascular leukocyte migration through platelet thrombi. *Blood* **2013**, *121*, 4555–4566. [CrossRef]

159. Orn, S.; Breland, U.M.; Mollnes, T.E.; Manhenke, C.; Dickstein, K.; Aukrust, P.; Ueland, T. The Chemokine Network in Relation to Infarct Size and Left Ventricular Remodeling Following Acute Myocardial Infarction. *Am. J. Cardiol.* **2009**, *104*, 1179–1183. [CrossRef]

160. Abiyounes, S.; Sauty, A.; Mach, F.; Sukhova, G.K.; Libby, P.; Luster, A.D. The Stromal Cell–Derived Factor-1 Chemokine Is a Potent Platelet Agonist Highly Expressed in Atherosclerotic Plaques. *Circ. Res.* **2000**, *86*, 131–138. [CrossRef]

161. Merckelbach, S.; Der Vorst, E.P.C.V.; Kallmayer, M.; Rischpler, C.; Burgkart, R.; Doring, Y.; De Borst, G.; Schwaiger, M.; Eckstein, H.H.; Weber, C. Expression and Cellular Localization of CXCR4 and CXCL12 in Human Carotid Atherosclerotic Plaques. *Thromb. Haemost.* **2018**, *118*, 195–206. [CrossRef] [PubMed]

162. Chatterjee, M.; Von Ungernsternberg, S.N.I.; Seizer, P.; Schlegel, F.; Buttcher, M.; Sindhu, N.A.; Muller, S.; Mack, A.F.; Gawaz, M. Platelet-derived CXCL12 regulates monocyte function, survival, differentiation into macrophages and foam cells through differential involvement of CXCR4–CXCR7. *Cell Death Dis.* **2015**, *6*, e1989. [CrossRef]

163. Akhtar, S.; Gremse, F.; Kiessling, F.; Weber, C.; Schober, A. CXCL12 Promotes the Stabilization of Atherosclerotic Lesions Mediated by Smooth Muscle Progenitor Cells in Apoe -Deficient Mice. *Arterioscler. Thromb. Vasc. Biol.* **2013**, *33*, 679–686. [CrossRef]

164. Andrae, J.; Gallini, R.; Betsholtz, C. Role of platelet-derived growth factors in physiology and medicine. *Genes Dev.* **2008**, *22*, 1276–1312. [CrossRef] [PubMed]

165. Raines, E.W. PDGF and cardiovascular disease. *Cytokine Growth Factor Rev.* **2004**, *15*, 237–254. [CrossRef]

166. Raica, M.; Cimpean, A.M. Platelet-Derived Growth Factor (PDGF)/PDGF Receptors (PDGFR) Axis as Target for Antitumor and Antiangiogenic Therapy. *Pharmaceuticals* **2010**, *3*, 572–599. [CrossRef] [PubMed]

167. Folestad, E.; Kunath, A.; Wågsäter, D. PDGF-C and PDGF-D signaling in vascular diseases and animal models. *Mol. Asp. Med.* **2018**, *62*, 1–11. [CrossRef] [PubMed]

168. Ricci, C.; Ferri, N. Naturally occurring PDGF receptor inhibitors with potential anti-atherosclerotic properties. *Vasc. Pharmacol.* **2015**, *70*, 1–7. [CrossRef]

169. Hu, W.; Huang, Y. Targeting the platelet-derived growth factor signalling in cardiovascular disease. *Clin. Exp. Pharmacol. Physiol.* **2015**, *42*, 1221–1224. [CrossRef]

170. Sano, H.; Sudo, T.; Yokode, M.; Murayama, T.; Kataoka, H.; Takakura, N.; Nishikawa, S.; Nishikawa, S.; Kita, T. Functional Blockade of Platelet-Derived Growth Factor Receptor-β but Not of Receptor-α Prevents Vascular Smooth Muscle Cell Accumulation in Fibrous Cap Lesions in Apolipoprotein E–Deficient Mice. *Circulation* **2001**, *103*, 2955–2960. [CrossRef]

171. Kozaki, K.; Kaminski, W.E.; Tang, J.; Hollenbach, S.; Lindahl, P.; Sullivan, C.M.; Yu, J.C.; Abe, K.; Martin, P.J.; Ross, R. Blockade of Platelet-Derived Growth Factor or Its Receptors Transiently Delays but Does Not Prevent Fibrous Cap Formation in ApoE Null Mice. *Am. J. Pathol.* **2002**, *161*, 1395–1407. [CrossRef]

172. He, C.; Medley, S.C.; Hu, T.; Hinsdale, M.E.; Lupu, F.; Virmani, R.; Olson, L.E. PDGFRβ signalling regulates local inflammation and synergizes with hypercholesterolaemia to promote atherosclerosis. *Nat. Commun.* **2015**, *6*, 7770. [CrossRef] [PubMed]

173. Rouhiainen, A.; Imai, S.; Rauvala, H.; Parkkinen, J. Occurrence of Amphoterin (HMG1) as an Endogenous Protein of Human Platelets that Is Exported to the Cell Surface upon Platelet Activation. *Thromb. Haemost.* **2000**, *84*, 1087–1094. [PubMed]

174. Ahrens, I.; Chen, Y.; Topcic, D.; Bode, M.; Haenel, D.; Hagemeyer, C.E.; Seeba, H.; Duerschmied, D.; Bassler, N.; Jandeleitdahm, K. HMGB1 binds to activated platelets via the receptor for advanced glycation end products and is present in platelet rich human coronary artery thrombi. *Thromb. Haemost.* **2015**, *114*, 994–1003. [PubMed]

175. Vogel, S.; Bodenstein, R.; Chen, Q.; Feil, S.; Feil, R.; Rheinlaender, J.; Schaffer, T.E.; Bohn, E.; Frick, J.; Borst, O. Platelet-derived HMGB1 is a critical mediator of thrombosis. *J. Clin. Investig.* **2015**, *125*, 4638–4654. [CrossRef] [PubMed]

176. Maugeri, N.; Campana, L.; Gavina, M.; Covino, C.; De Metrio, M.; Panciroli, C.; Maiuri, L.; Maseri, A.; Dangelo, A.; Bianchi, M. Activated platelets present high mobility group box 1 to neutrophils, inducing autophagy and promoting the extrusion of neutrophil extracellular traps. *J. Thromb. Haemost.* **2014**, *12*, 2074–2088. [CrossRef] [PubMed]

177. Coppinger, J.A.; Cagney, G.; Toomey, S.; Kislinger, T.; Belton, O.; Mcredmond, J.P.; Cahill, D.J.; Emili, A.; Fitzgerald, D.J.; Maguire, P.B. Characterization of the proteins released from activated platelets leads to localization of novel platelet proteins in human atherosclerotic lesions. *Blood* **2004**, *103*, 2096–2104. [CrossRef] [PubMed]

178. Nigro, P.; Satoh, K.; Odell, M.R.; Soe, N.N.; Cui, Z.; Mohan, A.; Abe, J.I.; Alexis, J.D.; Sparks, J.D.; Berk, B.C. Cyclophilin A is an inflammatory mediator that promotes atherosclerosis in apolipoprotein E–deficient mice. *J. Exp. Med.* **2011**, *208*, 53–66. [CrossRef] [PubMed]

179. Seizer, P.; Von Ungernsternberg, S.N.I.; Schonberger, T.; Borst, O.; Munzer, P.; Schmidt, E.; Mack, A.F.; Heinzmann, D.; Chatterjee, M.; Langer, H.F. Extracellular Cyclophilin A Activates Platelets Via EMMPRIN (CD147) and PI3K/Akt Signaling, which Promotes Platelet Adhesion and Thrombus Formation In Vitro and In Vivo. *Arterioscler. Thromb. Vasc. Biol.* **2015**, *35*, 655–663. [CrossRef] [PubMed]

180. Barrett, T.J.; Schlegel, M.; Zhou, F.; Gorenchtein, M.; Bolstorff, J.; Moore, K.J.; Fisher, E.A.; Berger, J.S. Platelet regulation of myeloid suppressor of cytokine signaling 3 accelerates atherosclerosis. *Sci. Transl. Med.* **2019**, *11*, eaax0481. [CrossRef] [PubMed]

181. Schaffner, A.; Rhyn, P.; Schoedon, G.; Schaer, D.J. Regulated expression of platelet factor 4 in human monocytes—Role of PARs as a quantitatively important monocyte activation pathway Abstract: Human mononuclear phagocytes have recently been shown to express constitutively and even more so, upon stimul. *J. Leukoc. Biol.* **2005**, *78*, 202–209. [CrossRef] [PubMed]

182. Gaertner, F.; Ahmad, Z.; Rosenberger, G.; Fan, S.; Nicolai, L.; Busch, B.; Yavuz, G.; Luckner, M.; Ishikawa-Ankerhold, H.; Hennel, R.; et al. Migrating Platelets Are Mechano-scavengers that Collect and Bundle Bacteria. *Cell* **2017**, *171*, 1368–1382.e23. [CrossRef] [PubMed]

183. Pitchford, S.C.; Momi, S.; Baglioni, S.; Casali, L.; Giannini, S.; Rossi, R.; Page, C.P.; Gresele, P. Allergen induces the migration of platelets to lung tissue in allergic asthma. *Am. J. Respir Crit. Care Med.* **2008**, *177*, 604–612. [CrossRef] [PubMed]

184. Kraemer, B.F.; Borst, O.; Gehring, E.M.; Schoenberger, T.; Urban, B.; Ninci, E.; Seizer, P.; Schmidt, C.; Bigalke, B.; Koch, M. PI3 kinase-dependent stimulation of platelet migration by stromal cell-derived factor 1 (SDF-1). *J. Mol. Med.-JMM* **2010**, *88*, 1277–1288. [CrossRef]

185. Witte, A.; Rohlfing, A.-K.; Dannenmann, B.; Dicenta, V.; Nasri, M.; Kolb, K.; Sudmann, J.; Castor, T.; Rath, D.; Borst, O. The chemokine CXCL14 mediates platelet function and migration via direct interaction with CXCR4. *Cardiovasc. Res.* **2020**, *80*, cvaa080. [CrossRef]

186. Witte, A.; Chatterjee, M.; Lang, F.; Gawaz, M. Platelets as a Novel Source of Pro-Inflammatory Chemokine CXCL14. *Cell Physiol. Biochem.* **2017**, *41*, 1684–1696. [CrossRef]

187. Bradfield, P.F.; Scheiermann, C.; Nourshargh, S.; Ody, C.; Luscinskas, F.W.; Rainger, G.E.; Nash, G.B.; Miljkovic-Licina, M.; Aurrand-Lions, M.; Imhof, B.A. JAM-C regulates unidirectional monocyte transendothelial migration in inflammation. *Blood* **2007**, *110*, 2545–2555. [CrossRef]

188. Gils, J.M.V.; Martins, P.A.D.C.; Mol, A.; Hordijk, P.L.; Zwaginga, J.J. Transendothelial migration drives dissociation of plateletmonocyte complexes. *Thromb. Haemost.* **2008**, *99*, 271–279.

3

Adaptive Immune Responses in Human Atherosclerosis

Silvia Lee [1,2,*], **Benjamin Bartlett** [1,3] **and Girish Dwivedi** [1,3,4]

1   Department of Advanced Clinical and Translational Cardiovascular Imaging, Harry Perkins Institute of
    Medical Research, Murdoch 6150, Australia; benjamin.bartlett@research.uwa.edu.au (B.B.);
    girish.dwivedi@perkins.uwa.edu.au (G.D.)
2   Department of Microbiology, Pathwest Laboratory Medicine, Murdoch 6150, Australia
3   School of Medicine, University of Western Australia, Nedlands 6009, Australia
4   Department of Cardiology, Fiona Stanley Hospital, Murdoch 6150, Australia
*   Correspondence: silvia.lee@uwa.edu.au

Abstract: Atherosclerosis is a chronic inflammatory disease that is initiated by the deposition and accumulation of low-density lipoproteins in the artery wall. In this review, we will discuss the role of T- and B-cells in human plaques at different stages of atherosclerosis and the utility of profiling circulating immune cells to monitor atherosclerosis progression. Evidence supports a proatherogenic role for intraplaque T helper type 1 (Th1) cells, $CD4^+CD28^{null}$ T-cells, and natural killer T-cells, whereas Th2 cells and regulatory T-cells (Treg) have an atheroprotective role. Several studies indicate that intraplaque T-cells are activated upon recognition of endogenous antigens including heat shock protein 60 and oxidized low-density lipoprotein, but antigens derived from pathogens can also trigger T-cell proliferation and cytokine production. Future studies are needed to assess whether circulating cellular biomarkers can improve identification of vulnerable lesions so that effective intervention can be implemented before clinical manifestations are apparent.

Keywords: human atherosclerosis; adaptive immune response; T-cells; B-cells

1. Introduction

Atherosclerosis is a chronic vascular disease involving endothelial dysfunction following the deposition and accumulation of lipoproteins (e.g., low-density lipoproteins (LDL)) in the arterial intima. Plaque rupture and subsequent arterial occlusion can lead to myocardial infarction and stroke, which are the leading causes of death worldwide. The initiation and progression of atherosclerosis involve inflammatory pathways, with the recruitment and activation of several immune cell types and the release of soluble mediators [1]. Cells of the innate immune system, primarily macrophages, can take up modified oxidized LDL (oxLDL) and transform into foam cells to form fatty streaks ("early plaques") [2]. Further lipid accumulation and leukocyte infiltration into established atherosclerotic plaques ("advanced") create a core region with a collagen-rich fibrous cap established by vascular smooth muscle cells [2]. Plaques can be categorized into two broad categories: stable or unstable. Stable plaques are characterized by a small lipid core, few inflammatory immune cells, and a thick fibrous cap. Unstable (also known as "vulnerable") plaques often have a very large lipid core, a thin fibrous cap, and intraplaque hemorrhage [2].

Cells of the innate and adaptive immune system are present in the different layers (intima, media, and adventitia) of the artery walls throughout the development of atherosclerotic plaques in mice and humans [3,4]. Studies using gene knockout mice have enabled detailed analyses of immune cells involved in atherogenesis [4], whilst human studies are more limited. However, it is important to highlight that different genetic and environmental factors affect atherogenesis in mice and humans. It is well established that different subsets of monocytes and macrophages play a crucial role in the atherosclerotic plaque establishment and disease progression [4]. In this review, we will summarize the roles of adaptive immune cells in human atherosclerotic plaques and review the clinical utility of profiling circulating immune cells in this context.

2. Development of T-Cell Subsets

Following antigen presentation by antigen-presenting cells (e.g., dendritic cells) and recognition by T-cell receptors, naive CD4$^+$ and CD8$^+$ T-cells (T$_N$) differentiate into central memory (T$_{CM}$) or effector memory T-cells (T$_{EM}$) [5] (Figure 1A). T$_{CM}$ generally reside in lymphoid tissues and are primed for rapid response to a previously encountered antigen. Following activation, T$_{CM}$ undergo clonal expansion and differentiate into T$_{EM}$. T$_{EM}$ can be defined by their expression of the cell surface receptor, CD45RO, and low levels of costimulatory receptors (e.g., CD28). Furthermore, these cells display loss of chemokine receptors (e.g., CCR7) necessary for cells to migrate to secondary lymphoid tissues such as lymph nodes and spleen, whilst there is upregulation of receptors required for migration to peripheral sites of inflammation (e.g., CCR5 and CXCR3). In response to antigens, both T$_{CM}$ and T$_{EM}$ can produce effector cytokines, but T$_{CM}$ possess higher proliferative capacities. Chronic exposure to antigens results in the generation of terminal effector T-cells (T$_{TE}$) that proliferate poorly but have strong cytokine-producing and cytotoxic capabilities.

(A)

Antigen	Function	T$_N$	T$_{CM}$	T$_{EM}$	T$_{TE}$
CD45RA		+++	–	–	++
CD45RO		–	+++	+++	–
CD28	Co-stimulatory	+++	+++	+	+
CD27	Co-stimulatory	+++	+++	–/+	–
CD69	Early activation marker	–	–/+	–/+	–/+
HLA-DR	Late activation marker	–	–/+	–/+	–/+

CCR7	Lymphoid tissue homing
Ki67	Proliferation
CX3CR1	Homing to inflamed tissue
CCR5	Homing to inflamed tissue
CXCR3	Homing to inflamed tissue
Perforin	Pore forming
Granzyme	Cleavage of proteins

(B)

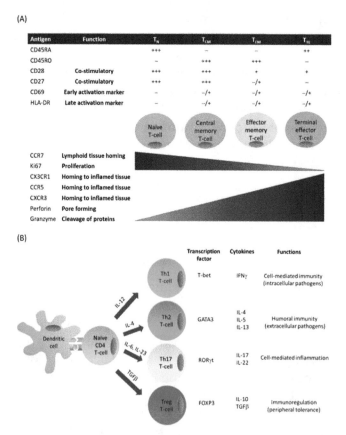

Figure 1. T-cell differentiation. (**A**) Following antigen presentation by antigen-presenting cells such as dendritic cells, naïve T-cells can differentiate to central memory or effector T-cells. This process is associated with the presence (+) or absence (−) of cell surface receptor expression on T-cells including costimulatory molecules and chemokine receptors, and functions including proliferation and cytotoxicity. (**B**) Depending on the costimulatory signals and the cytokines produced by antigen-presenting cells in the surrounding microenvironment, CD4$^+$ T-cells express specific transcription factors that favor the differentiation into the different T-cell subsets. These subsets can be characterized by their distinctive cytokine secretion profile and associated effector functions.

Depending on the antigen, costimulatory signals, and cytokine milieu of the microenvironment, naïve CD4+ T-cells differentiate into distinct T helper (Th) lineages (Figure 1B). T helper 1 (Th1) cells produce predominantly interferon (IFN)γ, Th2 cells produce interleukin (IL)-4, IL-5, and IL-13, and Th17 cells secrete IL-17 and IL-22 [5]. Differentiation into Th1, Th2, or Th17 subsets is controlled by specific transcription factors: T-bet, GATA3, and RORγt, respectively. Each Th cell subset possesses a unique expression profile and specific functions during an immune response.

Macrophages play a crucial role in regulating Th1/Th2 immune responses and can be broadly classified into two main subtypes: classically activated M1 macrophages and alternatively activated M2 macrophages [4]. M1 macrophages direct T-cells to produce Th1 cytokines to stimulate cytolytic activity and recruit more M1 macrophages and are considered proinflammatory. In contrast, M2 macrophages stimulate T-cells to produce Th2 cytokines to induce B-cell proliferation and amplify M2 macrophage responses and are considered anti-inflammatory. An imbalance of macrophage M1-M2 polarization can lead to inflammation and disease.

Human regulatory T-cells (Treg) can suppress the activation of immune cells through cell-to-cell contact and/or the secretion of inhibitory cytokines (e.g., transforming growth factor (TGF)-β and IL-10) [6]. They are characterized by the expression of the transcription factor forkhead box P3 (FOXP3) and the IL-2 receptor α subunit, CD25.

3. T-Cells in Atherosclerotic Plaques

3.1. CD3+ T-Cells

CD3 is a cell surface molecule that associates with the T-cell receptor (TCR) and is critical for the activation of CD4+ and CD8+ T-cells. It is commonly used as a pan T-cell marker in immunostaining protocols. In 1986, Jonasson et al. first demonstrated the presence of CD3+ T-cells in carotid plaques that were predominately located in the fibrous cap and constituted 20% of the total infiltrating cells [7]. A study of samples from autopsies revealed large numbers of CD3+ T-cells in the intimal and adventitial layers of coronary arteries displaying fatty streaks, with the highest numbers reported in advanced plaques with intimal thickening or necrotic cores [8]. A comprehensive histological study of human aortic tissues encompassing the entire spectrum of atherosclerotic disease confirmed the presence of CD3+ T-cells in the intima at all stages of atherosclerosis whereas CD3+ T-cells were present only in the medial layer of arteries displaying intimal thickening or in vulnerable plaques [9]. The authors also observed reduced numbers of CD3+ T-cells in the intima of healed ruptures and fibrotic calcified plaques [9]. Similarly, Rohm et al. reported higher numbers of CD3+ T cells in unstable plaques compared to stable plaques or vessels with no evidence of atherosclerosis [10].

Initial studies suggested that approximately 5–35% of CD3+ T-cells within plaques were activated and involved in the inflammatory response [11,12]. Immunofluorescent staining demonstrated increased expression of the chemokine CX3CL1 and its receptor CX3CR1 in the fibrous cap of coronary and carotid plaques [13]. The staining colocalized with CD3+ T-cells, suggestive of active recruitment of immune cells to inflamed tissues [13].

Previous studies using immunohistochemical or immunofluorescent staining investigated the location of immune cells within the plaque but do not reveal dynamic changes, assess the whole tissue, or provide detailed phenotypes of infiltrating cells. Flow cytometry allows unbiased quantitation and characterization of T-cells in affected tissues. For example, most cells isolated from endarterectomy specimens after collagenase digestion were found to be CD3+ T-cells, displayed a memory phenotype, and expressed markers of immune activation (e.g., CD25, HLA-DR) [12,14]. Combining flow cytometry and an ex vivo model of plaques, Lebedeva et al. confirmed the predominance of T-cells within carotid plaques [15].

3.2. CD4$^+$ T-Cells

CD4$^+$ T-cells have been shown to be more abundant in unstable plaques compared to stable plaques or arteries with no evidence of atherosclerosis [10]. Van Dijk et al. reported an absence of CD4$^+$ T-cells in the intimal and medial layers of early plaques whereas their numbers were increased in late fibrous plaques but then decreased in healed plaque ruptures [9]. CD4$^+$ T-cells with an effector memory or terminally differentiated phenotype have been found to predominate within plaques [16]. Additionally, intraplaque CD4$^+$ T-cells displayed a more activated profile (i.e., increased HLA-DR expression) [16], suggesting the presence of foreign antigens within plaques. Using mass cytometry and single-cell RNA sequencing analyses, CD4$^+$ T-cells in atherosclerotic plaques from symptomatic (stroke) patients displayed gene expression profiles consistent with activation, differentiation, and exhaustion whereas CD4$^+$ T-cells were mostly activated in plaques from asymptomatic (no recent stroke) patients [17].

There is compelling evidence pointing to a role for Th1 CD4$^+$ T-cells in promoting inflammation and atherosclerosis in humans. Using immunohistochemical and polymerase chain reaction techniques, Frostegard et al. demonstrated that Th1 CD4$^+$ T-cells predominated in advanced plaques, whereas Th2 cytokines including IL-4 and IL-5 were rarely detected [18]. Other investigators confirmed the Th1 bias of infiltrating CD4$^+$ T-cells in aortic or carotid plaques [19,20]. Intraplaque CD4$^+$ T-cells have been shown to express the chemokine receptor CXCR3 and this was associated with expression of IFNγ-inducible CXC chemokines—IFN-inducible protein 10 (IP-10), monokine induced by IFNγ (MIG), and IFN-inducible T-cell α chemoattractant (I-TAC) in endothelial cells, smooth muscle cells, and macrophages within the plaques [21]. This study revealed a role for chemokine signaling through CXCR3 in promoting recruitment and homing of Th1 cells to the site of plaque development. Furthermore, the proinflammatory cytokines IL-12 and IL-18, which act synergistically to promote T-cell differentiation along the Th1 lineage, have been identified in atherosclerotic plaques [22–24]. IFNγ is known to activate macrophages and dendritic cells, inhibit proliferation of vascular smooth muscle cells, and reduce production of collagen by these cells, leading to thinning of the fibrous cap and plaque destabilization [25].

Although plaque-infiltrating CD4$^+$ T-cells were shown to produce mainly IFNγ, other studies found some CD4$^+$ T-cells produce only IL-17 or both cytokines following polyclonal stimulation [16,26]. This may explain the increased plasma levels of IL-17 from patients with acute myocardial infarction or unstable angina compared to patients with stable angina or healthy controls [27–29]. Furthermore, positive associations have been observed between IL-17 levels and severity of carotid artery plaques [30].

A subset of CD4$^+$ T-cell lacking CD28 expression (representing 5–23% of all CD4$^+$ T-cells) and producing high levels of IFNγ and tumor necrosis factor (TNF)α have been found in the plaques from patients with acute coronary syndrome (ACS) [31,32]. CD28 is a costimulatory receptor necessary for T-cell activation and proliferation, so the loss of CD28 has been suggested to reflect repeated antigenic exposure [33]. CD4$^+$CD28^{null} T-cells have been shown to accumulate in unstable ruptured coronary plaque [31], and express high levels of OX40 and 4-1BB costimulatory proteins, which regulate degranulation and release of molecules involved in cytotoxicity including perforin and granzyme B [32]. These findings suggest that CD4$^+$CD28^{null} T-cells may damage cells in the vascular wall, thereby affecting the stability of plaques.

3.3. CD8$^+$ T-Cells

CD8$^+$ T-cells have been found to be more abundant in unstable plaques compared to stable plaques [10]. CD8$^+$ T-cells in advanced plaques resided mainly in the shoulder region and fibrous cap of the plaques [34]. Van Dijk et al. demonstrated CD8$^+$ T-cells in the intimal layer throughout the progression of atherosclerosis, but these cells predominated in the medial layer of advanced unstable plaques and numbers decreased in stable lesions [9]. Plaques were found to be enriched for CD8$^+$ T-cells that were primarily T$_{EM}$ cells, displayed an activated phenotype, and expressed IFNγ, IL-2, or IL-17 [16]. Likewise, using mass cytometry and single-cell RNA sequencing analyses, Fernandez et al. reported plaque-derived CD8$^+$ T-cells were predominantly differentiated and activated and displayed evidence of clonal expansion [17]. A recent study demonstrated an inverse correlation between percentages of CD8[+] T-cells and macrophages in advanced plaques [35]. As this was not evident with CD4[+] T-cells, the authors inferred that CD8[+] T-cells may play a protective role by reducing macrophage accumulation [35]. Granzyme B has been shown to localize to CD8[+] T-cells near the necrotic core of advanced plaques with a fibrous cap [36] and may be responsible for the apoptosis of macrophage-derived foam cells [37].

3.4. Treg Cells

Frequencies of FOXP3[+] Treg cells have been shown to be higher in the intima of lipid-rich advanced plaques compared to early lesions [38]. Furthermore, Patel et al. found that increased number of FOXP3[+] Treg cells and the Treg-associated cytokine IL-10 in carotid plaques were associated with symptomatic disease [39]. However, other investigators evaluating the plaque shoulder, which is prone to infiltrating immune cells, reported lower numbers of Treg cells in unstable plaques that correlated inversely with the number of dendritic cells [10,40]. Furthermore, unstable plaques were shown to have reduced mRNA expression of TGF-β [40], a Treg cell-associated cytokine that possess atheroprotective roles including suppression of lymphocyte and endothelial cell proliferation [41]. Results from experimental models have also identified several other potential mechanisms by which Treg cells and TGF-β production can affect plaque development and stability. These include inhibition of T- and B-cell effector functions, modulation of dendritic cell function and maturation, and inhibition of macrophage inflammation [42,43].

3.5. $\gamma\delta$ T-Cells

$\gamma\delta$ T-cells are important innate-like T-cells with a role in inflammation, infectious diseases, tumor surveillance, and autoimmunity. They represent 1–5% of circulating T-cells in the blood and recognize nonpeptide antigens such as lipids and phosphorylated nucleotides [44]. In apolipoprotein E knockout mice, $\gamma\delta$ T-cells were found to be the major T-cell subset in early aortic root and arch lesions [45,46] and produced predominantly IL-17 [45]. Human studies of $\gamma\delta$ T-cells in atherosclerotic lesions are limited. In humans, $\gamma\delta$ T-cells have been demonstrated in plaques [47,48], with high frequencies observed in the aorta during the early stages (i.e., fatty streaks with infiltration of macrophages and lymphocytes but no foam cells) of atherosclerosis [47]. Further human studies are required to address the precise role of $\gamma\delta$ T-cells in atherosclerosis.

3.6. NKT Cells

Natural killer T (NKT) cells are a unique subset of T-cells that express markers of NK and T-cells [49]. They can be classified as type 1 (invariant) or type 2 (CD1d-restricted) NKT cells. Invariant NKT cells express a restricted TCR repertoire comprising a Vα24-Jα18 TCRα chain that is preferentially paired with a Vβ11 TCRβ chain, whereas type 2 NKT cells have more variable TCRs. Invariant NKT cells recognize glycolipid antigens presented by the major histocompatibility complex (MHC) class I-like molecule CD1d expressed on antigen-presenting cells. Using flow cytometry, high percentages of NKT cells were identified in advanced plaques from patients with atherosclerosis [50]. Bobryshev et al. demonstrated NKT cells in the rupture-prone shoulders of advanced plaques that colocalized with CD1d-expressing dendritic cells [51]. Similarly, in plaques from patients with symptomatic atherosclerosis, Kyriakakis et al. revealed that up to 3% of infiltrating CD3[+] T-cells stained for Vβ11 or Vα24 and confirmed the colocalization of NKT cells with CD1d[+] cells [52]. Using immunohistochemical staining, an increased number of NKT cells were demonstrated in unstable plaques compared to stable lesions [10]. Plaque-derived NKT cells exhibited high sensitivity to antigen stimulation and also proangiogenic and pro-inflammatory activity, suggesting a role for these cells in plaque neovascularization and destabilization [52]. Furthermore, NKT cells isolated from atherosclerotic plaques in patients with abdominal aortic aneurysm promoted apoptosis of vascular smooth muscle cells via Fas, IFNγ production, and CD40 signaling which may affect stability of plaques [53].

4. B-Cells in Atherosclerotic Lesions

Compared to murine studies, evidence for a role of B-cells in human atherosclerosis is limited. In whole blood gene expression profiles from the Framingham Heart Study, genes associated with B-cell activation were reported to be expressed at higher levels in healthy controls compared to patients with coronary heart disease, suggesting a protective role [54]. However, B-cells have been demonstrated to be rare or undetectable by immunohistochemical staining [7,11] or constituted <1% of cells in plaques using flow cytometry [15]. Using polymerase chain reaction (PCR), Hamze et al. demonstrated the presence of IgG- and IgA-expressing B-cells in the arterial wall and showed that they produced proinflammatory cytokines including IL-6, TNF-α, and granulocyte-macrophage colony-stimulating factor (GM-CSF) [55].

5. Activation of T-Cells in Atherosclerotic Plaques

As mentioned previously, T-cells in atherosclerotic plaques mainly display an activated profile. Analysis of the T-cell repertoire in coronary plaques from patients with ACS or chronic stable angina revealed increased T-cells and specific T-cell clonotype expansions in unstable plaques but not in the peripheral blood, suggesting antigen-driven recruitment of T-cells to unstable plaques [56].

Several studies indicate that intraplaque T-cells are activated upon recognition of endogenous antigens. Heat shock proteins (HSP) are stress proteins that are conserved in prokaryotic and eukaryotic cells. Of these, HSP60 has been extensively studied in human atherosclerosis. Benagiano et al. found that in vivo activated CD4$^+$ (but not CD8$^+$) T-cells isolated from carotid plaques could be stimulated with human HSP60 to secrete IFNγ and TNFα [57]. Plaque-derived T-cells displayed increased reactivity against human HSP60 compared to peripheral blood-derived T-cells from the same individual and exhibited an oligoclonally restricted T-cell receptor repertoire, suggestive of antigen-driven proliferation within the plaque [58]. Furthermore, cocultures of HSP60-stimulated myeloid dendritic cells with T-cells isolated from plaques from the same individual were found to induce T-cell activation [59]. The authors also detected IFNγ, IL-6, TNFα, and IL-17 in myeloid dendritic cell–T-cell coculture supernatants and increased expression of the transcription factors T-bet (Th1) and RORγt (Th17) [59].

Production of reactive oxygen species and nitrogen species by endothelial cells mediates LDL oxidation in the vascular wall [60]. Scavenger receptors on macrophages have a high affinity for oxLDL resulting in lipid accumulation and the formation of foam cells. T-cell clones derived from plaques have been shown to become activated upon recognition of oxLDL [61]. Proliferation was observed when T-cells isolated from plaques were cultured with oxLDL-stimulated blood-derived dendritic cells [62,63]. This effect was abolished by atorvastatin (lipid-lowering medication) treatment [63] or reduced by inhibition of proprotein convertase subtilisin/kexin type 9 (PCSK9) [62].

Genetic studies have shown that a variant of bactericidal/permeability-increasing fold-containing family B member 4 (BPIFB4), a gene associated with longevity, may confer protection from cardiovascular diseases [64,65]. Mechanistically, Ciaglia et al. demonstrated that BPIFB4 promoted M2 polarization [66] and decreased activation of T-cells [67]. Further studies are warranted to determine whether BPIFB4 can be utilized as a novel therapeutic target in the management of atherosclerosis.

6. Role of Pathogens in the Pathogenesis of Atherosclerosis

Several pathogens have been implicated in the increased risk of cardiovascular disease. These pathogens, both bacteria and viruses, can infect several different cell types important in the pathogenesis of atherosclerosis, including monocytes and macrophages. Inflammation induced by these infectious agents may accelerate atherosclerotic plaque progression.

Cytomegalovirus (CMV) is a beta herpesvirus with a seroprevalence of 50–90% depending on age and geographic and socioeconomic status [68]. The association between CMV seropositivity and increased risk of cardiovascular disease is evident in epidemiological studies [69] of immunocompetent individuals, HIV-infected patients [70], and solid-organ transplant recipients [71].

Direct effects of CMV on atherosclerosis have been established in vivo by the detection of the virus in endothelial cells, smooth muscle cells, and monocytes/macrophages. CMV DNA has been identified in 63% of plaques obtained during coronary artery bypass graft surgery [72]. Compared to tissues with no evidence of atherosclerosis, CMV antigen and DNA were detected more frequently in atherosclerotic plaques from patients [73,74]. However, other investigators reported no differences in the detection of CMV DNA in atherosclerotic plaques compared to healthy vessels [75,76]. This may depend on the stage of atherosclerosis as one study identified CMV DNA in fatty streaks and early plaques, but it was rare in advanced plaques [77]. In contrast, another study reported higher CMV DNA and antigen in advanced plaques compared to early plaques [78]. CMV-positive cells were found to be mainly localized in the shoulder regions of the plaques but also in areas adjacent to the necrotic core and in the fibrous cap [79].

Nitiskaya et al. reported that 82% of plaques obtained from patients who underwent carotid endarterectomy had detectable CMV DNA and levels positively correlated with proportions of infiltrating T_{EM} CD4$^+$ and CD8$^+$ T-cells [80]. Similarly, Yaiw et al. demonstrated plaques positive for CMV had increased infiltration of CD3$^+$ T-cells [79], suggesting that the virus may be involved in the inflammatory process. Indeed, in vitro studies showed that soluble factors (IFNγ, TNFα) secreted by CMV-specific T-cells can activate endothelial cells to produce chemokines (IP-10, fractalkine) and adhesion molecules that promote further recruitment of effector CD4$^+$ and CD8$^+$ T-cells [81,82] and induce apoptosis in activated endothelial cells [81].

Izadi et al. reported an association between the presence of CMV DNA in coronary atherosclerotic plaques with a history of unstable angina and myocardial infarction [83]. Furthermore, detection rate of CMV by immunohistochemistry in coronary plaques was higher in patients with ACS compared to patients with no ACS [84].

Epstein–Barr virus (EBV) is a common pathogen, with more than 90% of adults infected worldwide. EBV DNA has been detected in 17/30 plaques obtained during coronary artery bypass graft surgery [72]. Another study found EBV-specific cytotoxic T-cells and EBV DNA in 11/19 plaques from patients undergoing carotid endarterectomy [85]. The authors implicated EBV-specific T-cells in plaque inflammation as these cells were found throughout the intimal layer of the arteries, expressed the activation markers CD40L and CD25, and produced IFNγ and granzymes [85].

Epidemiological studies and randomized clinical trials have demonstrated an association between influenza infection and cardiovascular disease [86]. Influenza infection increased the risks of ACS and stroke, whereas vaccination against influenza reduced the risk of these major adverse cardiovascular events. Despite the absence of influenza A viral genome in atherosclerotic plaques, plaque-derived T-cells demonstrated high proliferative responses that were virus-specific and mainly involved CD4$^+$ T-cells [87].

Chlamydia pneumoniae (*C. pneumoniae*) is a common pathogen in human respiratory tract infection and several studies have identified the bacteria in unstable plaques taken from patients who underwent carotid endarterectomy [88,89]. T-cell lines derived from carotid tissues have been found to proliferate in response to *C. pneumoniae* antigens, comprise predominantly CD4$^+$ T-cells, and primarily display a Th1 cytokine profile [88]. Furthermore, the majority of the *C. pneumoniae*-specific cell lines were shown to be also responsive to HSP60 [88]. Symptomatic carotid plaques positive for *C. pneumoniae* demonstrated increased CD4$^+$, CD8$^+$, and CD45RO$^+$ T-cells compared to asymptomatic plaques [90]. However, in symptomatic plaques without *C. pneumoniae*, CD4$^+$ T-cells and CD45RO$^+$ memory T-cells were increased, but not CD8$^+$ T-cells when compared with asymptomatic plaques [90].

7. Clinical Utility of Profiling Circulating Cells of the Adaptive Immune System to Monitor Atherosclerosis

To date, there are no reliable biomarkers that can predict risk of major adverse cardiovascular events in individuals with subclinical atherosclerosis due to the difficulties in identifying unstable atherosclerotic plaques that are prone to rupture. Similar to noninvasive imaging modalities that are currently used to evaluate atherosclerotic plaque burden and composition, profiling T- and B-cells in blood specimens may provide vital information on disease progression. The development of multicolor flow cytometry technologies has facilitated detailed phenotypic and functional analyses of circulating immune cell subpopulations. Recent studies are summarized in Table 1.

Table 1. Clinical utility of profiling circulating cells of the adaptive immune system to monitor atherosclerosis progression.

Immune Cell/s	Patient Group	Findings	Ref
CD4$^+$CD28^{null}	CAD, Controls	• ↑ frequencies of CD4$^+$CD28^{null} T-cells expressing the CX3CR1 in patients with CAD compared to controls	[13]
CD4$^+$ T-cells (Th1, Th17)	Acute MI ($n = 26$), UA ($n = 16$), SA ($n = 16$), Controls ($n = 16$)	• ↑ frequencies of Th1 and Th17 CD4$^+$ T-cells in acute MI and UA patients compared with SA patients and healthy controls	[29]
NKT cells	Asymptomatic atherosclerosis patients ($n = 10$), Symptomatic atherosclerosis patients ($n = 10$), Controls ($n = 10$)	• ↓ frequencies of NKT cells in patients with atherosclerosis, with the lowest percentages reported in patients with symptomatic (defined as having a previous CV event) atherosclerosis	[52]
CD4$^+$ T-cells	Chronic SAP ($n = 30$), Acute MI ($n = 60$), Controls ($n = 40$)	• ↑ frequencies of T$_{EM}$ and HLA-DR CD4$^+$ T-cells in chronic SAP and acute MI patients compared to controls • Proportions of T$_{EM}$ and HLA-DR CD4$^+$ T-cells were similar in chronic SAP and acute MI patients • Percentages of T$_{EM}$ and HLA-DR CD4$^+$ T-cells correlated with IMT	[91]

Table 1. *Cont.*

Immune Cell/s	Patient Group	Findings	Ref
CD4$^+$ T-cells, CD8$^+$ T-cells, B-cells	Nonobstructive CAD ($n = 21$), ACS ($n = 52$), Controls ($n = 50$)	• Absolute numbers of CD4$^+$ T-cells and CD19$^+$ B-cells similar in the three groups • ↑ numbers of CD8$^+$ T-cells in ACS patients compared to controls and nonobstructive CAD patients • ↑ frequencies of highly differentiated CD4$^+$ and CD8$^+$ T-cells subsets in ACS patients • Percentages of highly differentiated CD4$^+$ and CD8$^+$ T-cells were associated with worse SYNTAX score, greater number of affected vessels, lower LVEF, and increased number of prior ACS events	[92]
CD4$^+$ T-cells (Th1, Th2, Th17, Tregs)	Acute MI ($n = 19$), UA ($n = 25$), SA ($n = 20$), Controls ($n = 24$)	• ↑ frequencies of Th1 cells in acute MI and UA patients compared to SA patients and controls • Frequencies of Th17 and Th2 were similar in the four groups • ↓ frequencies of Tregs (CD25$^+$FOXP3$^+$) in acute MI and UA patients compared with SA patients and controls	[93]
CD4$^+$ T-cells (Th1, Th2)	Stable CAD ($n = 35$), STE ($n = 30$), NSTE ($n = 35$), Controls ($n = 33$)	• ↑ frequencies of Th1 cells and Th1/Th2 ratio in STE and NSTE patients compared to patients with stable CAD and controls • Proportions of Th1 T-cells and Th1/Th2 ratio also correlated with the number of affected coronary arteries, the degree of coronary artery stenosis, and lengths of lesions	[94]
Tregs	CAD (SAP and previous MI) ($n = 73$), Controls ($n = 64$)	• ↓ frequencies of Tregs (FOXP3$^+$) and T_{reg}/T_{eff} ratio in CAD patients compared to controls • ↑ expression of activation markers CD25 and CTLA4 on Tregs from CAD patients compared to controls • T_{reg}/T_{eff} ratio correlated inversely with levels of hs-HRP in CAD patients	[95]

Table 1. *Cont.*

Immune Cell/s	Patient Group	Findings	Ref
CD8$^+$ T-cells	SAP ($n = 34$), ACS ($n = 30$), Controls ($n = 36$)	• ↑ numbers and percentages of CD8$^+$CD56$^+$ T-cells were higher in ACS and SAP patients compared to controls	[96]
CD8$^+$ T-cells	Subjects with a coronary event ($n = 84$), stroke ($n = 54$), or no event ($n = 549$) during the 15-year follow-up	• High frequencies of CD8$^+$ T-cells at baseline were associated with increased incidence of coronary events but not ischemic stroke • High frequencies of CD8$^+$CD56$^-$ T-cells producing IFNγ at baseline were associated with increased incidence of ischemic stroke	[97]
CD8$^+$ T-cells	Stable CAD ($n = 66$), ACS ($n = 34$)	• ↓ frequencies of T$_N$ and ↑ frequencies of T$_{EM}$ CD8$^+$ T-cells in ACS patients compared to stable CAD patients	[98]
CD8$^+$ T-cells	Patients with nonsignificant lesions ($n = 41$), Patients with severe lesions ($n = 37$), Controls ($n = 36$)	• ↓ frequencies of T$_N$ CD8$^+$ T-cells in patients with severe lesions than controls • Percentages of T$_N$ CD8$^+$ T-cells correlated inversely with Gensini score • Proportions of T$_N$ CD8$^+$ T-cells correlated inversely with PWV in controls but not in patients with atherosclerosis	[99]
Tregs	Chronic SAP ($n = 36$), NSTE ACS ($n = 50$), ST acute MI ($n = 39$), Controls ($n = 75$)	• ↓ frequencies of Tregs (CD25^{high}CD127^{low}) in non-ST ACS patients and ↑ frequencies of Tregs in ST acute MI patients compared to chronic SAP patients and controls	[100]
Tregs	ACS ($n = 26$), Post-ACS ($n = 57$, 24 STE, and 33 NSTE), Controls ($n = 41$)	• ↓ frequencies of naïve Tregs (FOXP3$^+$ or CD25^{high}CD127^{low}) in ACS and post-ACS patients compared with controls • Proportion of naïve Tregs correlated inversely with the presence of plaques on the right and left carotid and also with right carotid IMT	[101]

Table 1. *Cont.*

Immune Cell/s	Patient Group	Findings	Ref
Tregs	ACS (n = 48), SAP (n = 24), Controls (n = 24)	• ↓ frequencies of Tregs (CD25$^+$CD127^{low}) in ACS patients compared with SAP patients and controls • Frequencies of Tregs correlated inversely with levels of hs-CRP	[102]
Tregs	PCI with no disease progression (n = 32), PCI with new stenosis (n = 24), Patients with three-vessel coronary disease (n = 34), No atherosclerosis (n = 27)	• ↓ frequencies of Tregs (FOXP3$^+$ or CD25^{high}CD127^{low}) in patients with multivessel atherosclerosis compared to individuals with no atherosclerosis • Percentages of Tregs were similar in the three groups of patients • Frequencies of Tregs correlated inversely with Gensini score in patients with multivessel atherosclerosis	[103]
Tregs	SAP (n = 34), ACS (n = 37), Controls (n = 35)	• ↓ frequencies of Tregs (CD25$^+$CD127−) in ACS patients compared to SAP patients and controls • Similar percentages of Tregs in SAP patients and controls	[104]
CD4$^+$ T-cells, CD8$^+$ T-cells, B-cells, Tregs	SAP (n = 13), ACS (n = 13)	• No differences in percentages of CD4$^+$ and CD8$^+$ T-cells, activated (CD69$^+$ or HLA-DR$^+$) T-cells, B-cells, and Tregs (CD25$^+$ and/or FOXP3$^+$) between SAP and ACS patients	[105]
B-cells	Patients with advanced atherosclerosis who did not experience a secondary CV event during 3-year follow-up (n = 118) and those who did (n = 54)	• ↓ frequencies of CD19$^+$ B-cells, unswitched (expressing IgM) and switched (expressing IgA or IgG) memory cells in patients who experienced a secondary CVD event compared to those who did not	[106]
B-cells	Individuals (n = 700) with a coronary event (n = 84), stroke (n = 66), or no event (n = 549) during 15-year follow-up	• ↓ proportions of suppressive CD19$^+$CD40$^+$ B-cells but ↑ frequencies of activated (CD19$^+$CD86$^+$) B-cells at baseline in individuals with a later incidence of stroke compared to those with no event • B-cell subsets were not associated with increased risk of CAD	[107]

Table 1. *Cont.*

Immune Cell/s	Patient Group	Findings	Ref
NKT cells	STE acute MI (PCI and follow-up) ($n = 52$)	• Percentage and absolute number of NKT cells did not change during acute MI and at follow-up	[108]

Tregs, regulatory T-cells; T_{EM}, effector memory T-cells; T_N, naïve T-cells; ACS, acute coronary syndrome; LVEF, left ventricular ejection fraction; STE, ST elevation; NSTE, non-ST elevation; IMT, intima–media thickness; SAP, stable angina pectoris; UA, unstable angina; hs-CRP, high-sensitivity C-reactive protein; CAD, coronary artery disease; MI, myocardial infarction; PCI, percutaneous coronary intervention; CV, cardiovascular; CMV, cytomegalovirus; PBMC, peripheral blood mononuclear cells; PWV, pulse wave velocity; ↑, increased; ↓, decreased.

7.1. CD4$^+$ T-Cells

In multiple regression analyses, age, creatinine, and T_{EM} CD4$^+$ T-cells were reported to be independent predictors of carotid intima–media thickness, a noninvasive measure of subclinical atherosclerosis [91]. The authors also observed increased frequencies of T_{EM} and activated CD4$^+$ T-cells in patients with acute myocardial infarction or chronic stable angina compared with controls, whereas no differences were detected for CD4$^+$ T-cells expressing the chemokine receptors, CCR5 or CXCR3 [91]. Increased percentages of highly differentiated CD4$^+$ T-cells were found in ACS patients compared to patients with nonobstructive coronary artery disease (CAD) and healthy controls. Furthermore, higher degree of CD4$^+$ T-cell differentiation correlated with more diseased vessels, lower left ventricular ejection fraction, increased number of prior ACS events, and worse SYNTAX score, which is an angiographic grading tool to determine the complexity of the CAD [92]. Together, these studies suggest ACS is associated with aging of the adaptive immune system and this correlates with measurements of disease pathology.

In patients with acute myocardial infarction or unstable angina, proportions of Th1 CD4$^+$ T-cells were found to be higher compared to patients with stable angina with no differences observed for frequencies of Th2 and Th17 CD4$^+$ T-cells between the two groups [93]. In a recent study, Li et al. reported increased percentages of Th1 CD4$^+$ T-cells and Th1/Th2 ratio in patients with acute myocardial infarction compared to patients with stable CAD [94]. Proportions of Th1 T-cells and Th1/Th2 ratio also correlated with the number of affected coronary arteries, the degree of coronary artery stenosis, and lengths of lesions [94].

CD4$^+$CD28^{null} T-cells have been shown to be increased in individuals with CAD compared to those without CAD [95]. Expression of the chemokine receptor CX3CR1 on CD4$^+$CD28^{null} T-cells was also higher in patients with CAD than the control group [13] and this could explain the recruitment and accumulation of these cells within atherosclerotic plaques. Interestingly, CMV infection has been found to drive the accumulation of proatherogenic CD4$^+$CD28^{null} T-cells in the circulation and these cells have the ability to recognize CMV antigens [109].

7.2. CD8$^+$ T-Cells

Bergstrom et al. reported higher numbers and percentages of CD8$^+$ T-cells expressing the natural killer cell marker CD56 in ACS and stable angina patients than in healthy controls independent of age, sex, and CMV seropositivity [96]. The authors also demonstrated higher proportions of CD8$^+$CD56$^+$ T-cells expressing IFNγ compared to CD8$^+$CD56$^-$ T-cells following stimulation, indicating a potential role for these cells in atherosclerosis progression and plaque instability [96]. In another study, Kolbus et al. investigated two subsets of activated CD8$^+$ T-cells (CD8$^+$CD25$^+$ and CD8$^+$CD56$^-$ T-cells expressing IFNγ) as a predictor of acute myocardial infarction and ischemic stroke during 15-year follow-up [97]. They found that high frequencies of CD8$^+$ T-cells were associated with increased incidence of coronary events but not ischemic stroke after adjustments for other cardiovascular risk factors [97]. Furthermore, proportions of CD8$^+$CD25$^+$ T-cells positively correlated with the degree of stenosis whereas inverse correlations were observed between the percentages of CD8$^+$CD56$^-$

T-cells expressing IFNγ and the degree of stenosis and carotid intima–media thickness, suggestive of differential roles of CD8$^+$ T-cell populations in disease progression [97].

Frequencies of circulating CD8$^+$ T-cells expressing CXCR3 have been reported to be increased in CAD patients [110]. These effector CD8$^+$ T-cells can home to inflammatory sites via the chemokine IP-10, MIG, and I-TAC, which are expressed by endothelial cells, smooth muscle cells, and macrophages in human carotid atherosclerotic plaques [25]. Furthermore, production of IFNγ, perforin, and granzyme B by CD8$^+$ T-cells can contribute to plaque rupture by promoting apoptosis of cells within lesions [111].

Percentages of T_{EM} CD8$^+$ T-cells have been found to be increased in ACS patients compared to stable CAD patients [98] and in patients with CAD compared to healthy controls [112]. Detailed analyses of T_{EM} CD8$^+$ T-cells revealed that they lacked the receptor for the proinflammatory cytokine IL-6 and possessed cytotoxic capabilities including the expression of perforin and granzyme B that can contribute to disease pathology [112]. Podolec et al. confirmed reduced frequencies of T_N CD8$^+$ T-cells in patients with significant narrowing of the coronary arteries compared to individuals with no atherosclerosis [99]. Moreover, proportions of these cells correlated inversely with pulse wave velocity, a measure of arterial stiffness and a predictor of cardiovascular risk, in individuals without atherosclerosis, but not in patients with extensive coronary artery narrowing [99]. The authors suggested that monitoring of this cell subset may be useful during the early stages of coronary atherosclerosis.

Decreased circulating T_N CD8$^+$ T-cells have also been reported in patients with ACS compared to individuals with stable CAD [99]. The authors showed that these cells displayed characteristics of immune exhaustion including impaired IL-12 production and upregulation of programmed cell death (PD)-1 molecule, and in vitro experiments indicated that oxLDL may contribute to this phenotype [99]. CD8$^+$ T-cells that recognize and respond to oxLDL and HSP60 have been identified in patients with non-ST elevation myocardial infarction or stable angina but not in healthy controls [113]. This suggests that antigen-specific T-cells in atherosclerotic lesions can re-enter the circulation and therefore may be a useful indicator of plaque stability.

7.3. Treg Cells

The clinical utility of Treg cells as a metric of atherosclerosis progression has been complicated due to the different cell surface markers used to define these cells. Frequencies of Treg cells identified as CD4$^+$CD25^{high}CD127^{low} were found not to be associated with carotid intima–media thickness or progression of atherosclerosis [100]. In contrast, Hasib et al. demonstrated that naive but not memory Treg (defined using the markers CD4, FOXP3, and CD45RA) correlated inversely with right carotid intima–media thickness and also with the presence of atherosclerotic plaques [101].

Using FOXP3 and CD45RA, frequencies of resting and activated Treg cells were reported to be increased in patients with myocardial infarction or stable angina compared to individuals without cardiovascular disease [95]. However, several other investigators found reduced or no differences in the percentages of CD4$^+$CD25^{high}CD127^{low} and CD4$^+$CD25^{high}FOXP3$^+$ Treg cells in patients with ACS compared to normal controls or patients with stable angina [93,101–105]. Peripheral blood cells from ACS patients cultured in vitro with simvastatin have been shown to increase the number and suppressive function of CD4$^+$CD25$^+$FOXP3$^+$ Treg cells, suggesting a beneficial role for statins in stabilizing vulnerable atherosclerosis plaques [114].

7.4. B-Cells and NKT Cells

Frequencies of different B-cell subsets including CD19$^+$ B-cells, unswitched (expressing IgM) and switched (expressing IgG or IgA) memory B-cells have been found to be reduced in patients who experienced a secondary cardiovascular event compared to those who did not [106]. A study of 700 individuals followed for 15 years in the Malmo Diet and Cancer Study showed lower baseline percentages of suppressive CD19$^+$ B-cells expressing CD40 but higher activated CD19$^+$ B-cells expressing CD86 in individuals with a later incidence of stroke [107]. However, these B-cell subsets were not associated with increased risk of CAD [107]. In patients undergoing percutaneous coronary intervention, proportions of iNKT cells were stable during acute myocardial infarction and follow-up [108].

8. Conclusions

Compelling evidence implicates adaptive immune cells in all phases of human atherosclerosis, from plaque initiation to destabilization (Figure 2). More extensive studies utilizing plaque tissues are necessary to characterize the effector cells and map critical pathways during atherogenesis. Studies in patients with different stages of atherosclerosis are now providing valuable insight, but heterogeneity of plaque characteristics hampers direct comparison between plaque features and circulating immune cells. Early detection of vulnerable lesions remains the main goal of biomarker discovery. Future studies including circulating cellular biomarkers are warranted to improve identification of vulnerable lesions so that effective intervention can be implemented before clinical manifestations are apparent.

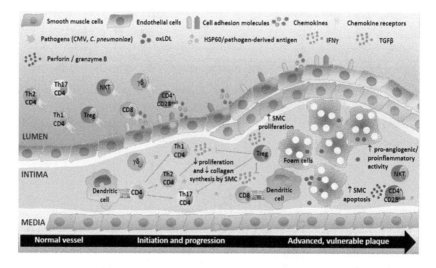

Figure 2. Adaptive immune cells are involved in all stages of human atherosclerosis. Endothelial cells activation upregulates cell adhesion molecules and secretion of chemokines and so directs T-cells to the site of inflammation. T helper (Th)1 cells produce interferon-γ (IFNγ), a proatherogenic cytokine able to activate macrophages, inhibit proliferation, and reduce collagen production by smooth muscle cells. Th2 cells produce interleukin (IL)-4 and may be atheroprotective as they can inhibit Th1 cells. CD4$^+$CD28^{null} T-cells may damage cells in the vascular wall via the release of perforin and granzyme B. CD8$^+$ T-cells may be proatherogenic via the production of IFNγ or protective by reducing macrophage content in the plaque. Treg cells can suppress Th1 and Th17 responses and increase smooth muscle cell proliferation through the secretion of cytokines (e.g., transforming growth factor (TGF)-β). Natural killer (NK)T cells exhibit proangiogenic and proinflammatory activities suggesting an involvement in plaque destabilization. Th17 and γδ T-cells are present in lesions but their roles are not well characterized. T-cells can be activated by heat shock proteins (e.g., HSP60), oxidized lipoproteins (oxLDL), or antigens derived from pathogens (e.g., cytomegalovirus (CMV) and *Chlamydia pneumoniae* (*C. pneumoniae*)).

Author Contributions: Writing, S.L.; writing—review and editing, B.B. and G.D. All authors have read and agreed to the published version of the manuscript.

Acknowledgments: We thank Patricia Price for comments and proofreading of the manuscript.

Abbreviations

ACS	Acute coronary syndrome
BPIFB4	Bactericidal/permeability-increasing fold-containing family B member 4
CAD	Coronary artery disease
CMV	Cytomegalovirus
CV	Cardiovascular
DNA	Deoxyribonucleic acid
EBV	Epstein–Barr virus
FOXP3	Forkhead box 3
GM-CSF	Granulocyte-macrophage colony-stimulating factor
HIV	Human immunodeficiency virus
Hs-CRP	High-sensitivity C-reactive protein
HSP	Heat shock protein
IFNγ	Interferon gamma
IL	Interleukin
IMT	Intima–media thickness
IP-10	IFN-inducible protein 10
I-TAC	IFN-inducible T-cell α chemoattractant
LDL	Low-density lipoproteins
LVEF	Left ventricular ejection fraction
MHC	Major histocompatibility complex
MI	Myocardial infarction
MIG	Monokine induced by IFNγ
NKT	Natural killer T-cells
NSTE	Non-ST elevation
oxLDL	Oxidized low-density lipoproteins
PBMC	Peripheral blood mononuclear cells
PCI	Percutaneous coronary intervention
PCR	Polymerase chain reaction
PCSK9	Proprotein convertase subtilisin/kexin type 9
PD-1	Programmed cell death 1
PWV	Pulse wave velocity
RNA	Ribonucleic acid
SAP	Stable angina pectoris
STE	ST elevation
TCR	T-cell receptor
TGFβ	Transforming growth factor beta
Th	T helper
TNFα	Tumor necrosis factor alpha
Treg	Regulatory T-cells
T_{CM}	Central memory T-cells
T_{EM}	Effector memory T-cells
T_N	Naïve T-cells
T_{TE}	Terminal effector T-cells
UA	Unstable angina

References

1. Wong, B.W.; Meredith, A.; Lin, D.; McManus, B.M. The Biological Role of Inflammation in Atherosclerosis. *Can. J. Cardiol.* **2012**, *28*, 631–641. [CrossRef]
2. Moore, K.J.; Tabas, I. Macrophages in the Pathogenesis of Atherosclerosis. *Cell* **2011**, *145*, 341–355. [CrossRef] [PubMed]
3. Fatkhullina, A.R.; Peshkova, I.O.; Koltsova, E.K. The role of cytokines in the development of atherosclerosis. *Biochemistry* **2016**, *81*, 1358–1370. [CrossRef] [PubMed]

4. Bartlett, B.; Ludewick, H.P.; Misra, A.; Lee, S.; Dwivedi, G. Macrophages and T cells in atherosclerosis: A translational perspective. *Am. J. Physiol. Circ. Physiol.* **2019**, *317*, H375–H386. [CrossRef] [PubMed]

5. Farber, D.L.; Yudanin, N.A.; Restifo, N.P. Human memory T cells: Generation, compartmentalization and homeostasis. *Nat. Rev. Immunol.* **2014**, *14*, 24–35. [CrossRef] [PubMed]

6. Von Boehmer, H. Mechanisms of suppression by suppressor T cells. *Nat. Immunol.* **2005**, *6*, 338–344. [CrossRef] [PubMed]

7. Jonasson, L.; Holm, J.; Skalli, O.; Bondjers, G.; Hansson, G.K. Regional accumulations of T cells, macrophages, and smooth muscle cells in the human atherosclerotic plaque. *Arter. Off. J. Am. Heart Assoc. Inc.* **1986**, *6*, 131–138. [CrossRef] [PubMed]

8. Kortelainen, M.-L.; Porvari, K. Adventitial macrophage and lymphocyte accumulation accompanying early stages of human coronary atherogenesis. *Cardiovasc. Pathol.* **2014**, *23*, 193–197. [CrossRef]

9. Van Dijk, R.A.; Duinisveld, A.J.F.; Schaapherder, A.F.; Mulder-Stapel, A.; Hamming, J.F.; Kuiper, J.; De Boer, O.J.; Van Der Wal, A.C.; Kolodgie, F.D.; Virmani, R.; et al. A Change in Inflammatory Footprint Precedes Plaque Instability: A Systematic Evaluation of Cellular Aspects of the Adaptive Immune Response in Human Atherosclerosis. *J. Am. Heart Assoc.* **2015**, *4*, e001403. [CrossRef]

10. Rohm, I.; Atiskova, Y.; Drobnik, S.; Fritzenwanger, M.; Kretzschmar, D.; Pistulli, R.; Zanow, J.; Krönert, T.; Mall, G.; Figulla, H.R.; et al. Decreased Regulatory T Cells in Vulnerable Atherosclerotic Lesions: Imbalance between Pro- and Anti-Inflammatory Cells in Atherosclerosis. *Mediat. Inflamm.* **2015**, *2015*, 1–13. [CrossRef]

11. De Boer, O.J.; Hirsch, F.; Van Der Wal, A.C.; Van Der Loos, C.M.; Das, P.K.; Becker, A.E. Costimulatory molecules in human atherosclerotic plaques: An indication of antigen specific T lymphocyte activation. *Atherosclerosis* **1997**, *133*, 227–234. [CrossRef]

12. Stemme, S.; Holm, J.; Hansson, G.K. T lymphocytes in human atherosclerotic plaques are memory cells expressing CD45RO and the integrin VLA-1. *Arter. Thromb. A J. Vasc. Biol.* **1992**, *12*, 206–211. [CrossRef]

13. Zhang, X.; Feng, X.; Cai, W.; Liu, T.; Liang, Z.; Sun, Y.; Yan, C.; Han, Y. Chemokine CX3CL1 and its receptor CX3CR1 are associated with human atherosclerotic lesion volnerability. *Thromb. Res.* **2015**, *135*, 1147–1153. [CrossRef] [PubMed]

14. Bonanno, E.; Mauriello, A.; Partenzi, A.; Anemona, L.; Spagnoli, L.G. Flow cytometry analysis of atherosclerotic plaque cells from human carotids: A validation study. *Cytometry* **2000**, *39*, 158–165. [CrossRef]

15. Lebedeva, A.; Vorobyeva, D.; Vagida, M.; Ivanova, O.; Felker, E.; Fitzgerald, W.; Danilova, N.; Gontarenko, V.; Shpektor, A.; Vasilieva, E.; et al. Ex vivo culture of human atherosclerotic plaques: A model to study immune cells in atherogenesis. *Atherosclerosis* **2017**, *267*, 90–98. [CrossRef] [PubMed]

16. Villa, F.; Carrizzo, A.; Ferrario, A.; Maciag, A.; Cattaneo, M.; Spinelli, C.C.; Montella, F.; Damato, A.; Ciaglia, E.; Puca, A.A. A Model of Evolutionary Selection: The Cardiovascular Protective Function of the Longevity Associated Variant of BPIFB4. *Int. J. Mol. Sci.* **2018**, *19*, 3229. [CrossRef] [PubMed]

17. Dossena, M.; Ferrario, A.; Lopardo, V.; Ciaglia, E.; Puca, A.A. New Insights for BPIFB4 in Cardiovascular Therapy. *Int. J. Mol. Sci.* **2020**, *21*, 7163. [CrossRef]

18. Ciaglia, E.; Montella, F.; Lopardo, V.; Scala, P.; Ferrario, A.; Cattaneo, M.; Carrizzo, A.; Malovini, A.; Madeddu, P.; Vecchione, C.; et al. Circulating BPIFB4 Levels Associate With and Influence the Abundance of Reparative Monocytes and Macrophages in Long Living Individuals. *Front. Immunol.* **2020**, *11*. [CrossRef]

19. Ciaglia, E.; Montella, F.; Maciag, A.; Scala, P.; Ferrario, A.; Banco, C.; Carrizzo, A.; Spinelli, C.C.; Cattaneo, M.; De Candia, P.; et al. Longevity-Associated Variant of BPIFB4 Mitigates Monocyte-Mediated Acquired Immune Response. *J. Gerontol. Ser. A Boil. Sci. Med Sci.* **2019**, *74*, S38–S44. [CrossRef]

20. Grivel, J.-C.; Ivanova, O.; Pinegina, N.; Blank, P.S.; Shpektor, A.; Margolis, L.B.; Vasilieva, E. Activation of T Lymphocytes in Atherosclerotic Plaques. *Arter. Thromb. Vasc. Biol.* **2011**, *31*, 2929–2937. [CrossRef]

21. Fernandez, D.M.; Rahman, A.H.; Fernandez, N.F.; Chudnovskiy, A.; Amir, E.-A.D.; Amadori, L.; Khan, N.S.; Wong, C.K.; Shamailova, R.; Hill, C.A.; et al. Single-cell immune landscape of human atherosclerotic plaques. *Nat. Med.* **2019**, *25*, 1576–1588. [CrossRef] [PubMed]

22. Frostegård, J.; Ulfgren, A.-K.; Nyberg, P.; Hedin, U.; Swedenborg, J.; Andersson, U.; Hansson, G.K. Cytokine expression in advanced human atherosclerotic plaques: Dominance of pro-inflammatory (Th1) and macrophage-stimulating cytokines. *Atherosclerosis* **1999**, *145*, 33–43. [CrossRef]

23. De Boer, O.J.; Van Der Wal, A.C.; Verhagen, C.E.; Becker, A.E. Cytokine secretion profiles of cloned T cells from human aortic atherosclerotic plaques. *J. Pathol.* **1999**, *188*, 174–179. [CrossRef]

24. Oliveira, R.T.D.; Silva, R.M.; Teo, F.H.; Mineiro, M.F.; Ferreira, M.C.; Altemani, A.; Mamoni, R.L.; Menezes, F.H.; Blotta, M.H.S.L. Detection of TCD4+ subsets in human carotid atheroma. *Cytokine* **2013**, *62*, 131–140. [CrossRef] [PubMed]

25. Mach, F.; Sauty, A.; Iarossi, A.S.; Sukhova, G.K.; Neote, K.; Libby, P.; Luster, A.D. Differential expression of three T lymphocyte-activating CXC chemokines by human atheroma-associated cells. *J. Clin. Investig.* **1999**, *104*, 1041–1050. [CrossRef]

26. Mallat, Z.; Corbaz, A.; Scoazec, A.; Besnard, S.; Leseèche, G.; Chvatchko, Y.; Tedgui, A. Expression of Interleukin-18 in Human Atherosclerotic Plaques and Relation to Plaque Instability. *Circulation* **2001**, *104*, 1598–1603. [CrossRef]

27. Pigarevskii, P.V.; Maltseva, S.V.; Snegova, V.; Davydova, N.G. Role of Interleukin-18 in Destabilization of the Atherosclerotic Plaque in Humans. *Bull. Exp. Biol. Med.* **2014**, *157*, 821–824. [CrossRef]

28. Uyemura, K.; Demer, L.L.; Castle, S.C.; Jullien, D.; Berliner, J.A.; Gately, M.K.; Warrier, R.R.; Pham, N.; Fogelman, A.M.; Modlin, R.L. Cross-regulatory roles of interleukin (IL)-12 and IL-10 in atherosclerosis. *J. Clin. Investig.* **1996**, *97*, 2130–2138. [CrossRef]

29. Voloshyna, I.; Littlefield, M.J.; Reiss, A.B. Atherosclerosis and interferon-gamma: New insights and therapeutic targets. *Trends Cardiovasc. Med.* **2014**, *24*, 45–51. [CrossRef]

30. Eid, R.E.; Rao, D.A.; Zhou, J.; Lo, S.L.; Ranjbaran, H.; Gallo, A.; Sokol, S.I.; Pfau, S.; Pober, J.S.; Tellides, G. Interleukin-17 and interferon-gamma are produced concomitantly by human coronary artery-infiltrating T cells and act synergistically on vascular smooth muscle cells. *Circulation* **2009**, *119*, 1424–1432. [CrossRef]

31. Cheng, X.; Yu, X.; Ding, Y.-J.; Fu, Q.-Q.; Xie, J.-J.; Tang, T.-T.; Yao, R.; Chen, Y.; Liao, Y.-H. The Th17/Treg imbalance in patients with acute coronary syndrome. *Clin Immunol.* **2008**, *127*, 89–97. [CrossRef] [PubMed]

32. Hashmi, S.; Zeng, Q.T. Role of interleukin-17 and interleukin-17-induced cytokines interleukin-6 and interleukin-8 in unstable coronary artery disease. *Coron. Artery Dis.* **2006**, *17*, 699–706. [CrossRef] [PubMed]

33. Zhang, L.; Wang, T.; Wang, X.Q.; Du, R.Z.; Zhang, K.N.; Liu, X.G.; Ma, D.X.; Yu, S.; Su, G.H.; Li, Z.H.; et al. Elevated frequencies of circulating Th22 cell in addition to Th17 cell and Th17/Th1 cell in patients with acute coronary syndrome. *PLoS ONE* **2013**, *8*, e71466. [CrossRef] [PubMed]

34. Liu, Z.; Lu, F.; Pan, H.; Zhao, Y.; Wang, S.; Sun, S.; Li, J.; Hu, X.; Wang, L. Correlation of peripheral Th17 cells and Th17-associated cytokines to the severity of carotid artery plaque and its clinical implication. *Atherosclerosis* **2012**, *221*, 232–241. [CrossRef]

35. Liuzzo, G.; Goronzy, J.J.; Yang, H.; Kopecky, S.L.; Holmes, D.R.; Frye, R.L.; Weyand, C.M. Monoclonal T-Cell Proliferation and Plaque Instability in Acute Coronary Syndromes. *Circulation* **2000**, *101*, 2883–2888. [CrossRef]

36. Dumitriu, I.E.; Baruah, P.; Finlayson, C.J.; Loftus, I.M.; Antunes, R.F.; Lim, P.; Bunce, N.; Kaski, J.C. High Levels of Costimulatory Receptors OX40 and 4-1BB Characterize CD4+CD28null T Cells in Patients With Acute Coronary Syndrome. *Circ. Res.* **2012**, *110*, 857–869. [CrossRef]

37. Dumitriu, I.E. The life (and death) of CD4+CD28null T cells in inflammatory diseases. *Immunology* **2015**, *146*, 185–193. [CrossRef]

38. Paul, V.S.V.; Paul, C.M.P.; Kuruvilla, S. Quantification of Various Inflammatory Cells in Advanced Atherosclerotic Plaques. *J. Clin. Diagn. Res.* **2016**, *10*, EC35–EC38. [CrossRef]

39. Van Duijn, J.; Kritikou, E.; Benne, N.; Van Der Heijden, T.; Van Puijvelde, G.H.; Kröner, M.J.; Schaftenaar, F.H.; Foks, A.; Wezel, A.; Smeets, H.; et al. CD8+ T-cells contribute to lesion stabilization in advanced atherosclerosis by limiting macrophage content and CD4+ T-cell responses. *Cardiovasc. Res.* **2018**, *115*, 729–738. [CrossRef]

40. Hendel, A.; Cooper, D.; Abraham, T.; Zhao, H.; Allard, M.F.; Granville, D.J. Proteinase inhibitor 9 is reduced in human atherosclerotic lesion development. *Cardiovasc. Pathol.* **2012**, *21*, 28–38. [CrossRef]

41. Choy, J.C.; McDonald, P.C.; Suarez, A.C.; Hung, V.H.Y.; Wilson, J.E.; McManus, B.M.; Granville, D.J. Granzyme B in Atherosclerosis and Transplant Vascular Disease: Association with Cell Death and Atherosclerotic Disease Severity. *Mod. Pathol.* **2003**, *16*, 460–470. [CrossRef]

42. De Boer, O.J.; Van Der Meer, J.J.; Teeling, P.; Van Der Loos, C.M.; Van Der Wal, A.C. Low Numbers of FOXP3 Positive Regulatory T Cells Are Present in all Developmental Stages of Human Atherosclerotic Lesions. *PLoS ONE* **2007**, *2*, e779. [CrossRef]

43. Patel, S.; Chung, S.; White, G.; Bao, S.; Celermajer, D. The "atheroprotective" mediators apolipoproteinA-I and Foxp3 are over-abundant in unstable carotid plaques. *Int. J. Cardiol.* **2010**, *145*, 183–187. [CrossRef] [PubMed]

44. Dietel, B.; Cicha, I.; Voskens, C.J.; Verhoeven, E.; Achenbach, S.; Garlichs, C.D. Decreased numbers of regulatory T cells are associated with human atherosclerotic lesion vulnerability and inversely correlate with infiltrated mature dendritic cells. *Atherosclerosis* **2013**, *230*, 92–99. [CrossRef] [PubMed]

45. Toma, I.; McCaffrey, T.A. Transforming growth factor-β and atherosclerosis: Interwoven atherogenic and atheroprotective aspects. *Cell Tissue Res.* **2012**, *347*, 155–175. [CrossRef] [PubMed]

46. Foks, A.C.; Lichtman, A.H.; Kuiper, J. Treating Atherosclerosis with Regulatory T Cells. *Arter. Thromb. Vasc. Biol.* **2015**, *35*, 280–287. [CrossRef] [PubMed]

47. Ou, H.-X.; Guo, B.-B.; Liu, Q.; Li, Y.-K.; Yang, Z.; Feng, W.-J.; Mo, Z.-C. Regulatory T cells as a new therapeutic target for atherosclerosis. *Acta Pharmacol. Sin.* **2018**, *39*, 1249–1258. [CrossRef]

48. Lawand, M.; Déchanet-Merville, J.; Dieu-Nosjean, M.-C. Key Features of Gamma-Delta T-Cell Subsets in Human Diseases and Their Immunotherapeutic Implications. *Front. Immunol.* **2017**, *8*, 761. [CrossRef]

49. Vu, D.M.; Tai, A.; Tatro, J.B.; Karas, R.H.; Huber, B.T.; Beasley, D. gammadeltaT cells are prevalent in the proximal aorta and drive nascent atherosclerotic lesion progression and neutrophilia in hypercholesterolemic mice. *PLoS ONE* **2014**, *9*, e109416. [CrossRef]

50. Cheng, H.-Y.; Wu, R.; Hedrick, C.C. Gammadelta ($\gamma\delta$) T lymphocytes do not impact the development of early atherosclerosis. *Atherosclerosis* **2014**, *234*, 265–269. [CrossRef]

51. Kleindienst, R.; Xu, Q.; Willeit, J.; Waldenberger, F.R.; Weimann, S.; Wick, G. Immunology of atherosclerosis. Demonstration of heat shock protein 60 expression and T lymphocytes bearing alpha/beta or gamma/delta receptor in human atherosclerotic lesions. *Am. J. Pathol.* **1993**, *142*, 1927–1937. [PubMed]

52. Millonig, G.; Malcom, G.T.; Wick, G. Early inflammato.ry-immunological lesions in juvenile atherosclerosis from the Pathobiological Determinants of Atherosclerosis in Youth (PDAY)-study. *Atherosclerosis* **2002**, *160*, 441–448. [CrossRef]

53. Van Puijvelde, G.H.; Kuiper, J. NKT cells in cardiovascular diseases. *Eur. J. Pharmacol.* **2017**, *816*, 47–57. [CrossRef] [PubMed]

54. Rombouts, M.; Ammi, R.; Van Brussel, I.; Roth, L.; De Winter, B.Y.; Vercauteren, S.R.; Hendriks, J.M.; Lauwers, P.; Van Schil, P.E.; De Meyer, G.R.Y.; et al. Linking CD11b+ Dendritic Cells and Natural Killer T Cells to Plaque Inflammation in Atherosclerosis. *Mediat. Inflamm.* **2016**, *2016*, 1–12. [CrossRef] [PubMed]

55. Bobryshev, Y.V.; Lord, R.S. Co-accumulation of Dendritic Cells and Natural Killer T Cells within Rupture-prone Regions in Human Atherosclerotic Plaques. *J. Histochem. Cytochem.* **2005**, *53*, 781–785. [CrossRef] [PubMed]

56. Kyriakakis, E.; Cavallari, M.; Andert, J.; Philippova, M.; Koella, C.; Bochkov, V.; Erne, P.; Wilson, S.B.; Mori, L.; Biedermann, B.C.; et al. Invariant natural killer T cells: Linking inflammation and neovascularization in human atherosclerosis. *Eur. J. Immunol.* **2010**, *40*, 3268–3279. [CrossRef] [PubMed]

57. Chan, W.L.; Pejnovic, N.; Hamilton, H.; Liew, T.V.; Popadić, S.; Poggi, A.; Khan, S.M. Atherosclerotic Abdominal Aortic Aneurysm and the Interaction Between Autologous Human Plaque-Derived Vascular Smooth Muscle Cells, Type 1 NKT, and Helper T Cells. *Circ. Res.* **2005**, *96*, 675–683. [CrossRef]

58. Huan, T.; Zhang, B.; Wang, Z.; Joehanes, R.; Zhu, J.; Johnson, A.D.; Ying, S.; Munson, P.J.; Raghavachari, N.; Wang, R.; et al. A Systems Biology Framework Identifies Molecular Underpinnings of Coronary Heart Disease. *Arter. Thromb. Vasc. Biol.* **2013**, *33*, 1427–1434. [CrossRef]

59. Hamze, M.; Desmetz, C.; Berthe, M.L.; Roger, P.; Boulle, N.; Brancherau, P.; Picard, E.; Guzman, C.; Tolza, C.; Guglielmi, P. Characterization of Resident B Cells of Vascular Walls in Human Atherosclerotic Patients. *J. Immunol.* **2013**, *191*, 3006–3016. [CrossRef]

60. De Palma, R.; Del Galdo, F.; Abbate, G.; Chiariello, M.; Calabrò, R.; Forte, L.; Cimmino, G.; Papa, M.F.; Russo, M.G.; Ambrosio, G.; et al. Patients with Acute Coronary Syndrome Show Oligoclonal T-Cell Recruitment Within Unstable Plaque. *Circulation* **2006**, *113*, 640–646. [CrossRef]

61. Benagiano, M.; D'Elios, M.M.; Amedei, A.; Azzurri, A.; Van Der Zee, R.; Ciervo, A.; Rombolà, G.; Romagnani, S.; Cassone, A.; Del Prete, G. Human 60-kDa Heat Shock Protein Is a Target Autoantigen of T Cells Derived from Atherosclerotic Plaques. *J. Immunol.* **2005**, *174*, 6509–6517. [CrossRef]

62. Rossmann, A.; Henderson, B.; Heidecker, B.; Seiler, R.; Fraedrich, G.; Singh, M.; Parson, W.; Keller, M.; Grubeck-Loebenstein, B.; Wick, G. T-cells from advanced atherosclerotic lesions recognize hHSP60 and have a restricted T-cell receptor repertoire. *Exp. Gerontol.* **2008**, *43*, 229–237. [CrossRef]

63. Rahman, M.; Steuer, J.; Gillgren, P.; Hayderi, A.; Liu, A.; Frostegård, J. Induction of Dendritic Cell–Mediated Activation of T Cells From Atherosclerotic Plaques by Human Heat Shock Protein 60. *J. Am. Hear. Assoc.* **2017**, *6*, e006778. [CrossRef] [PubMed]

64. Di Pietro, N.; Formoso, G.; Pandolfi, A. Physiology and pathophysiology of oxLDL uptake by vascular wall cells in atherosclerosis. *Vasc. Pharmacol.* **2016**, *84*, 1–7. [CrossRef] [PubMed]

65. Stemme, S.; Faber, B.; Holm, J.; Wiklund, O.; Witztum, J.L.; Hansson, G.K. T lymphocytes from human atherosclerotic plaques recognize oxidized low density lipoprotein. *Proc. Natl. Acad. Sci. USA* **1995**, *92*, 3893–3897. [CrossRef] [PubMed]

66. Liu, A.; Frostegård, J. PCSK9 plays a novel immunological role in oxidized LDL-induced dendritic cell maturation and activation of T cells from human blood and atherosclerotic plaque. *J. Intern. Med.* **2018**, *284*, 193–210. [CrossRef]

67. Frostegård, J.; Zhang, Y.; Sun, J.; Yan, K.; Liu, A. Oxidized Low-Density Lipoprotein (OxLDL)–Treated Dendritic Cells Promote Activation of T Cells in Human Atherosclerotic Plaque and Blood, Which Is Repressed by Statins: MicroRNA let-7c Is Integral to the Effect. *J. Am. Hear. Assoc.* **2016**, *5*, e003976. [CrossRef]

68. Cannon, M.J.; Schmid, D.S.; Hyde, T.B. Review of cytomegalovirus seroprevalence and demographic characteristics associated with infection. *Rev. Med Virol.* **2010**, *20*, 202–213. [CrossRef]

69. Lv, Y.; Han, F.-F.; Gong, L.-L.; Liu, H.; Ma, J.; Yu, W.-Y.; Wan, Z.-R.; Jia, Y.-J.; Zhang, W.; Shi, M.; et al. Human cytomegalovirus infection and vascular disease risk: A meta-analysis. *Virus Res.* **2017**, *227*, 124–134. [CrossRef]

70. Lichtner, M.; Cicconi, P.; Vita, S.; Cozzi-Lepri, A.; Galli, M.; Caputo, S.L.; Saracino, A.; De Luca, A.; Moioli, M.; Maggiolo, F.; et al. Cytomegalovirus Coinfection Is Associated With an Increased Risk of Severe Non–AIDS-Defining Events in a Large Cohort of HIV-Infected Patients. *J. Infect. Dis.* **2015**, *211*, 178–186. [CrossRef]

71. Courivaud, C.; Bamoulid, J.; Chalopin, J.-M.; Gaiffe, E.; Tiberghien, P.; Saas, P.; Ducloux, D. Cytomegalovirus Exposure and Cardiovascular Disease in Kidney Transplant Recipients. *J. Infect. Dis.* **2013**, *207*, 1569–1575. [CrossRef] [PubMed]

72. Priyanka, S.; Kaarthikeyan, G.; Nadathur, J.D.; Mohanraj, A.; Kavarthapu, A. Detection of cytomegalovirus, Epstein–Barr virus, and Torque Teno virus in subgingival and atheromatous plaques of cardiac patients with chronic periodontitis. *J. Indian Soc. Periodontol.* **2017**, *21*, 456–460. [PubMed]

73. Heybar, H.; Alavi, S.M.; Nejad, M.F.; Latifi, M. Cytomegalovirus Infection and Atherosclerosis in Candidate of Coronary Artery Bypass Graft. *Jundishapur J. Microbiol.* **2015**, *8*, e15476. [CrossRef] [PubMed]

74. Cao, J.; Mao, Y.; Dong, B.; Guan, W.; Shi, J.; Wang, S. Detection of specific Chlamydia pneumoniae and cytomegalovirus antigens in human carotid atherosclerotic plaque in a Chinese population. *Oncotarget* **2017**, *8*, 55435–55442. [CrossRef] [PubMed]

75. Bayram, A.; Erdoğan, M.B.; Ekşi, F.; Yamak, B. Demonstration of Chlamydophila pneumoniae, Mycoplasma pneumoniae, Cytomegalovirus, and Epstein-Barr virus in atherosclerotic coronary arteries, nonrheumatic calcific aortic and rheumatic stenotic mitral valves by polymerase chain reaction. *Anadolu Kardiyol. Dergisi/Anatol. J. Cardiol.* **2011**, *11*, 237–243. [CrossRef] [PubMed]

76. Xenaki, E.; Hassoulas, J.; Apostolakis, S.; Sourvinos, G.; Spandidos, D.A. Detection of Cytomegalovirus in Atherosclerotic Plaques and Nonatherosclerotic Arteries. *Angiology* **2009**, *60*, 504–508. [CrossRef]

77. Pampou, S.Y.; Gnedoy, S.N.; Bystrevskaya, V.B.; Smirnov, V.N.; Chazov, E.I.; Melnick, J.L.; DeBakey, M.E. Cytomegalovirus genome and the immediate-early antigen in cells of different layers of human aorta. *Virchows Arch.* **2000**, *436*, 539–552. [CrossRef]

78. Yi, L.; Wang, D.-X.; Feng, Z.-J. Detection of Human Cytomegalovirus in Atherosclerotic Carotid Arteries in Humans. *J. Formos. Med. Assoc.* **2008**, *107*, 774–781. [CrossRef]

79. Yaiw, K.-C.; Ovchinnikova, O.; Taher, C.; Mohammad, A.-A.; Davoudi, B.; Shlyakhto, E.V.; Rotar, O.P.; Konradi, A.; Wilhelmi, V.; Rahbar, A.; et al. High prevalence of human cytomegalovirus in carotid atherosclerotic plaques obtained from Russian patients undergoing carotid endarterectomy. *Herpesviridae* **2013**, *4*, 3. [CrossRef]

80. Nikitskaya, E.; Lebedeva, A.; Ivanova, O.; Maryukhnich, E.; Shpektor, A.; Grivel, J.; Margolis, L.; Vasilieva, E. Cytomegalovirus-Productive Infection Is Associated With Acute Coronary Syndrome. *J. Am. Heart Assoc.* **2016**, *5*, e003759. [CrossRef]

81. Van De Berg, P.J.E.J.; Yong, S.-L.; Remmerswaal, E.B.M.; Van Lier, R.A.W.; Berge, I.J.M.T. Cytomegalovirus-Induced Effector T Cells Cause Endothelial Cell Damage. *Clin. Vaccine Immunol.* **2012**, *19*, 772–779. [CrossRef] [PubMed]

82. Sacre, K.; Hunt, P.W.; Hsue, P.Y.; Maidji, E.; Martin, J.N.; Deeks, S.G.; Autran, B.; McCune, J.M. A role for cytomegalovirus-specific CD4+CX3CR1+ T cells and cytomegalovirus-induced T-cell immunopathology in HIV-associated atherosclerosis. *AIDS* **2012**, *26*, 805–814. [CrossRef] [PubMed]

83. Izadi, M.; Fazel, M.; Saadat, S.H.; Naseri, M.H.; Ghasemi, M.; Dabiri, H.; Aryan, R.S.; Esfahani, A.; Ahmadi, A.; Kazemi-Saleh, D.; et al. Cytomegalovirus Localization in Atherosclerotic Plaques Is Associated with Acute Coronary Syndromes: Report Of 105 Patients. *Methodist DeBakey Cardiovasc. J.* **2012**, *8*, 42–46. [CrossRef]

84. Liu, R.; Moroi, M.; Yamamoto, M.; Kubota, T.; Ono, T.; Funatsu, A.; Komatsu, H.; Tsuji, T.; Hara, H.; Hara, H.; et al. Presence and Severity of Chlamydia pneumoniae and Cytomegalovirus Infection in Coronary Plaques Are Associated With Acute Coronary Syndromes. *Int. Heart J.* **2006**, *47*, 511–519. [CrossRef]

85. De Boer, O.J.; Teeling, P.; Idu, M.M.; Becker, A.E.; Van Der Wal, A.C. Epstein Barr virus specific T-cells generated from unstable human atherosclerotic lesions: Implications for plaque inflammation. *Atherosclerosis* **2006**, *184*, 322–329. [CrossRef] [PubMed]

86. Ciszewski, A. Cardioprotective effect of influenza and pneumococcal vaccination in patients with cardiovascular diseases. *Vaccine* **2018**, *36*, 202–206. [CrossRef] [PubMed]

87. Keller, T.T.; Van Der Meer, J.J.; Teeling, P.; Van Der Sluijs, K.; Idu, M.M.; Rimmelzwaan, G.F.; Levi, M.; Van Der Wal, A.C.; De Boer, O.J. Selective Expansion of Influenza A Virus-Specific T Cells in Symptomatic Human Carotid Artery Atherosclerotic Plaques. *Stroke* **2008**, *39*, 174–179. [CrossRef]

88. Mosorin, M.; Surcel, H.-M.; Laurila, A.; Lehtinen, M.; Karttunen, R.; Juvonen, J.; Paavonen, J.; Morrison, R.P.; Saikku, P.; Juvonen, T. Detection ofChlamydia pneumoniae–Reactive T Lymphocytes in Human Atherosclerotic Plaques of Carotid Artery. *Arter. Thromb. Vasc. Biol.* **2000**, *20*, 1061–1067. [CrossRef]

89. De Boer, O.J.; Van Der Wal, A.C.; Houtkamp, M.A.; Ossewaarde, J.M.; Teeling, P.; Becker, A.E. Unstable atherosclerotic plaques contain T-cells that respond to Chlamydia pneumoniae. *Cardiovasc. Res.* **2000**, *48*, 402–408. [CrossRef]

90. Nadareishvili, Z.G.; Koziol, D.E.; Szekely, B.; Ruetzler, C.; Labiche, R.; McCarron, R.; DeGraba, T.J. Increased CD8+T Cells Associated With Chlamydia pneumoniae in Symptomatic Carotid Plaque. *Stroke* **2001**, *32*, 1966–1972. [CrossRef]

91. Ammirati, E.; Cianflone, D.; Vecchio, V.; Banfi, M.; Vermi, A.C.; de Metrio, M.; Grigore, L.; Pellegatta, F.; Pirillo, A.; Garlaschelli, K.; et al. Effector Memory T cells Are Associated with Atherosclerosis in Humans and Animal Models. *J. Am. Heart Assoc.* **2012**, *1*, 27–41. [CrossRef] [PubMed]

92. Moro-García, M.A.; Iglesias, F.L.; Avanzas, P.; Echeverría, A.; López-Larrea, C.; de la Tassa, C.M.; Alonso-Arias, R. Disease complexity in acute coronary syndrome is related to the patient's immunological status. *Int. J. Cardiol.* **2015**, *189*, 115–123. [CrossRef] [PubMed]

93. Zhao, Z.; Wu, Y.; Cheng, M.; Ji, Y.; Yang, X.; Liu, P.; Jia, S.; Yuan, Z.-Y. Activation of Th17/Th1 and Th1, but not Th17, is associated with the acute cardiac event in patients with acute coronary syndrome. *Atherosclerosis* **2011**, *217*, 518–524. [CrossRef] [PubMed]

94. Li, C.; Zong, W.; Zhang, M.; Tu, Y.; Zhou, Q.; Ni, M.; Li, Z.; Liu, H.; Zhang, J. Increased Ratio of Circulating T-Helper 1 to T-Helper 2 Cells and Severity of Coronary Artery Disease in Patients with Acute Myocardial Infarction: A Prospective Observational Study. *Med. Sci. Monit.* **2019**, *25*, 6034–6042. [CrossRef]

95. Emoto, T.; Sasaki, N.; Yamashita, T.; Kasahara, K.; Yodoi, K.; Sasaki, Y.; Matsumoto, T.; Mizoguchi, T.; Hirata, K.-I. Regulatory/effector T-cell ratio is reduced in coronary artery disease. *Circ. J.* **2014**, *78*, 2935–2941. [CrossRef]

96. Bergstrom, I.; Backteman, K.; Lundberg, A.; Ernerudh, J.; Jonasson, L. Persistent accumulation of interferon-gamma-producing CD8+CD56+ T cells in blood from patients with coronary artery disease. *Atherosclerosis* **2012**, *224*, 515–520. [CrossRef]

97. Kolbus, D.; Ljungcrantz, I.; Andersson, L.; Hedblad, B.; Fredrikson, G.N.; Björkbacka, H.; Nilsson, J. Association between CD8+ T-cell subsets and cardiovascular disease. *J. Intern. Med.* **2013**, *274*, 41–51. [CrossRef]

98. Zidar, D.A.; Mudd, J.C.; Juchnowski, S.; Lopes, J.P.; Sparks, S.; Park, S.S.; Ishikawa, M.; Osborne, R.; Washam, J.B.; Chan, C.; et al. Altered Maturation Status and Possible Immune Exhaustion of CD8 T Lymphocytes in the Peripheral Blood of Patients Presenting With Acute Coronary Syndromes. *Arter. Thromb. Vasc. Biol.* **2016**, *36*, 389–397. [CrossRef]

99. Podolec, J.; Niewiara, L.; Skiba, D.S.; Siedlinski, M.; Baran, J.; Komar, M.; Guzik, B.; Kablak-Ziembicka, A.; Kopeć, G.; Guzik, T.; et al. Higher levels of circulating naïve CD8+CD45RA+ cells are associated with lower extent of coronary atherosclerosis and vascular dysfunction. *Int. J. Cardiol.* **2018**, *259*, 26–30. [CrossRef]

100. Ammirati, E.; Cianflone, D.; Banfi, M.; Vecchio, V.; Palini, A.; De Metrio, M.; Marenzi, G.; Panciroli, C.; Tumminello, G.; Anzuini, A.; et al. Circulating CD4 + CD25 hi CD127 lo Regulatory T-Cell Levels Do Not Reflect the Extent or Severity of Carotid and Coronary Atherosclerosis. *Arter. Thromb. Vasc. Biol.* **2010**, *30*, 1832–1841. [CrossRef]

101. Hasib, L.; Lundberg, A.K.; Zachrisson, H.; Ernerudh, J.; Jonasson, L. Functional and homeostatic defects of regulatory T cells in patients with coronary artery disease. *J. Intern. Med.* **2015**, *279*, 63–77. [CrossRef] [PubMed]

102. Liu, M.; Xu, L.-J.; Wu, J.-X. Changes of circulating CD4+CD25+CD127low regulatory T cells in patients with acute coronary syndrome and its significance. *Genet. Mol. Res.* **2015**, *14*, 15930–15936. [CrossRef] [PubMed]

103. Potekhina, A.V.; Pylaeva, E.; Provatorov, S.; Ruleva, N.; Masenko, V.; Noeva, E.; Krasnikova, T.; Arefieva, T. Treg/Th17 balance in stable CAD patients with different stages of coronary atherosclerosis. *Atherosclerosis* **2015**, *238*, 17–21. [CrossRef] [PubMed]

104. Huang, L.; Zheng, Y.; Yuan, X.; Ma, Y.; Xie, G.; Wang, W.; Chen, H.; Shen, L. Decreased frequencies and impaired functions of the CD31+subpopulation in Tregcells associated with decreased FoxP3 expression and enhanced Tregcell defects in patients with coronary heart disease. *Clin. Exp. Immunol.* **2016**, *187*, 441–454. [CrossRef]

105. Backteman, K.; Andersson, C.; Dahlin, L.-G.; Ernerudh, J.; Jonasson, L. Lymphocyte Subpopulations in Lymph Nodes and Peripheral Blood: A Comparison between Patients with Stable Angina and Acute Coronary Syndrome. *PLoS ONE* **2012**, *7*, e32691. [CrossRef]

106. Meeuwsen, J.A.L.; Van Duijvenvoorde, A.; Gohar, A.; Kozma, M.O.; Van De Weg, S.M.; Gijsberts, C.M.; Haitjema, S.; Björkbacka, H.; Fredrikson, G.N.; De Borst, G.J.; et al. High Levels of (Un)Switched Memory B Cells Are Associated With Better Outcome in Patients With Advanced Atherosclerotic Disease. *J. Am. Heart Assoc.* **2017**, *6*. [CrossRef]

107. Mantani, P.T.; Ljungcrantz, I.; Andersson, L.; Alm, R.; Hedblad, B.; Björkbacka, H.; Nilsson, J.-Å.; Fredrikson, G.N. Circulating CD40 + and CD86 + B Cell Subsets Demonstrate Opposing Associations With Risk of Stroke. *Arter. Thromb. Vasc. Biol.* **2014**, *34*, 211–218. [CrossRef]

108. Novak, J.; Dobrovolny, J.; Tousek, P.; Kočka, V.; Teringova, E.; Nováková, L.; Widimský, P. Potential role of invariant natural killer T cells in outcomes of acute myocardial infarction. *Int. J. Cardiol.* **2015**, *187*, 663–665. [CrossRef]

109. Pera, A.; Caserta, S.; Albanese, F.; Blowers, P.; Morrow, G.; Terrazzini, N.; Smith, H.E.; Rajkumar, C.; Reus, B.; Msonda, J.R.; et al. CD28null pro-atherogenic CD4 T-cells explain the link between CMV infection and an increased risk of cardiovascular death. *Theranostics* **2018**, *8*, 4509–4519. [CrossRef]

110. Athanassopoulos, P.; Vaessen, L.M.B.; Balk, A.H.M.M.; Weimar, W.; Sharma, H.S.; Bogers, A.J.J.C. Altered Chemokine Receptor Profile on Circulating Leukocytes in Human Heart Failure. *Cell Biophys.* **2006**, *44*, 083–102. [CrossRef]

111. Kyaw, T.; Tipping, P.; Toh, B.-H.; Bobik, A. Killer cells in atherosclerosis. *Eur. J. Pharmacol.* **2017**, *816*, 67–75. [CrossRef] [PubMed]

112. Hwang, Y.; Yu, H.T.; Kim, N.-H.; Jang, J.; Kim, H.Y.; Kang, I.; Kim, H.C.; Park, S.; Lee, W.-W. Expansion of CD8+ T cells lacking the IL-6 receptor α chain in patients with coronary artery diseases (CAD). *Atherosclerosis* **2016**, *249*, 44–51. [CrossRef] [PubMed]

113. Ghio, M.; Fabbi, P.; Contini, P.; Fedele, M.; Brunelli, C.; Indiveri, F.; Barsotti, A. OxLDL- and HSP-60 antigen-specific CD8+ T lymphocytes are detectable in the peripheral blood of patients suffering from coronary artery disease. *Clin. Exp. Med.* **2013**, *13*, 251–255. [CrossRef] [PubMed]

114. Meng, X.; Zhang, K.; Li, J.; Dong, M.; Yang, J.; An, G.; Qin, W.; Gao, F.; Zhang, C.; Zhang, Y. Statins Induce the Accumulation of Regulatory T Cells in Atherosclerotic Plaque. *Mol. Med.* **2012**, *18*, 598–605. [CrossRef]

4

Diabetes and Hypertension Consistently Predict the Presence and Extent of Coronary Artery Calcification in Symptomatic Patients

Rachel Nicoll [1], Ying Zhao [2], Pranvera Ibrahimi [1], Gunilla Olivecrona [3] and Michael Henein [1],*

[1]   Department of Public Health and Clinical Medicine, Umea University and Heart Centre, Umea SE-901-87, Sweden; rachelnicoll25@gmail.com (R.N.); pranvera_i86@hotmail.com (P.I.)

[2]   Department of Ultrasound, Beijing Anzhen Hospital, Capital Medical University, Beijing 100029, China; yingzhaoecho@163.com

[3]   Department of Medical Biosciences, Umea University, Umea SE-901-87, Sweden; gunilla.olivecrona@medbio.umu.se

*   Correspondence: michael.henein@umu.se;

Academic Editor: Joseph Moxon

Abstract: Background: The relationship of conventional cardiovascular risk factors (age, gender, ethnicity, diabetes, dyslipidaemia, hypertension, obesity, exercise, and the number of risk factors) to coronary artery calcification (CAC) presence and extent has never before been assessed in a systematic review and meta-analysis. Methods: We included only English language studies that assessed at least three conventional risk factors apart from age, gender, and ethnicity, but excluded studies in which all patients had another confirmed condition such as renal disease. Results: In total, 10 studies, comprising 15,769 patients, were investigated in the systematic review and seven studies, comprising 12,682 patients, were included in the meta-analysis, which demonstrated the importance of diabetes and hypertension as predictors of CAC presence and extent, with age also predicting CAC presence. Male gender, dyslipidaemia, family history of coronary artery disease, obesity, and smoking were overall not predictive of either CAC presence or extent, despite dyslipidaemia being a key risk factor for coronary artery disease (CAD). Conclusion: Diabetes and hypertension consistently predict the presence and extent of CAC in symptomatic patients.

Keywords: meta-analysis; systematic review; coronary calcification; risk factors

1. Introduction

The presence of conventional cardiovascular (CV) risk factors (hypertension, diabetes, dyslipidaemia, smoking, obesity, and family history of coronary artery disease) have been shown to predict the 10-year coronary event risk [1–3]. In patients at intermediate risk, coronary artery calcification (CAC) is described as a subclinical form of atherosclerosis, often occurring as calcified atheroma or spotty calcification within a lipid core. Its measurement is commonly used clinically to avoid an invasive angiogram or as a marker for atherosclerosis in studies [4]. Similarly, the conventional CV risk factors may be used clinically to assess the likelihood of coronary calcification. Since both the CV risk factors and the presence and extent of CAC are predictive of coronary event risk [5,6], we investigated for the first time, in a systematic review and meta-analysis, whether conventional risk factors were also predictive of CAC presence, extent or progression in symptomatic patients. We hoped this would also throw more light on the phenomenon of coronary calcification, which in severe form could represent a clinical challenge as patients tend not to respond to conventional anti-anginal therapy [7]. Furthermore, as there is currently no specific treatment for arterial calcification, with atherosclerosis therapy such as statins and vasodilators having little effect [8], we hope that identifying specific predictive risk factors may point the way towards a remedy which could help prevent or even slow the process of coronary calcification.

2. Methods

The methodology for this systematic review and meta-analysis conforms to the Preferred Reporting Items for Systematic Reviews and Meta-Analyses statement [9].

2.1. Information Search and Data Collection

We systematically searched electronic databases (PubMed, MEDLINE, EMBASE, and Cochrane Centre Register) for observational human studies, assessing CAC and conventional CV risk factors. Articles were selected if the title or abstract indicated that the paper analysed original associations between CAC and CV risk factors using different combinations of the Medical Subject Headings (MeSH): "coronary calcification" or "coronary calcium" and "risk factors", "hypertension", "dyslipidaemia", "hyperlipidaemia obesity", "diabetes", "smoking", "family history", "exercise" or "physical activity". No date limit was applied to article selection. Since computed tomographic scanning for CAC was first introduced in the early 1990s, the study dates range from then to the present date. Two researchers performed the literature search, study selection and data extraction independently of each other, with the results placed in a spreadsheet; disagreements were resolved by discussion between the two researchers and a third adjudicated in case of disagreement. The selected reports were manually searched and other relevant articles, obtained from the reference lists, were retrieved. We also performed a quality assessment of each study included in the meta-analysis.

2.2. Study Eligibility Criteria

Any clinical studies that reported the presence, extent, new development or progression of CAC, assessed by electron beam computed tomography (EBCT), multi-detector computed tomography (MDCT), or coronary angiography, were eligible, regardless of whether or not the study objective was an assessment of the association of risk factors with CAC.

Study inclusion criteria were:

(a) English language articles published in peer-reviewed journals;

(b) In addition to age, gender, and ethnicity (where applicable), the study must include assessment of at least three risk factors out of dyslipidaemia, hypertension, obesity, diabetes, smoking, family history of premature CVD, or exercise. In some cases surrogate markers were used to indicate the presence of a risk factor, such as elevated low density lipoprotein (LDL) cholesterol to indicate hyperlipidaemia or elevated systolic blood pressure (SBP) consistent with hypertension. Any differences in risk factor criteria between studies are discussed in the narrative;

(c) The ability of risk factors to predict CAC presence, extent, new development, or progression must be displayed in a table rather than as a narrative. This criterion was included because narrative results in some studies did not adequately reflect the tabular results, for example, where a risk factor shown as significant in a table was not mentioned in the narrative. Studies also varied in their treatment of a p-value of 0.05, with some taking it as borderline and others as significant but the exact p-value may not be shown in the narrative; for our purposes only $p < 0.05$ is taken as significant,

(d) The patients must be symptomatic (complaining of chest pain or any other typical or atypical angina symptoms); and

(e) For the systematic review only, the study results must show risk factors as multivariate predictors of CAC presence, extent, or progression.

Study exclusion criteria were:

Those involving patients with a specific diagnosis, such as Type 1 diabetes or renal disease, which had no healthy control group.

There were no specified requirements for the control groups, where applicable.

2.3. Statistical Analysis

The data was extracted from each study and analysed using the Revman software 5.3 (Copenhagen, Denmark: The Nordic Cochrane Centre, The Cochrane Collaboration, 2014). The publication bias was tested using Egger's regression interception test and funnel plot by comprehensive meta-analysis software. The unadjusted odds ratios (ORs) of each risk factors were estimated from the exposure distributions for CAC presence or absence. The ORs and 95% confidence intervals (CIs) were converted into Log OR and standard error (SE) using the calculator and the Revman software in order to obtain the forest plots for each risk factor. The statistical heterogeneity was evaluated using the I^2 statistical test. When the I^2 was greater than 50%, the analysis was considered significantly heterogeneous and the random effect model was applied. When the I^2 was less than 50%, the analysis was considered not heterogeneous and the fixed effect meta-analysis model was applied. A p-value of <0.05 was regarded as significant.

3. Results

3.1. Data Extraction

A total of 884 studies were identified. After exclusion of duplicates and review of the retrieved papers for the above criteria (the selection process is shown in Figure 1), 10 studies comprising 15,769 symptomatic patients [10–19] were eligible for inclusion in the systematic review, while seven studies comprising 12,682 patients [10–12,14,16–18] were eligible for inclusion in the meta-analysis. All are listed in Table 1. A risk factor was included in the meta-analysis when at least three papers had provided data on that risk factor. The papers were then divided according to CAC assessment type (i.e., CAC presence, extent or progression). One study, Lai et al. [10], assessed both CAC presence and extent and is, consequently, shown twice in both the systematic review and meta-analysis, while studies by Mayer et al. [11] and Mitsutake et al. [12] could be used for both CAC presence and extent in the meta-analysis but were used only for CAC extent in the systematic review.

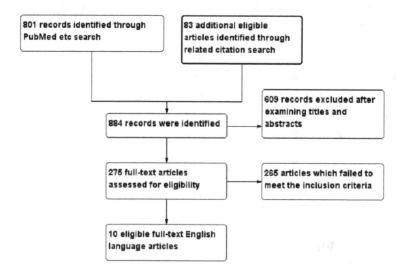

Figure 1. Flowchart showing selection of eligible studies.

Table 1. Study characteristics.

CAC Measurement	Author, Year	Reference No.	Study Population CAC = 0 CAC > 0 or Total Population If No Data Provided		Mean Age (Years)	Means of CAC Assessment	Notable Patient Characteristics
CAC Extent	Lai et al., 2015 as above	[10]	91	120	71.1	64-slice GE scanner	Chinese ethnicity, males aged ≥ 65
	Mayer et al., 2007	[11]	333	544	59.7	Angiographic, CAC observed in the coronary vessels could be none, mild-moderate or severe.	Males
	Mitsutake et al., 2007	[12]	245	290	64	16- or 64-slice Toshiba CT scanner	Japanese ethnicity
	Tanaka et al., 2012	[13]	1363		68	64-slice Toshiba CT scanner	Japanese ethnicity
	Atar et al., 2013	[14]	382	60	53.6	64-slice Phillips CT scanner	Turkish ethnicity
CAC Presence	Greif et al., 2013	[15]	Males	1123	55.4	16-slice Siemens CT scanner	European ethnicity
			Females	437	63.2		
	Kovacic et al., 2012	[16]	8553	1440	66.6	Angiographic, CAC on stenotic lesion undergoing PCI, could be none, mild, moderate or severe.	All with coronary stenosis ≥ 60%
	Lai et al., 2015	[10]	91	120	71.1	64-slice GE scanner	Chinese ethnicity, males aged ≥ 65
	Maragiannis et al., 2015	[17]	65	49	56.1	16-slice Phillips CT scanner	US study
	Qing et al., 2015	[18]	146	364	56.0	64-slice GE CT scanner	Chinese ethnicity
CAC Progression	Okada et al., 2013	[19]	164 (all with CAC > 0)		68.7	64-slice Toshiba CT scanner	Japanese ethnicity

All studies of CAC presence and extent were case-control studies, while the one study of CAC progression (Okada et al. [19]) was a cohort study.

CAC presence was defined as any CAC score >0. CAC extent was defined as the amount of the CAC score in studies which did not use a CAC score threshold or, in studies which did use a CAC score threshold, CAC extent was defined as any CAC score >100 compared to CAC = 0; any study with a CAC score threshold ≤100 was taken as a study of CAC presence. Similarly in angiographic studies, where moderate/severe calcification was compared with mild/no calcification, this was also taken as a study of CAC presence. CAC progression was defined as an increase in the CAC score over time.

Ten studies fitted our inclusion criteria [10–19], comprising 15,769 symptomatic patients, as outlined in Table 1. The number of patients ranged from 114 in Maragiannis et al. [17], to 1560 in Greif et al. [15], with one study of CAC presence by Kovacic et al. [16] comprising 9993 patients; due to the large numbers in this study, it will be separately mentioned in the analysis unless its results conform to those of all other studies. Three studies had a solely Japanese population [12,13,19], two studies were Chinese [10,18], while one was Turkish [14]. All studies were mixed gender, except for Lai et al. [10] and Mayer et al. [11], which investigated exclusively male patients. One study, Greif et al. [15], separately investigated males and females and, consequently, this was treated as two separate studies [15] in the analysis. All studies investigated a wide age range except Lai et al. [10], whose patients were aged ≥65. All patients in the study by Kovacic et al. [16] had coronary stenosis ≥60%, while those in the study by Mayer et al. [11] had CAD and a close relative who had suffered a myocardial infarction before the age of 60 years. Eight of the 10 studies had CAC assessed by CT scanner, either 16- or 64-slice, but the remaining two were investigated angiographically. Kovacic et al. [16] assessed the extent of CAC on the stenotic lesion undergoing percutaneous coronary intervention (PCI), with CAC being graded as none, mild, moderate or severe, while Mayer et al. [11] assessed the CAC observed in the coronary vessels as none, mild-moderate, or severe. Kovacic et al. [16] assessed predictors for calcification as moderate-severe calcification compared to no calcification; we have included this in the analysis as a study of CAC presence rather than CAC extent.

3.1.1. Systematic Review

We analysed the following numbers of studies in each category:

CAC presence cross-sectional	six studies	12,830 patients
CAC extent cross-sectional	four studies	2986 patients
CAC progression	one study	164 patients
Total symptomatic patients	15,980 patients	

However, Lai et al. [10], with 211 patients, was included in both CAC presence and extent.

3.1.2. Meta-Analyses

We analysed the following numbers of studies in each category, with three studies providing data for both CAC presence and extent:

CAC presence cross-sectional	seven studies	12,682 patients
CAC extent cross-sectional	three studies	1623 patients

The unadjusted ORs of each risk factors were estimated from the exposure distributions for CAC presence or absence [20,21], with the exception of the ORs from the study by Kovacic et al. [16], which directly showed the univariate ORs in the results. Since age was a continuous parameter, the OR for age was pooled from multivariate results. For the remaining risk factors, few papers provided the multivariate ORs, so consequently the pooled ORs from multivariate results were not analysed. In the three papers which provided the ORs for both CAC presence and extent [10–12], we extracted the exposure distributions for moderate and severe CAC and combined them as CAC presence. In these three papers, the ORs for the comparison between mild to moderate CAC and zero CAC and the comparison between severe CAC and zero CAC were pooled from the exposure distribution separately to assess the risk factors which predicted CAC extent.

3.2. Systematic Review

The papers were then analysed by age, gender, ethnicity, diabetes, dyslipidaemia, family history, hypertension, obesity, and smoking (Table 2). In none of the studies was physical activity assessed. In several studies the definition of the risk factor comprised multiple components for example, dyslipidaemia could include any of elevated total, LDL cholesterol or the total/HDL cholesterol ratio, or decreased HDL cholesterol. For the purposes of analysis for the systematic review, a risk factor was assessed if any one of its components was present (so dyslipidaemia was predictive if only LDL cholesterol was elevated and all other components were in normal range). Analysis of the precise risk factor components is also provided in each relevant section, where any modifying effect of age is also considered.

Table 2. Systematic Review: analysis of the number and type of studies investigating risk factors for CAC.

Risk Factors	CAC Presence		CAC Extent		CAC Progression	
	Predictive	Not Predictive	Predictive	Not Predictive	Predictive	Not Predictive
Age	5	1	3	1	0	1
Gender	2	2	2	0	0	0
Ethnicity	1	0	0	0	0	0
Diabetes	3	4	1	3	1	0
Dyslipidaemia	3	4	1	3	0	1
Hypertension	2	5	3	1	1	0
Family history	0	1	1	1	0	0
Obesity	1	5	0	3	0	1
Smoking	1	5	0	4	0	0

Age: There are five studies showing that age is predictive of CAC presence [14–18], compared to one which is not predictive [10], although in this study all patients were as ≥65. Three studies showed that age was predictive of CAC extent [11–13] and the same study of patients aged ≥65 found age not to be predictive [10]. The only study of CAC progression found that age was not predictive [19].

Male gender: two studies of CAC presence showed that gender was not predictive [14,16], including the angiographic study of 9993 patients [16], although in two studies of CAC presence [17,18] and two studies of CAC extent it was predictive [12,13].

Ethnicity: The study of 9993 patients was the only one to consider ethnicity and this found that being white was predictive of CAC presence [16].

Diabetes mellitus: The two Greif et al. studies [15] and the angiographic study of 9993 patients [16] found diabetes to be predictive of CAC presence, although four smaller studies showed that it is not [10,14,17,18]. Although one study of 1363 patients found diabetes to be predictive of CAC extent [13], three studies with a total of 1623 patients showed that it was not predictive [10–12]. The only study of CAC progression showed that diabetes was predictive [19].

When the studies are analysed by markers for diabetes:

- Blood glucose was not predictive of CAC presence [14] or extent [12].
- Insulin was not predictive in one study of CAC presence and extent [10].
- HbA1c was not predictive of CAC presence [15,18] or extent [11,12], although it did show predictive ability for CAC progression [19].
- Oral hypoglycaemic medication was not predictive in one study of CAC presence and extent [10].
- Homeostatic Model Assessment-Insulin Resistance (HOMA-IR) was not predictive of CAC presence [15].

Dyslipidaemia: Thee studies showed that dyslipidaemia was predictive of CAC presence [15,18], while four studies, including the study of 9333 patients, shows that it is not predictive [10,14,16,17]. For CAC extent, however, one study showed that dyslipidaemia was predictive [11] but three studies, with more than twice as many patients, found it not to be predictive [10,12,13]. The one study of CAC progression [19] showed that it was not predictive.

When the studies are analysed by markers and biomarkers for dyslipidaemia:

- Elevated LDL cholesterol was not predictive in all four studies of CAC presence [14–16] and in two studies of CAC extent [11,12].
- Elevated total cholesterol was not predictive in two studies of CAC presence [14,18], two studies of CAC extent [11,12], and one study of CAC progression [19].
- Decreased HDL was not predictive in three studies of CAC presence [14,15] and one study of CAC extent [12], but was predictive of severe CAC extent in one study [11].
- Lipid-lowering medication was predictive in three studies of CAC presence [15,18], but was not predictive in one study of CAC presence [10] and two studies of CAC extent [10,12].

Hypertension: Although two studies, including the study of 9993 patients, [16,17] found that hypertension was predictive of CAC presence, the remaining studies showed that it had no predictive ability for CAC presence [10,13,15,18]. Three studies of CAC extent found that it was predictive [11–13], but one study found it not to be predictive [10]; the one study of CAC progression was also predictive [19].

When the studies are analysed by markers for hypertension:

- Systolic blood pressure (SBP) was not predictive in three studies of CAC presence [10,15] and two studies of CAC extent [10,12] but one angiographic study showed it was predictive of severe CAC extent [11]. SBP was also predictive of CAC progression [19].
- Diastolic blood pressure (DBP) was not predictive in three studies of CAC presence [10,15] and three studies of CAC extent [10–12].
- Antihypertensive medications were not predictive in four studies of CAC presence [10,15,18] and one of CAC extent [10].
- Pulse pressure was not predictive in one study of CAC extent [11] and the study of CAC progression [19].

Family history of premature CHD: The only study to assess predictive ability for CAC presence was the study of 9993 patients [16], which found it was not predictive. Among those investigating CAC extent, one was predictive, with 877 patients, [11] but another was not, with 535 patients [12]. The one predictive study of CAC extent was angiographic and investigated a family history of CAC since the population was preselected to comprise males with a family history of CAD [11].

Obesity: Five studies found no ability for obesity to predict CAC presence [10,15,17,18], although the large study by Kovacic et al. found that there was an inverse predictive ability between obesity and CAC presence, making obesity protective against CAC [16]. No study of CAC extent, found that obesity was predictive [10–12]. The only study of CAC progression did not find obesity to be predictive [19].

When the studies are analysed by markers for obesity:

- Body mass index (BMI) was inversely predictive in the angiographic study of CAC presence involving 9993 patients [16], but not in a further three studies of CAC presence [10,17,18] and one of CAC extent [10]. BMI was not predictive in one study of CAC progression [19].
- Weight was not predictive in one study of CAC extent [16].

Smoking: With respect to CAC presence, only one small study found it to be predictive [14], while the remainder, including the study of 9993 patients, found that smoking was not predictive of CAC presence [10,15,16,18]. None of the four studies of CAC extent [10–13] found smoking to be predictive.

When the studies are analysed by markers for smoking, current smoking was not predictive in two studies of CAC presence [15].

3.3. Meta-Analysis

Out of the ten papers that were eligible for the systematic review [10–19], seven were also suitable for the meta-analysis: Lai et al. [10], Mayer et al. [11], Mitsutake et al. [12], Atar et al. [14], Kovacic et al. [16], Maragiannis et al. [17], and Qing et al. [18].

The meta-analysis investigated the predictive ability of age, male gender, diabetes, dyslipidaemia, hypertension, and smoking for CAC presence and extent (Supplementary Materials, Figure S1). It was not possible to include ethnicity, obesity, exercise, or number of risk factors, although family history of CAD was not predictive; since no other study assessed these two risk factors, they have not been entered in the meta-analysis. As mentioned above, data from three studies investigating CAC extent in the systematic review (Lai et al. [10], Mayer et al. [11], and Mitsutake et al. [12]) have been re-analysed to identify potential risk factor predictors of CAC presence in the meta-analysis.

3.3.1. Predictors of CAC Presence

Table 3 gives the pooled results from the meta-analysis. The predictors of CAC presence in order of importance were hypertension (OR = 1.71, $p < 0.00001$), male gender (OR = 1.47, $p = 0.02$), diabetes (OR = 1.34, $p = 0.03$), and age (OR = 1.07, $p = 0.04$). Smoking and dyslipidaemia were not predictive of CAC presence. The Egger's regression interception test was not significant suggesting no significant publication bias (Table 3). Age, being a continuous variable, could not be entered into the Egger test. The funnel plots for each risk factor are provided in the supplementary Figure S2 and, similarly, show no publication bias.

Table 3. Meta-analysis: pooled risk factors and their ORs predicting CAC presence.

Risk Factors	Pooled or (95% CI)	*p* for Overall Effect	Studies	Patient Numbers	Egger's Test		
					Intercept	*t*-Value	*p*-Value
Age (years)	1.07 (1.00–1.04)	0.04	[10,14,18]	1163			
Male gender	1.47 (1.05–2.06)	0.02	[12,14,16–18]	11,594	2.29	2.42	0.09
Hypertension	1.71 (1.51–1.94)	<0.00001	[10–12,14,16–18]	12,682	0.94	0.78	0.47
Diabetes mellitus	1.34 (1.02–1.75)	0.03	[10–12,14,16–18]	12,682	0.81	0.83	0.44
Smoking	1.42 (0.90–2.22)	0.13	[10–12,14,16–18]	12,682	3.39	1.84	0.12
Dyslipidaemia	1.25 (0.81–1.94)	0.31	[10,12,16,17]	10,853	1.09	0.64	0.59

Due to the disproportionately large number of patients in the study by Kovavic et al. [16], we repeated the meta-analysis after excluding this paper (shown in the supplementary data, Table S1). This slightly increased the ORs for hypertension to 1.89 ($p < 0.00001$), male gender to 1.74 ($p < 0.00001$), diabetes to 1.45 ($p < 0.00001$). Smoking and dyslipidaemia were still not significant.

3.3.2. Predictors of CAC Extent

Only three studies (Lai et al. [10], Mayer et al. [11], and Mitsutake et al. [12]) analysed the predictors of CAC extent, among which Mayer et al. was an angiographic study classifying CAC as either "no calcification", "mild to moderate calcification", or "severe calcification". Mitsutake et al. [12] used CAC scoring and classified the lowest group (taken to be CAC = 0) as a CAC score of 0–12, the mild-moderate group as a CAC score of 13–445, and the severe calcification group as a CAC score of >445, while Lai et al. [10] used a threshold CAC score of ≥400 The results are shown in Table 4.

Table 4. Meta-analysis: pooled risk factors and their ORs predicting CAC extent.

Risk Factors	Mild to Moderate CAC or CACS 13-445 vs. CACS = 0		Severe CAC or CACS > 445 vs. CACS = 0		Patient Numbers
	OR	*p*-Value	OR	*p*-Value	
Hypertension	1.61 (1.28–2.03)	<0.0001	2.09 (1.09–4.03)	0.0100	1623
Diabetes mellitus	1.22 (0.93–1.60)	0.1600	1.55 (1.14–2.10)	0.0050	1623
Dyslipidaemia	0.75 (0.52–1.00)	0.1300	1.03 (0.65–1.63)	0.9000	746
Smoking	0.93 (0.72–1.20)	0.6000	1.07 (0.68–1.67)	0.7700	1623

CACS = Coronary artery calcification score; Studies used in CAC extent meta-analysis: Lai et al. [10], Mayer et al. [11], and Mitsutake et al. [12]. Lai et al. [10], a study using a threshold of >400, was included as severe CAC.

The presence of mild-moderate CAC, compared with zero CAC, was independently predicted only by hypertension (OR 1.61, $p < 0.0001$), with diabetes, dyslipidaemia, and smoking proving not to be predictive of mild-moderate CAC. The presence of severe CAC, compared with zero CAC, was predicted by hypertension (OR 2.09, $p = 0.01$) and diabetes (OR 1.55, $p = 0.005$); dyslipidaemia and smoking were not independently predictive of severe CAC. It was not possible to analyse age or male gender as predictors of CAC extent.

A summary of the studies showing the predictive ability of the risk factors from the systematic review and meta-analysis are shown at Table 5.

Table 5. Summary of studies showing risk factor predictive ability for CAC presence, extent, or progression.

Risk Factors	SYSTEMATIC REVIEW References			Meta-Analysis References	
	CAC Presence	CAC Extent	CAC Progression	CAC Presence	CAC Extent
Age	[10,14–18]	10, 11–13	19	[10,14,18]	Not assessed
Male gender	[14,16–18]	12, 13	Not assessed	[12,14,16–18]	Not assessed
Ethnicity	[16]	Not assessed	Not assessed	Not assessed	Not assessed
Diabetes	[10,14–18]	13–10	19	[10–12,14,16–18]	10; 11
Dyslipidaemia	[10,14–18]	13–10	19	[10,12,16,17]	10; 11
Hypertension	[10,13,15–18]	13–10	19	[10–12,14,16–18]	10; 11
Family history	[16]	11,12	Not assessed	Not assessed	Not assessed
Obesity	[10,15–18]	12–10	19	Not assessed	Not assessed
Smoking	[10,14–16,18]	13–10	Not assessed	[10–12,14,16–18]	10; 11

Reference key: [10]: Lai et al., 221 Chinese males aged ≥65; [11]: Mayer et al., 877 males with CAD, angiographic study; [12]: Mitsutake et al., 535 patients, Japanese ethnicity; [13]: Tanaka et al., 1363 patients, Japanese ethnicity; [14]: Atar et al., 442 patients, Turkish ethnicity; [15]: Greif et al., 1123 males, European ethnicity; [15]: Greif et al., 437 females, European ethnicity; [16]: Kovacic et al., 9993 patients, angiographic study; [17]: Maragiannis et al., 114 patients, US study; [18]: Qing et al., 510 patients, Chinese ethnicity; [19]: Okada et al., 164 patients with CAC, Japanese ethnicity.

3.3.3. Quality Assessment

We carried out a MINORS evaluation of the studies included in the meta-analysis, as shown at Table 6. The items are scored 0 (not reported), 1 (reported but inadequate), or 2 (reported and adequate), with the global ideal score being 16 for non-comparative studies. Most studies scored 2 for all parameters, except follow-up data and prospectivity, which were obviously not in the design for our case-control studies. These results were considered quite satisfactory.

Table 6. Quality assessment of studies included in the meta-analysis.

Study	Clearly Stated Aim	Consecutive Patients Inclusion	Prospective Collection of Data	Endpoints Appropriate	Unbiased Assessment of the Study Endpoint	Follow-up Period Appropriate to the Aim of the Study	Loss to Follow up Less than 5%	Prospective Calculation of the Study Size	Total Score
Atar et al., 2013 [14]	2	2	2	2	2	0	0	0	10
Greif et al., 2013 [15]	2	2	2	2	2	0	0	0	10
Kovacic et al., 2012 [16]	1	2	0	1	2	0	0	0	6
Mayer et al., 2007 [11]	2	2	2	2	2	0	0	0	10
Mitsutake et al., 2007 [12]	2	2	2	2	2	0	0	0	10
Okada et al., 2013 [19]	2	2	2	2	2	2	1	0	13
Tanaka et al., 2012 [13]	2	2	2	2	2	0	0	0	10
Lai et al., 2015 [10]	2	2	2	2	2	0	0	0	10
Maragiannis et al., 2015 [17]	2	1	2	2	2	0	0	0	9
Qing et al., 2015 [18]	2	2	2	2	2	0	0	0	10

Evaluation of meta-analysis studies using the Methodological Index for Non-Randomized Studies (MINORS) [22]. Elements are scored 0 (not reported), 1 (reported but inadequate), or 2 (reported and adequate).

4. Discussion

4.1. Findings

In the Systematic Review, age was strongly predictive of both CAC presence and extent, but not of CAC progression. The results for other risk factors for CAC presence are not as clear cut, largely due to the Kovacic et al. [16] study of 9993 patients, which overwhelmed the analysis. This study found that white ethnicity, diabetes, hypertension, and obesity were predictive of CAC presence, but not male gender, dyslipidaemia, family history, or smoking. These results do not necessarily accord with the totality of the studies, in which a broadly equal number showed that male gender, diabetes, and dyslipidaemia were predictive of CAC presence as not predictive. Only two studies (including Kovacic et al. [16]) found that hypertension was predictive of CAC presence, compared to five studies finding that it was not predictive, while only Kovacic et al. [16] found that obesity was predictive (albeit inversely), whereas five studies found that it was not predictive of CAC presence. Smoking was, overall, not predictive. No study of CAC presence, other than Kovacic et al. [16], assessed ethnicity (predictive) or family history of CAD (not predictive). With respect to CAC extent, male gender, hypertension, and possibly a family history of CAC were predictive, but diabetes, dyslipidaemia, obesity, and smoking were, overall, not predictive. For diabetes there were an almost equal amount of patient numbers in the three studies which found diabetes to be predictive as not predictive of CAC extent. In the one study of CAC progression, diabetes and hypertension were predictive, but not age, dyslipidaemia, or obesity.

Among the risk factor markers, only use of lipid-lowering medication and higher BMI were broadly predictive of CAC presence, with possibly decreased HDL and increased SBP being predictive of CAC extent, although these results were found in only one study. In the single study of CAC progression, HbA1c and SBP were predictive.

The meta-analysis included seven studies, rather than the ten in the systematic review, although two studies of CAC extent also provided sufficient statistical data to be used to assess CAC presence, while another study provided data for both CAC presence and extent. This analysis shows that hypertension followed by male gender, diabetes, and age were predictive of CAC presence, while smoking and dyslipidaemia were not predictive. For CAC extent, however, mild-moderate CAC was predicted by hypertension alone, whereas severe CAC was predicted by hypertension followed by diabetes. The MINORS scores were quite satisfactory for all included studies which adds to the strength of the data analysis.

4.2. Areas of Difference between Results from the Systematic Review and Meta-Analysis

The most striking difference between the results from the systematic review and the meta-analysis is the minimal importance of age as a predictor of CAC in the meta-analysis, whereas it is a consistent predictor of both CAC presence and extent in the systematic review. However, this may largely be accounted for, firstly, by the fact that age is a continuous variable and, secondly, that a different mix of studies of CAC presence were used for the systematic review and meta-analysis. We have previously shown the important predictive value of age in a large cohort of symptomatic patients [23].

With respect to CAC presence, there were no other clear predictive risk factors based on the numbers of studies but when considering numbers of patients then the Kovacic et al. [16] study of 9993 patients, which found that diabetes and hypertension were predictive, was broadly in agreement with the meta-analysis. In the systematic review, CAC extent was predicted by male gender and hypertension, whereas in the meta-analysis CAC extent was predicted by hypertension and diabetes; this can be explained by the different mix of studies between the two methods. The main limitation of the systematic review is its qualitative analysis with many contributory factors, such as the power of the study, the number of studies, and the number of patients. These limitations are overcome by the quantitative pooling of the meta-analysis.

4.3. Comparison with Other Studies

Although we have found that in symptomatic patients the predictive risk factors for CAC presence, extent, and progression are hypertension and diabetes, this is not the case in asymptomatic subjects where dyslipidaemia, smoking, obesity, and family history of CAD have also been shown to be predictive of CAC presence and progression in large population studies, such as the Multi-Ethnic Study of Atherosclerosis and Heinz Nixdorf Recall [24,25]. No systematic review or meta-analysis of risk factor predictors for CAC in asymptomatic subjects has been carried out. Although the two conditions, hypertension and diabetes, are different in their clinical presentation and means of treatment, their effect on the arterial wall seems to be phenotypically similar, suggesting a shared mechanism such as oxidative stress [26,27]. Arterial calcification represents segmental ossification which is known to be progressive even after controlling risk factors, thus suggesting a perpetual effect, through a biochemical and/or histopathological mechanism, of those risk factors rather than just a triggering effect that subsides with their optimum control. Nevertheless, there is no inherent reason why the conventional CV risk factors, which were identified as predictors of 10-year coronary event risk [28,29], should predict CAC presence or extent, merely because CAC can also predict the 10-year event risk [3].

Curiously, the expected predictive risk of dyslipidaemia did not feature strongly in either the systematic review or the meta-analysis. While some studies have shown that dyslipidaemia can be predictive of arterial calcification presence or extent in asymptomatic subjects, this is not always the case, previously seen in a systematic review and meta-analysis of predictors of breast arterial calcification which found no relationship with dyslipidaemia [30]. In addition, dyslipidaemia is a particularly Caucasian problem [31] and it may be that the high number of studies with a Chinese or Japanese population included in the meta-analysis has impacted the results. Nevertheless, we have previously found that lipid-lowering medication has no effect on reducing coronary or aortic valve calcification [32,33], while other studies have found that rather than the treatment group, it is the placebo group that has less calcium progression [22,34]. It may, however, be the case that by the time calcification is established, the association with dyslipidaemia has been lost.

4.4. Limitations

A number of limitations deserve mention. Firstly, although we attempted to identify and include all relevant studies, there will inevitably be some that we have overlooked. Secondly, our search was restricted to studies in English, so it may be possible that some studies in other languages have been missed. Thirdly, the studies included in this systematic review and meta-analysis varied in design, population (e.g., eligibility by age), definition and duration of risk factor, and year of publication. As expected, we observed considerable heterogeneity between studies, so it is arguable whether a summary estimate should be presented. However, our objective was not to provide this but rather to present a general approximation of the prevalence of these risk factors to facilitate the message. In particular, two studies assessed CAC angiographically, which is not sensitive to CAC detection, while the remainder used 16- or 64-slice CT scanning. Fourthly, analysis of studies of CAC presence was overwhelmed by the study of 9333 patients, while the next largest study had only 1560. Fifthly, the lack of standardisation of definitions of risk factors limits our ability to provide summary estimates and we had no information on the duration of risk factors, which might have impacted the analysis. Sixthly, we were confined to those risk factors commonly measured in a clinical setting and, inevitably, there are others which might have been relevant.

5. Conclusions

Our meta-analysis showed that hypertension followed by diabetes were the most important risk factors for prediction of CAC presence and extent, with age and male gender also showing predictive ability for CAC presence. The results from the systematic review were more equivocal, but the two forms of analysis were in general agreement that dyslipidaemia, obesity, and smoking were not predictive of CAC presence or extent. Irrespective of the mechanism for arterial endothelial damage, hypertension and diabetes seem to result in a common phenotypic arterial wall damage in the form of calcification. Finally, despite CAC and the conventional CV risk factors both being predictive of 10-year coronary event risk, only a few of the CV risk factors appear predictive of CAC.

References

1. Assmann, G.; Cullen, P.; Schulte, H. Simple scoring scheme for calculating the risk of acute coronary events based on the 10-year follow-up of the Prospective Cardiovascular Muenster (PROCAM) study. *Circulation* **2002**, *105*, 310–315. [CrossRef] [PubMed]

2. The Second Joint Task Force of European and Other Societies. Prevention of coronary heart disease in clinical practice. Recommendations of the Second Joint Task Force of European and other Societies on Coronary Prevention. *Eur. Heart J.* **1998**, *19*, 1434–1503.

3. Grundy, S.M.; Cleeman, J.I.; Merz, C.N.; Brewer, H.B., Jr.; Clark, L.T.; Hunninghake, D.B.; Pasternak, R.C.; Smith, S.C., Jr.; Stone, N.J.; National Heart, Lung, and Blood Institute; et al. Implications of recent clinical trials for the National Cholesterol Education Program Adult Treatment Panel III guidelines. *Circulation* **2004**, *13*, 227–239. [CrossRef] [PubMed]

4. Rumberger, J.A.; Simons, D.B.; Fitzpatrick, L.A.; Sheedy, P.F.; Schwartz, R.S. Coronary artery calcium area by electron-beam computed tomography and coronary atherosclerotic plaque area. A histopathologic correlative study. *Circulation* **1995**, *92*, 2157–2162. [CrossRef] [PubMed]

5. National Cholesterol Education Program (NCEP) Expert Panel on Detection, Evaluation, and Treatment of High Blood Cholesterol in Adults (Adult Treatment Panel III). Third Report of the National Cholesterol Education Program (NCEP) Expert Panel on Detection, Evaluation, and Treatment of High Blood Cholesterol in Adults (Adult Treatment Panel III) final report. *Circulation* **2002**, *106*, 3143–3421.

6. Zeb, I.; Budoff, M. Coronary Artery Calcium Screening: Does it Perform Better than Other Cardiovascular Risk Stratification Tools? *Int. J. Mol. Sci.* **2015**, *16*, 6606–6620. [CrossRef] [PubMed]

7. Henein, M.; Nicoll, R. Atherosclerosis and extensive arterial calcification: The same condition? *Int. J. Cardiol.* **2010**, *141*, 1–2. [CrossRef] [PubMed]

8. Henein, M.; Owen, A. Statins moderate coronary atheroma but not coronary calcification: Results from meta-analyses. *Scand. Cardiovasc. J.* **2010**, *44*. [CrossRef]

9. Liberati, A.; Altman, D.G.; Tetzlaff, J.; Mulrow, C.; Gøtzsche, P.C.; Ioannidis, J.P.A.; Clarke, M.; Devereaux, P.J.; Kleijnen, J.; Moher, D. The PRISMA statement for reporting systematic reviews and meta-analyses of studies that evaluate health care interventions: Explanation and elaboration. *Ann. Intern. Med.* **2009**, *151*, W65–W94. [CrossRef] [PubMed]

10. Lai, J.; Ge, Y.; Shao, Y.; Xuan, T.; Xia, S.; Li, M. Low serum testosterone level was associated with extensive coronary artery calcification in elderly male patients with stable coronary artery disease. *Coron. Artery Dis.* **2015**, *26*, 437–441. [CrossRef] [PubMed]

11. Mayer, B.; Lieb, W.; Radke, P.W.; Götz, A.; Fischer, M.; Bässler, A.; Doehring, L.C.; Aherrahrou, Z.; Liptau, H.; Erdmann, J. Association between arterial pressure and coronary artery calcification. *J. Hypertens.* **2007**, *25*, 1731–1738. [CrossRef] [PubMed]

12. Mitsutake, R.; Miura, S.; Saku, K. Association between coronary artery calcification score as assessed by multi-detector row computed tomography and upstroke time of pulse wave. *Intern Med.* **2007**, *46*, 1833–1836. [CrossRef] [PubMed]

13. Tanaka, M.; Fukui, M.; Tomiyasu, K.; Akabame, S.; Nakano, K.; Yamasaki, M.; Hasegawa, G.; Oda, Y.; Nakamura, N. Eosinophil count is positively correlated with coronary artery calcification. *Hypertens. Res.* **2012**, *35*, 325–328. [CrossRef] [PubMed]

14. Atar, A.I.; Yilmaz, O.C.; Akin, K.; Selçoki, Y.; Er, O.; Eryonucu, B. Serum uric acid level is an independent risk factor for presence of calcium in coronary arteries: An observational case-controlled study. *Anadolu Kardiyol. Derg.* **2013**, *13*, 139–145. [CrossRef] [PubMed]

15. Greif, M.; Arnoldt, T.; von Ziegler, F.; Ruemmler, J.; Becker, C.; Wakili, R.; D'Anastasi, M.; Schenzle, J.; Leber, A.W.; Becke, A. Lipoprotein(a) is independently correlated with coronary artery calcification. *Eur. J. Intern. Med.* **2013**, *24*, 75–79. [CrossRef] [PubMed]

16. Kovacic, J.C.; Lee, P.; Baber, U.; Karajgikar, R.; Evrard, S.M.; Moreno, P.; Mehran, R.; Fuster, V.; Dangas, G.; Sharma, S.K.; et al. Inverse relationship between body mass index and coronary artery calcification in patients with clinically significant coronary lesions. *Atherosclerosis* **2012**, *221*, 176–182. [CrossRef] [PubMed]

17. Maragiannis, D.; Schutt, R.C.; Gramze, N.L.; Chaikriangkrai, K.; McGregor, K.; Chin, K.; Nabi, F.; Little, S.H.; Nagueh, S.F.; Chang, S.M. Association of Left Ventricular Diastolic Dysfunction with Subclinical Coronary Atherosclerotic Disease Burden Using Coronary Artery Calcium Scoring. *J. Atheroscler. Thromb.* **2015**, *22*, 1278–1286. [CrossRef] [PubMed]

18. Qing, P.; Li, X.L.; Zhang, Y.; Li, Y.L.; Xu, R.X.; Guo, Y.L.; Li, S.; Wu, N.Q.; Li, J.J. Association of Big Endothelin-1 with Coronary Artery Calcification. *PLoS ONE* **2015**, *10*, e0142458. [CrossRef] [PubMed]

19. Okada, H.; Fukui, M.; Tanaka, M.; Matsumoto, S.; Mineoka, Y.; Nakanishi, N.; Tomiyasu, K.; Nakano, K.; Hasegawa, G.; Nakamura, N. Visit-to-visit variability in systolic blood pressure is a novel risk factor for the progression of coronary artery calcification. *Hypertens. Res.* **2013**, *36*, 996–999. [CrossRef] [PubMed]

20. Greenland, S.; Longnecker, M.P. Methods for trend estimation from summarised dose-response data, with applications to meta-analysis. *Am. J. Epidemiol.* **1992**, *135*, 1301–1309. [PubMed]

21. Hamling, J.; Lee, P.; Weitkunat, R.; Ambuhl, M. Facilitating meta-analyses by deriving relative effect and precision estimates for alternative comparisons from a set of estimates presented by exposure level or disease category. *Stat. Med.* **2008**, *27*, 954–970. [CrossRef] [PubMed]

22. Slim, K.; Nini, E.; Forestier, D.; Kwiatkowski, F.; Panis, Y.; Chipponi, J. Methodological index for non-randomized studies (minors): Development and validation of a new instrument. *ANZ J. Surg.* **2003**, *73*, 712–716. [CrossRef] [PubMed]

23. Nicoll, R.; Wiklund, U.; Zhao, Y.; Diederichsen, A.; Mickley, H.; Ovrehus, K.; Zamorano, J.; Gueret, P.; Schmermund, A.; Maffei, E.; et al. Gender and age effects on risk factor-based prediction of coronary artery calcium in symptomatic patients: A Euro-CCAD study. *Atherosclerosis* **2016**. in press. [CrossRef] [PubMed]

24. Kronmal, R.A.; McClelland, R.L.; Detrano, R.; Shea, S.; Lima, J.A.; Cushman, M.; Bild, D.E.; Burke, G.L. Risk factors for the progression of coronary artery calcification in asymptomatic subjects: Results from the Multi-Ethnic Study of Atherosclerosis (MESA). *Circulation* **2007**, *115*, 2722–2730. [CrossRef] [PubMed]

25. Schmermund, A.; Lehmann, N.; Bielak, L.F.; Yu, P.; Sheedy, P.F.; Cassidy-Bushrow, A.E.; Turner, S.T.; Moebus, S.; Möhlenkamp, S.; Stang, A.; et al. Comparison of subclinical coronary atherosclerosis and risk factors in unselected populations in Germany and US-America. *Atherosclerosis* **2007**, *195*, e207–e216. [CrossRef] [PubMed]

26. Harvey, A.; Montezano, A.C.; Touyz, R.M. Vascular biology of ageing-Implications in hypertension. *J. Mol. Cell. Cardiol.* **2015**, *83*, 112–121. [CrossRef] [PubMed]

27. Gross, M.; Steffes, M.; Jacobs, D.R., Jr.; Yu, X.; Lewis, L.; Lewis, C.E.; Loria, C.M. Plasma F2-isoprostanes and coronary artery calcification: The CARDIA Study. *Clin. Chem.* **2005**, *51*, 125–131. [CrossRef] [PubMed]

28. Erbel, R.; Möhlenkamp, S.; Moebus, S.; Schmermund, A.; Lehmann, N.; Stang, A.; Dragano, N.; Grönemeyer, D.; Seibel, R.; Kälsch, H.; et al. Coronary risk stratification, discrimination, and reclassification improvement based on quantification of subclinical coronary atherosclerosis: The Heinz Nixdorf Recall study. *J. Am. Coll. Cardiol.* **2010**, *56*, 1397–1406. [CrossRef] [PubMed]

29. Polonsky, T.S.; McClelland, R.L.; Jorgensen, N.W.; Bild, D.E.; Burke, G.L.; Guerci, A.D.; Greenland, P. Coronary artery calcium score and risk classification for coronary heart disease prediction. *JAMA* **2010**, *303*, 1610–1616. [CrossRef] [PubMed]

30. Hendriks, E.J.; de Jong, P.A.; van der Graaf, Y.; Mali, W.P.; van der Schouw, Y.T.; Beulens, J.W. Breast arterial calcifications: A systematic review and meta-analysis of their determinants and their association with cardiovascular events. *Atherosclerosis* **2015**, *239*, 11–20. [CrossRef] [PubMed]

31. Budoff, M.J.; Nasir, K.; Mao, S.; Tseng, P.H.; Chau, A.; Liu, S.T.; Flores, F.; Blumenthal, R.S. Ethnic differences of the presence and severity of coronary atherosclerosis. *Atherosclerosis* **2006**, *187*, 343–350. [CrossRef] [PubMed]

32. Henein, M.Y.; Owen, A. Statins moderate coronary stenoses but not coronary calcification: Results from meta-analyses. *Int. J. Cardiol.* **2011**, *153*, 31–35. [CrossRef] [PubMed]

33.   Zhao, Y.; Nicoll, R.; He, Y.H.; Henein, M.Y. The effect of statins on valve function and calcification in aortic stenosis: A meta-analysis. *Atherosclerosis* **2016**, *246*, 318–324. [CrossRef] [PubMed]
34.   McCullough, P.A.; Chinnaiyan, K.M. Annual progression of coronary calcification in trials of preventive therapies: A systematic review. *Arch. Intern. Med.* **2009**, *169*, 2064–2070. [CrossRef] [PubMed]

5

Advances in the Study of the Antiatherogenic Function and Novel Therapies for HDL

Peiqiu Cao [1], Haitao Pan [1], Tiancun Xiao [2,3], Ting Zhou [3], Jiao Guo [1,*] and Zhengquan Su [1,*]

[1] Key Research Center of Liver Regulation for Hyperlipemia SATCM/Class III, Laboratory of Metabolism SATCM, Guangdong TCM Key Laboratory for Metabolic Diseases, Guangdong Pharmaceutical University, Guangzhou 510006, China; cpq_520@126.com (P.C.); pangel7835001@163.com (H.P.)

[2] Inorganic Chemistry Laboratory, University of Oxford, South Parks Road, Oxford OX1 3QR, UK; xiao.tiancun@chem.ox.ac.uk

[3] Guangzhou Boxabio Ltd., D-106 Guangzhou International Business Incubator, Guangzhou 510530, China; ting4677@126.com

* Correspondence: suzhq@scnu.edu.cn (Z.S.); wshxalb@163.com (J.G.);

Academic Editor: Michael Henein

Abstract: The hypothesis that raising high-density lipoprotein cholesterol (HDL-C) levels could improve the risk for cardiovascular disease (CVD) is facing challenges. There is multitudinous clear clinical evidence that the latest failures of HDL-C-raising drugs show no clear association with risks for CVD. At the genetic level, recent research indicates that steady-state HDL-C concentrations may provide limited information regarding the potential antiatherogenic functions of HDL. It is evident that the newer strategies may replace therapeutic approaches to simply raise plasma HDL-C levels. There is an urgent need to identify an efficient biomarker that accurately predicts the increased risk of atherosclerosis (AS) in patients and that may be used for exploring newer therapeutic targets. Studies from recent decades show that the composition, structure and function of circulating HDL are closely associated with high cardiovascular risk. A vast amount of data demonstrates that the most important mechanism through which HDL antagonizes AS involves the reverse cholesterol transport (RCT) process. Clinical trials of drugs that specifically target HDL have so far proven disappointing, so it is necessary to carry out review on the HDL therapeutics.

Keywords: HDL; biomarker; HDL function; reverse cholesterol transport; HDL therapies

1. Introduction

Hyperlipidemia, a risk factor for atherosclerosis (AS), is a serious consequence for people who have experienced coronary heart disease, stroke, and artery stenosis disease. AS, which is the leading cause of cardiovascular disease (CVD), is responsible for 50% of all mortality in many developed countries [1]. A persistent increase in circulating low-density lipoprotein cholesterol (LDL-C) levels in the body is one of the most important causes for the initiation and progression of AS [2]. It has been shown in epidemiological studies and clinical trials that LDL-C levels are directly related to the rate at which CVD events occur [2,3]. There are abundant antilipemic agents (Table 1) on the market, but the meta-analysis of intervention trials has shown that a per mmol/L decrease in LDL-C is associated with an approximate 22% reduction of CVD events and a 10% reduction of all-cause mortality [3]. There is a wealth of evidence showing that statins that play a beneficial role in lowering LDL-C levels and are efficient in preventing first cardiovascular events. However, a large residual disease burden remains, even in patients treated with a high dose of statins and other CVD risk-modifying interventions [1]. Furthermore, treatment with statins may lead to a significant increase of muscle toxicity and liver transaminase, and may not be suitable for all CVDs. Investigators are eagerly searching for novel therapeutic targets. Because high-density lipoprotein cholesterol (HDL-C) levels, a predictor of major cardiovascular events in patients, are inversely associated with risk for CVD [2,4], strategies for increasing HDL levels have been explored as a new approach for combatting CVD, which may overcome the significant residual cardiovascular risk remaining after treatment with statins [4]. However, a recent genetic analysis failed to show a causal association between genetically raised plasma HDL cholesterol levels and risk for myocardial infarction [5]. In addition, nicotinic acid and fibrates currently are used to increase HDL-C levels, both of which have some weaknesses (e.g., uricosuria, increased glucose tolerance and flushing for nicotinic acid and problematic pharmacokinetic interactions for fibrates) that impose restrictions on their use [6]. Moreover, raising HDL-cholesterol by the cholesteryl-ester transfer protein (CETP) inhibitor did not play its expected role in protection from CVD [7,8]. The goals of previous HDL therapy are currently being reassessed due to numerous difficulties validating the hypothesis. Therefore, HDL structure, composition and function are the focus of ongoing research efforts, as they might provide more valuable information than steady-state HDL-cholesterol levels [9]. From the study of the structure and composition of HDL, novel strategies for the treatment of hyperlipemia-induced AS are being developed. Apolipoprotein A-I (apoA-I) is the major structural protein component of HDL particles [10], and it has been shown to play a pivotal role in reverse cholesterol transport (RCT) [11]. ApoA-I has also been shown to exert direct anti-inflammatory effects [12]. Stimulating increased synthesis of endogenous apoA-I may be a promising approach. Regarding the function of HDL, the atheroprotective activities of HDL particles are attributed to their central role in anti-inflammatory, antithrombotic, and antioxidant processes and their ability to improve endothelial function [13,14]. In addition, RCT is currently understood as the physiological process by which cholesterol in peripheral tissues is transported by HDL to the liver for excretion in the bile and feces [15]. This process is complex and beneficial, and it has been known as a widely accepted mechanism for the protective effect of HDL.

This paper is aimed at looking for a better HDL biomarker to predict AS precisely and explaining how HDL functions in detail, then providing an overview of novel therapies that target HDL to enhance HDL's ability to reduce residual cardiovascular risk in the population. Finally, we carry out an assessment of a natural drug that has been linked to HDL, which represents a unique field in the treatment of AS that warrants exploration.

Table 1. Drugs of anti-hyperlipidemia in the current market. In recent years many cholesterol-lowering drugs are commonly used on the market, which mainly includes stains, fibrates, nicotinic acids, cholesterol absorption inhibitor and polyene unsaturated fatty acids.

Classification	Drug	Mechanism	TC	TG	VLDL	LDL	HDL	Advantage	Disadvantage
Stains	Atorvastatin Lovastatin	As inhibition of HMG CoA reductase, reduce cholesterol synthesis		↓	↓	↓↓	↑	The advantage of these drugs is a low incidence of adverse reaction, and can be suitable for a variety of hypercholesterolemia except hypertriglyceridemia , is a lipid-lowering drug with rapid development in recent years	Gastrointestinal symptoms and rash, and the residual risk
Fibrates	Gemfibrozil Fenofibrate	The drug can increase Lp(a) Lipase activity to remove VLDL, TG; Thus reducing VLDL and TG, TC and LDL can also be reduced		↓ ↓	↓	↓	↑	These drugs do not cause the increase of diabetic insulin resistance or affect the control of blood sugar, therefore this kind of drugs is the first choice for treating the diabetic patients with hyperlipidemia	Gastrointestinal reactions, allergic reaction, due the drugs increase the concentration of cholesterol in bile, it may cause gallstones, occasional eyesight obstacle and hematological abnormalities
Nicotinic Acids	Niacin; Inositol Aluminum Aluminum Nicotinate	The drug can prevent fat decomposition, prevent free fatty acid formation, inhibit synthesis of TG and secretion of VLDL in liver		↓	↓	↓ ↓	↑	Cheap, and it is the only lipid-lowering drug can also reduce risk and mortality of cardiovascular disease	It is not suitable for diabetes patients, overdose adverse reactions (toxic to the liver, high blood sugar) has a high incidence common adverse reactions are skin flushing, itching, rash
Cholesterol Absorption Inhibitor	Ezetimibe	The drug can combine with bile acid to block the bile acid absorption; Prompte the translation of the cholesterol into bile in the gallbladder, then bile binding to drug is eliminated from the body	↓ ↓	↓		↓	↑	This kind of medicine is recognized as TC lowering drugs, when treats together with statins, the risk of accidental heart disease related to decrease the occurrence of 50% or more	The common adverse reactions are mild nausea and abdominal distension, constipation, therefore, it is not suitable for intestinal diseases and intractable constipation patients
Polyene Unsaturated Fatty Acids	Duoxikang Ecosapeatanolic acid	This drug can combine with total cholesterol to be ester; Then promotes the degradation of bile acid excreted along with the bile, decreases plasma total cholesterol concentration	↓	↓ ↓		↓		These drugs in combination with statins can reduce the level of TG, and play an effective role in the prevention and treatment of coronary heart disease	This kind of medicaments is easy to be oxidized to atherogenic substance, has inhibitory effect on platelet aggregation, so it needs to be used with caution

2. HDL and AS

AS can be considered to be a form of chronic inflammation, beginning with increased endothelial permeability of monocytes under the influence of adhesion molecules [16]. It promotes endocytosis of oxidized LDL into the arterial wall and intima, which can be devoured by intimal macrophages to become foam cells. This is a key process in the development of atherosclerotic plaque. Along with an increase in macrophages and foam cells, the plaque becomes unstable. This progression can ultimately lead to the development of complex lesions, or plaques, that protrude into the arterial lumen. Plaque rupture and thrombosis result in the acute clinical complications of myocardial infarction and stroke [17,18]. Cardiovascular diseases are the leading cause of death and illness in developed countries, with AS being the most important contributor [13]. In recent years, there has been growing interest in finding a cardiovascular biomarker that provides prognostic and predictive information to act as a tool to influence treatment strategies [19]. The use of HDL-related indexes as biomarkers is undergoing predictive tests, and they represent the greatest promise of this technology and the shortest and most effective path to furthering our understanding.

2.1. HDL as the Biomarker for AS

2.1.1. HDL-C

Because trends relating high plasma levels of HDL-C and decreased incidence of CVD endpoints were observed in prospective epidemiological studies conducted in several countries many years ago, HDL-C levels have served as a significant predictor for relieving AS in the clinic. There have been several attempts to increase HDL-C levels using pharmacological intervention [3,17]. HDL-C levels have been reported to increase upon chronic administration of fibrates as agonists of the peroxisome proliferator activated receptor α (PPARα) in animals and in humans. Niacin is the first antidyslipidemic agent identified that has been available for patients to raise HDL-C. However, recent data from a Global Health outcomes (AIM-HIGH) trial with niacin did not show any significant improvement in the cardiovascular risk over statins, which are commonly used drugs for lipid management [20,21]. Recently a few attempts have been made to inhibit CETP to raise the levels of HDL-C. Torcetrapib, a cholesterol ester transferase inhibitor, reliably increased HDL (without countervailing effects on LDL) but ultimately increased cardiovascular mortality. Dalcetrapib, a new CETP inhibitor, also has unintended effects, and the outcomes are the same as those for torcetrapib [7,8]. As a result, CETP inhibitors continue to face safety hurdles, and no significant clinical benefits have resulted from these pharmacological regimens. A recent report suggested that the sole increase of HDL-C in humans would not necessarily improve the rate of cardiovascular events (all-cause mortality, coronary heart disease mortality, non-fatal myocardial infarction, and stroke) [22–25]. In justification for the use of statins in prevention: an Intervention Trial Evaluating Rosuvastatin (JUPITER), on-treatment HDL-C was not predictive of residual risk among statin-treated individuals, whereas HDL-C was predictive among those taking placebo [26]. Similarly, on-treatment apoA-I and triglycerides were not predictive of residual risk [27]. For these reasons, the use of the HDL-C biomarker as a surrogate end point remains a difficult and distant goal.

2.1.2. HDL Particle Size

Dyslipidemia may influence enzymes and transfer proteins needed for lipoprotein particle remodeling. HDL particle size may differ in the number of molecules of apo and free cholesterol, esterified cholesterol, and phospholipids content on the lipoprotein surface [28,29] due to the changes in activity of Lecithin-cholesterol acyltransferase (LCAT), CETP, phospholipid transfer protein (PLTP) plasma transfer proteins, and enzymes (e.g., lipoprotein lipase (LPL), hepatic lipase (HL)) in the process. Calculated indices and the evaluation of lipoprotein particle size have been widely used to predict cardiovascular risk. An evaluation of the association between HDL particle size and risk of incident coronary artery disease (CHD) in apparently healthy volunteers indicated that decreased

HDL particle size is associated with an adverse cardiometabolic risk profile [30]. Small HDL particle size was also associated with an increased CHD risk, which resulted from the different lipid transfer ability [31]. Another study found that the high TG-low HDL cholesterol dyslipidemia, which is found in viscerally obese subjects and characterized by hyperinsulinemia, was strongly correlated with reduced HDL particle size [32]. However, the latest finding is not consistent with previous conclusions. The HDL particle size (nm) values were not different between the dyslipidemia, normolipidemic and dyslipdemic groups without treatment with lipid-lowering drugs [33]. In addition, several studies using GGE-measured HDL size have reported that patients with CHD tend to have smaller HDL particles and that large HDL particles may protect against the development of AS. There are also other studies that show that only small HDL particles are atheroprotective, this is supported by the analysis of HDL subfraction data and carotid artery disease (CAAD) [34]. It is found that among HDL-C, HDL_2, and HDL_3, HDL_3 best predicts CAAD risk, and the remaining phenotypes do not add significant predictive power [34]. Although public opinions about HDL size are divergent, the propagation rate and maximal diene formation during total HDL oxidation correlated significantly with HDL mean particle size [30,32]. It is clear that proper HDL particle size may have advantages in the reduction of CVD events. In the future, we believe that HDL particle size will play an essential role in predicting the risk of AS.

2.1.3. HDL Particles Concentration (HDL-P)

Given the extreme heterogeneity of HDL, measuring the content of HDL particles will, at best, only partially reflect the potential role of HDL in cardiovascular risk assessment and therapeutic drug development. In this regard, the HDL-P may be a better marker of residual vascular risk after potent statin therapy in the JUPITER trial than chemically measured HDL-C or apoA-I [35]. HDL-P may be a promising metric of HDL that is more independent of other metabolic and lipoprotein risk factors than HDL cholesterol or HDL size [36]. In the European Prospective Investigation into Cancer and Nutrition (EPIC)-Norfolk study, HDL-P was inversely associated with CVD, consistent with the above-mentioned observations [37]. However, in the Women's Health Study, HDL-P was not associated with incident CVD events among healthy low-risk women in contrast with inverse associations seen for HDL size and HDL-C [38]. Moreover, an emerging outcome from a determinant of residual risk among statin-treated individuals suggests that overall HDL-P is not as important as the sub-type of HDL-P, which contains the lysosphingolipid sphingosine-1-phosphate (S1P) [36]. This conclusion is supported by the evidence that it is the S1P content of HDL, as opposed to the HDL particle itself, which is responsible for the beneficial antiatherothrombotic, anti-inflammatory, antioxidant, antiglycation, and profibrinolytic activities of these lipoproteins [36]. At present, two techniques, nuclear magnetic resonance (NMR) and ion mobility analysis (IMA) have been described for quantifying HDL-P in human plasma. However, the final HDL-P yield determined using these two methods differ by up to >5-fold. With the progress of science and technology, the accurate and reasonable use of ^1H NMR [39] and application of termed calibrated ion mobility analysis (calibrated IMA) [40] will greatly determine the feasibility of HDL-P as biomarker.

2.1.4. Other Biomarkers

The HDL-associated Apolipoprotein M (apoM) plays a role in the anti-atherogenic function in a variety of atherosclerotic models, making it interesting to investigate whether apoM is a predictor of AS [41–44]. With the discovery of apoM as an important carrier of S1P in HDL particles, it forms a new basis for investigations of apoM biology. An improved understanding of the role of the apoM/S1P axis in relation to AS may unravel new avenues for treatment or use of biomarkers for disease or risk evaluation [45].

The expression of serum amyloid A (SAA) protein was greater in the patients with AS, and it can be explained by high serum levels of SAA-predicted AS [45–49]. By means of two-dimensional electrophoresis (2-DE) coupled with mass spectrometry (MS) analysis on plasma-purified VLDL, LDL and HDL fractions from patients undergoing carotid endarterectomy, increased levels of acute-phase SAA (AP SAA) in all lipoprotein fractions helped to identify AP SAA as a potential marker of advanced carotid AS [50]. Studies in both mice and humans suggest that proinflammatory HDL may be a novel biomarker for increased risk of AS in patients with systemic lupus erythematosus (SLE) and rheumatoid arthritis (RA) [51]. Moreover, proinflammatory HDL-associated hemoglobin (Hb) was also found to be differentially associated with HDL from coronary heart disease patients compared with healthy controls [52,53]. Hb contributes to the proinflammatory nature of HDL in mouse and human models of AS and may serve as a novel biomarker for AS [52–54].

In addition, HDL has a wide range of functions, some of which are independent of its cholesterol content. Tests for HDL function as a biomarker may be useful for diagnosing the risk for patients with CHD. As a result, we elaborate the functions of HDL in the next section with the purpose of identifying the best biomarker of AS.

2.2. HDL in Anti-Atherosclerosis

HDLs have several well-documented functions with the potential to protect against AS. These functions include an ability to promote the efflux of cholesterol from macrophages in the artery wall, inhibit the oxidative modification of LDLs, inhibit vascular inflammation, inhibit thrombosis, promote endothelial repairing, promote angiogenesis, enhance endothelial function, improve diabetic control, and inhibit hematopoietic stem cell proliferation. Some of these functions have been mechanistically linked to the well-known ability of HDLs to induce the activation of cellular cholesterol efflux pathways, whereas many other functions of HDLs are independent of the effects of HDLs on cellular cholesterol homeostasis. Below, we will discuss the most relevant functions of HDLs for AS more specifically (Figure 1).

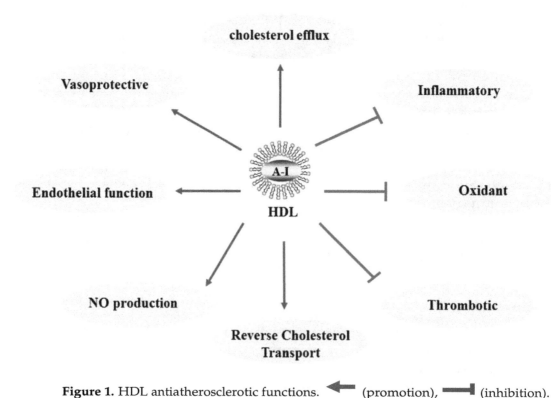

Figure 1. HDL antiatherosclerotic functions. ⬅ (promotion), ⊣ (inhibition).

2.2.1. Reverse Cholesterol Transport

In many studies, we found that the ability of HDL to promote cholesterol efflux from macrophages was strongly and inversely associated with both subclinical AS and obstructive coronary artery disease [55,56]. The efflux of cholesterol from a variety of cell types, including macrophages, to HDLs in the extracellular space is mediated by two distinct processes. One is the efflux of cholesterol induced by a specific cellular transporter [57–62], and the other is passive aqueous diffusion of cholesterol from cell membranes to HDLs [63,64]. Then, excess cholesterol from peripheral tissues will be transported back to the liver for excretion in the bile and ultimately the feces by HDL via a process called RCT. We herein would like to describe the importance of RCT in detail, and therefore, the multiplex RCT pathway has been described in the following four parts (Figure 2) [65].

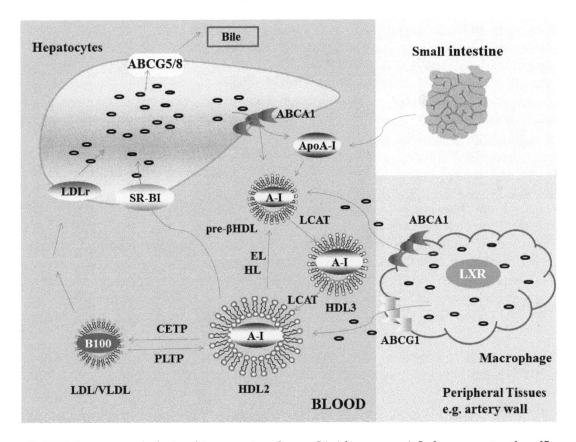

Figure 2. HDL in reverse cholesterol transport pathway. Lipid-poor apoA-I also promotes the efflux of free cholesterol from macrophages via ABCA1. LCAT esterifies free cholesterol to cholesteryl esters to form mature HDL, which promotes cholesterol efflux from macrophages via the ABCG1 transporter, as well as from other peripheral tissues by processes not fully defined. In macrophages, both ABCA1 and ABCG1 are regulated by Liver X receptors (LXR). Mature HDL can transfer its cholesterol to the liver directly via scavenger receptor class B type I (SR-BI) or indirectly via CETP-mediated transfer to ApoB-containing lipoproteins, with subsequent uptake by the liver via the LDL-r. Hepatic cholesterol can be excreted directly into the bile as cholesterol or after conversion to bile acids and, unless reabsorbed by the intestine, is ultimately excreted in the feces. HL, EL, and PLTP, play an indispensable role in remodeling HDL, thus, the RCT pathway is dependent on interaction with them [9].

Part One: The Formation of Nascent HDL

Lipid-free or lipid-poor apoA-I secreted in the liver can mediate cellular efflux of both cholesterol and phospholipids from macrophages via the ATP-binding cassette transporter A1 (ABCA1) and gather them on the surface of pre-β HDL, resulting in the rapid lipidation of apoA-I to generate mature α HDL, which is called nascent HDL particles [66,67]. Once loss of two ABCA1 genes occurs in the body, such as in the case of Tangier disease, the result is abnormally low levels of serum HDL-C, an acceleration of the accumulation of cholesterol in peripheral tissues, and the formation of premature AS [68]. The mature HDL particles can then serve as acceptors of cholesterol provided by ATP-binding cassette transporter G1 (ABCG1) [69] or SR-BI [70]. ABCG1 is another member of the ATP-binding cassette family that plays a critical role in the efflux of cellular phospholipid (PL) and free cholesterol (FC) to mature HDL, but not pre-β HDL. By intraperitoneal injection of mice with [³H]-cholesterol-labeled J774 macrophages with either increased or reduced ABCG1 expression and primary macrophages lacking ABCG1 expression, followed by measurement of the macrophage-derived [³H]-cholesterol levels in plasma and feces [71], it was shown that macrophages lacking ABCG1 cause damage and secretion of FC and excessive cholesterol accumulation in macrophages. Therefore, ABCG1 mediates cholesterol efflux [72]. In an investigation of extracellular cholesterol microdomains that form during the enrichment of macrophages with cholesterol, extracellular cholesterol microdomains did not develop when ABCG1-deficient mouse bone marrow-derived macrophages were enriched with cholesterol [69]. Many studies have demonstrated that ABCA1 and ABCG1 play a role in many aspects of cholesterol efflux from macrophages [69,71–73].

Liver X receptors (LXR), the members of the steroid nuclear receptor superfamily, are oxysterol-activated transcription factors that, after heterodimerization with the 9-*cis*-retinoic acid receptor (RXR), bind to specific LXR response elements (LXREs), thus regulating the expression of target genes involved in intra- and extracellular lipid metabolism [74]. In part by modulating cholesterol efflux from macrophages to apoA-I and HDL, LXRs induce the direct target genes ABCA1 and ABCG1/ABCG4 to promote reverse cholesterol transport. The oxidation of steroids from FC can activate LXR and regulate gene expression of ABCA1 and ABCG1 to strengthen the peripheral tissue cholesterol secretion. Meanwhile, the LXRs are also readily oxidized by PPARα. PPARαcontrols lipid and glucose metabolism in several tissues and cell types including liver, heart, kidneys, adipose tissue and macrophages. PPARα-activation suppresses chylomicron and increases HDL production by enterocytes [75,76]. In addition, its agonists promote secretion of macrophage cholesterol via stimulating expression of ABCA1 and LXR to increase reverse cholesterol transport [77].

Part Two: The Process of Cholesterol Esterified by LCAT

LCAT, a lipoprotein-associated enzyme, is a key player in the RCT pathway. LCAT has two different catalytic activities that account for its ability to esterify cholesterol. One is phospholipase A2 activity, and the other is its transesterification activity. It requires apoA-I and, to a lesser degree, other apolipoproteins, which most likely activate LCAT by modifying the presentation of its substrates, namely, phospholipids and cholesterol, on the surface of lipoproteins [78]. After FC efflux to pre-β HDL (the nascent, discoidal-shaped HDL), cholesterol in HDLs may be esterified by the enzymatic activity of LCAT. The LCAT reaction occurs in two steps. After binding to a lipoprotein, LCAT cleaves the fatty acid in the sn-2 position of phosphatidylcholine and transfers it onto a serine residue. Next, the fatty acid is transesterified to the 3-β-hydroxyl group on the A-ring of cholesterol to form cholesterol ester. Cholesteryl esters formed by LCAT partition, which are more hydrophobic than free cholesterol, are transferred from the surface of lipoproteins to the hydrophobic core. This process converts pre-β HDL to HDL_2 and HDL_3 particles, which are the major HDL species found in plasma and which represent larger, spherical-shaped α-migrating forms of HDL. LCAT is important in the process of RCT by generating a gradient of free cholesterol from cells to HDL [79]. This effect of LCAT prevents the back exchange of cholesterol by passive diffusion from HDL to peripheral cells and thus is believed to promote net removal of cholesterol from peripheral cells to HDL. Without ongoing esterification of cholesterol, the capacity of HDL to remove and bind additional cholesterol would eventually be diminished. Two lipases, endothelial lipase (EL) and HL, are the complete opposite of LCAT in HDL metabolism. HL and EL are members of the triglyceride lipase family, which also includes LPL [80,81]. EL has high phospholipase A1 activity and remodels HDL into small particles, whereas HL is more effective in hydrolyzing triglycerides [82]. Although HL causes a remodeling of HDL into smaller particles, it also promotes the release of lipid-poor apoA-I [83]. The combined functions of HL and EL have a significant effect on plasma HDL-C levels [84–87]. HL- and EL-deficient mice were studied to demonstrate that the magnitude of macrophage-derived [³H] cholesterol in feces was increased, which promoted macrophage-to-feces RCT, and its ability to protect against LDL oxidation was enhanced [88].

Part Three: The Exchange of CE (Cholesteryl Esters) Mediated by CETP

CETP is a hydrophobic glycoprotein that is synthesized in several tissues but mainly in the liver. It facilitates the exchange of cholesteryl esters and triglycerides between HDL and apoB-containing particles (LDL, IDL, VLDL) and represents a major branching point for RCT [7,8]. This results in the recycling of cholesterol and an increasing attenuation in blood circulation, with the potential to go back into the artery wall. Two major observations were made using many novel methods, such as innovative X-ray crystallographic, electron microscopic (EM), and bioinformatics observations: (i) CETP connects with or forms bridges between two lipoproteins, e.g., HDL and LDL, with resultant neutral lipid transfer; and (ii) CETP appears to contain a hydrophobic tunnel along its entire long axis capable of neutral lipid transfer. These observations may clearly explain the relationships between CETP interactions with lipoproteins and the lipid transfer processes [89]. Most CEs derived from LCAT do not return to the liver via the HDL SR-B1 pathway but, rather, through more atherogenic pathways. CETP mediates the transfer of most CE from HDL to VLDL or to other more atherogenic intermediate-density lipoproteins and remnants, and the transfer of triglycerides from VLDL-1 to HDL results in larger, relatively triglyceride-enriched LDL species [90]. Transfer of CE from HDL directly to LDL by CETP could also be antiatherogenic if the LDL is cleared by the liver LDL receptor. Another transfer protein in this part of RCT, PLTP, transfers phospholipids between VLDL and HDL [91]. PLTP is one of the main modulators of plasma HDL size, composition and function [92] and one of the major modulators of HDL metabolism in plasma [93]. The level of HDL or HDL production is dramatically decreased in PLTP⁻/⁻ mice [94,95], and PLTP deficiency attenuates plaque accumulation in different atherosclerotic models. This indicates that PLTP plays an important role in atherogenesis, and its function goes well beyond that of transferring phospholipids between lipoprotein particles [96,97].

Part Four: Catabolism of HDL Cholesterol in Biliary Pathway

After efflux, cholesterol in HDLs may be esterified by the enzymatic activity of LCAT whereupon HDLs can deliver the excess cholesterol from peripheral cells back to the liver in in distinct ways: HDL cholesteryl esters, but not the protein component of HDLs, are selectively taken up into the liver via SR-BI. Ultimately, cholesterol is excreted from the liver into the bile, either directly as free cholesterol or after conversion into bile acids, and eliminated from the body via the feces. In humans, HDL-C can be metabolized by the liver via another pathway: CETP exchanges of HDL CE for triglycerides in apoB-containing lipoproteins, followed by hepatic uptake mediated by LDL-r. An LDL-r deficiency in mice substantially decreases selective HDL CE uptake by liver and adrenals. Thus, LDL-r expression has a substantial impact on HDL metabolism in mice [98].

Via the classic RCT pathway, excessive cholesterol collected from peripheral tissues, which is delivered back to the liver, is followed by biliary secretion and elimination via the feces. In addition to the traditional RCT-mediated biliary pathway, in the last few years, direct trans-intestinal excretion of plasma-derived cholesterol (TICE) was shown to contribute substantially to fecal neutral sterol (FNS) excretion in mice, describing the transport of cholesterol from blood to the intestinal lumen directly via enterocytes. The TICE pathway was called a nonhepatobiliary-related route, which has been shown to have a high degree of correlation with the main contributors Niemann-Pick disease, type C1/2 (NPC1/2), ABCG5/G8, LDL-r, and LXR [99–101]. The application of PPAR δ agonist and LXR agonists, have been shown to stimulate the process of TICE [102]. In the RCT pathway, HDL plays an important role. In contrast, there is evidence from animal experiments that HDL plays an essential role in TICE [103].

2.2.2. Antioxidant Properties of High-Density Lipoprotein

LDL is one of the main causes of AS. Oxidation of LDL yields a more pro-atherogenic particle, and numerous studies have found that HDLs are capable of impeding oxidative changes in LDL. HDL exhibits potent antioxidant activity, which may arise from synergy in the inactivation of oxidized LDL lipids by enzymatic and nonenzymatic mechanisms, in part reflecting distinct intrinsic physicochemical properties [104]. The anti-oxidative properties of HDL critically involve HDL-associated enzymes, such as paraoxonase 1 (PON1), lipoprotein-associated phospholipase A2 (Lp-PLA2), and LCAT, which have been reported to hydrolyze oxidized phospholipids into lyso-phosphatidylcholine [105–109]. In addition, HDL carries glutathione selenoperoxidase, which can reduce lipid peroxide (LOOH) to the corresponding hydroxides and thereby detoxify them [110]. ApoA-I can remove oxidized lipids from LDL, suggesting that HDL can function as an acceptor of oxidized lipids. In cell culture experiments, apoA-I removes lipids from LDL and thereby makes LDL resistant to vascular cell-mediated oxidation and prevents oxidized LDL-induced monocyte adherence and chemotaxis [108]. Other HDL apolipoproteins, such as apoA-II, apoA-IV, apoE, and apoJ, also function as antioxidants *in vitro*.

2.2.3. HDL in the Endothelium

Traditionally, the endothelium has been considered to be an inert component of the vessel wall. Injury to the endothelium results in deleterious alterations of endothelial physiology, also referred to as endothelial dysfunction, which represents a key early step in the development of an atherosclerotic lesion and is implicated in the malignant development that follows. It has become evident that HDL from healthy subjects can exert direct potential atheroprotective effects on endothelial cells and can positively affect several endothelial functions in the regulation of vascular tone, inflammation [111] and endothelial oxidant stress [112], which is associated with activation of NO synthesis by HDL. NO is an endothelium-derived signaling molecule that activates guanylate cyclase in vascular smooth muscle cells (SMCs) to induce relaxation, which is generated by a constitutive eNOS. Notably, HDLs also beneficially affect the vasculature by promoting endothelial cell survival. In endothelial cells, HDLs still maintain anti-thrombotic functions, mainly inhibiting thrombin-induced tissue factor, mediating the extrinsic coagulation pathway, and stimulating the activation of the anticoagulant proteins C and S.

2.2.4. Anti-inflammatory Properties of HDL

HDL and apoA I are believed to protect against the development of AS, in part, which is closely related to their anti-inflammatory function. The anti-inflammatory properties of HDL encompass suppression of macrophage inflammatory cytokine production and inhibition of the expression of endothelial cell adhesion molecules that promote the entry of monocytes and neutrophils into arteries. HDLs potently block murine experimental endotoxinemia, indicating that HDLs bind lipopolysaccharides (LPS), which leads to lower systemic proinflammatory cytokine levels and improved survival rates [113]. Up-regulation of adhesion molecules (E-selectin, ICAM-1, and VCAM-1) and secretion of pro-inflammatory mediators (monocyte chemoattractant 1, MCP-1) lead to the activation of the vascular endothelium and induce AS.

3. Novel Therapies with HDL as the Key Components

3.1. Novel Pharmacotherapeutic Strategies in Increasing HDL

3.1.1. Infusions of Special HDL

One approach to increase the serum levels of HDL is to infuse reconstituted HDL (rHDL) or recombinant HDL particles into the circulation rather than by increasing HDL indirectly by modulating HDL metabolism. CSL-111 is a reconstituted HDL-particle comprising both human apoA-1 and soybean phosphatidylcholine. CSL-112 is being evaluated in phase II trials to improve the weakness of CSL-111. There is a benefit of CSL-111/CSL-112 infusions to increase HDL-C levels and up-regulation of cellular cholesterol efflux in patients with acute coronary syndrome (ACS). Some trials have demonstrated that infusions of recombinant HDL-containing apoA-I Milano and CER-001 significantly reduce or stabilize mean plaque atheroma volume and still exert greater anti-inflammatory effects in LDL-r$^{-/-}$ mice [114–116]. However, most clinical studies have demonstrated that rapid clearance of CER-001 leads to a requirement for repeated administration due to the inability to achieve effective plasma concentrations [117]. Pegylation of apoA-I in rHDL markedly increases its plasma half-life and enhances its antiatherogenic properties *in vivo* [118].

3.1.2. Autologous Delipidated HDL

Another novel approach to HDL therapeutics is to raise the levels of HDL particles by intravenous infusion with the use of autologous delipidated HDL. Preclinical evaluation of selective delipidated HDL in a nonhuman primate model of dyslipidemia achieved a significant 6.9% reduction in aortic atheroma volume, as assessed by intravenous ultrasound (IVUS) [119]. In a small clinical study in which 28 patients with ACS received five weekly infusions of delipidated HDL, the decreased total atheroma volume by 5.2% from baseline may be associated with selectively increased preβ-HDL [120].

3.2. Novel Pharmacotherapeutic Strategies in Four Steps of RCT

3.2.1. First Part of RCT

ApoA-I Mimetic Peptides

ApoA-I mimetics, which are short synthetic peptides, mimic the amphipathic a-helix of apoA-I. Because the first apoA-I mimetic consisted of 18 amino acids, additional improved peptides were generated by increasing the number of phenylalanine residues on the hydrophobic face (referred to as 2F, 3F, 4F, 5F, 6F, and 7F) of the polypeptide. Two different types of apoA-I mimetic peptide 4F were used in clinical trials, including L-4F (the 4F peptide synthesized from L-amino acids) and D-4F (the 4F peptide synthesized from all D-amino acids). Compared with high plasma L-4F levels not improving HDL anti-inflammatory function, a single dose of D-4F was found to have a significant effect on the inflammatory index of HDL with modest oral bioavailability [10]. ABCA1-independent lipid efflux played a major role in this aspect of RCT. Recently, 5A, an asymmetric bihelical peptide based on 2F, had increased ABCA1-dependent cholesterol efflux and decreased hemolysis compared with its parent compound [121]. Furthermore, ATI-5261 synthetic peptide, like apoA-I mimetic peptides, successfully enhances cholesterol efflux from macrophages and reduces aortic AS, which exerts its effects similar to that of the role of HDL in reverse cholesterol transport in mice. Reservelogix-208 (RVX-208), an apoA-I upregulator that increases endogenous synthesis of apoA-I, has a unique mechanism of action related to epigenetically influencing the accessibility of apoA-I gene by the transcription machinery. Encouragingly, there is a progressive discovery that nanolipid particles containing multivalent peptides (HDL-like nanoparticles) promoted efficient cellular cholesterol efflux and were functionally superior to those derived from monomeric apoA-I mimetic peptides [122].

Regulators of ABCA1 and ABCG1

LXR and miR-33 (similars: miR-758, miR-26 and miR-106b) have been demonstrated to regulate macrophages ABCA1 and ABCG1. The activation of the former can upregulate the expression of two genes, which promote macrophage cholesterol efflux and augment intestinal HDL generation, while the opposite is true of the latter. In the animal experiments, LXR agonists exhibit a significant decrease of atherosclerotic plaque formation and exert anti-inflammatory characteristics [123]. The negative effects caused by hepatic LXR agonists, such as a fatty liver, will be overcome by more intestine-specific LXRα agonists that are still under preclinical investigation [124]. As an alternative to LXR agonism, gene- silencing approaches involving microRNA 33 are being explored to control gene expression at the post-transcriptional level [125]. An antisense oligonucleotide has been developed that effectively silences miR-33 (miRNA-33a/b) and increases ABCA1 and ABCG1 expression in macrophages. Studies in nonhuman primates showed that antisense oligonucleotides to miRNA-33a/b that induce ABCA1 expression as well as the expression of other proteins involved in fatty acid metabolism result in a 50% increase in HDL-C and a decrease in VLDL [126]. Recent studies in PPARγ-activated macrophages demonstrated that treatment with miR-613 leads to inhibition of cholesterol efflux by downregulating LXRα and ABCA1 [127]. This study sheds new insights into the possibility that the miR-613 inhibitor may serve as a novel therapy for the treatment of cholesterol metabolism diseases. Similarly, PPAR agonists also increase ABCA1 gene expression and target the LXR gene. PPARα (K-877), PPARγ (INT131) and PPARα/δ (GFT505) modulators play pivotal roles in ABCA1 gene expression and apoA-I secretion, and increase HDL-C in patients with hyperlipidemia [126,127]. Growing evidence suggests that MBX-8025, a promising PPARδ agonist targeting the ABCA1 gene and LXRα gene, with a greater binding potency, is under development. Additional dual PPARα/γ and PPARβ/δ agonists that are under development may play an important role in RCT pathway [78].

3.2.2. Second Part of RCT

LCAT Agonists

LCAT plays a major role in this part of RCT, and mediates the esterification of free cholesterol located at the surface of lipoprotein particles. Several drug development approaches have recently been initiated for modulating LCAT activity. Recombinant human LCAT (rhLCAT) efficiently promotes the process of RCT, which induces a marked increase in HDL-C levels and the maturation of small preb-HDL into α-migrating particles in LCAT-deficient plasma [128]. Currently, recombinant LCAT (ACP-501) in Phase 1 clinical trials was shown to rapidly and substantially elevate the formation of cholesteryl esters, representing the promotion of RCT. It is reported that Apo AI-derived peptides present the ability to modulate LCAT activity, with a significant increase in 3H-cholesteryl ester production in a higher proportion at 0.3 mg/mL [129]. An early apoA-I mimetic peptide (ETC-642) promotes LCAT activation and has entered clinical development [130].

3.2.3. Third Part of RCT

CETP Inhibitor

Anacetrapib. The Determining Efficacy and Tolerability of Anacetrapib has shown a 138% increase in HDL-C, a 40% reduction in LDL-C, and a 36% decrease in Lp(a) of patients with CAD. This results from the ability of anacetrapib to inhibit both heterotypic and homotypic CE transfer. A large phase III study, Randomized EValuationof the Effects of Anacetrapib Through Lipid-modification (REVEAL), will be completed in January 2017 [131].

Evacetrapib. Evacetrapib has a similar structure and mechanism of action as torcetrapib but, based on IC_{50} values, appears to be a more potent CETP inhibitor than torcetrapib or anacetrapib [132]. It is the most recently developed CETP-inhibitor currently undergoing a phase III CVD outcome trial. In a phase II study, high doses of evacetrapib do not elevate blood pressure in rats and do not induce aldosterone or cortisol biosynthesis in a human adrenal cortical carcinoma cell line [133]. The Assessment of Clinical Effects of Cholesteryl Ester Transfer Protein Inhibition With Evacetrapib in Patients at a High-Risk for Vascular Outcomes (ACCELERATE) phase III CVD outcome trial is recruiting.

BAY 60-5521/TA-8995. BAY 60-5521 and TA-8995 are two potential inhibitors of CETP. The clinical results suggest that these two agents are safe and well tolerated, with effective inhibition of CETP activity and increased high HDL-C [134,135].

CETP ASO. Antisense oligonucleotide inhibitor of CETP (CETP ASO) is associated with reductions in CETP mRNA and also shows an enhanced effect on macrophage RCT. It is reported that the CETP ASO does not act through binding and inactivating CETP associated with the HDL particle. Instead, it specifically targets and degrades CETP mRNA. In hyperlipidemic, CETP transgenic, LDL-r$^{-/-}$ mice, CETP ASO provided comparable reductions in HDL cholesterol, decreases in CETP activity with an enhanced effect on macrophage RCT, and results in less accumulation of aortic cholesterol [136]. CETP ASO could produce a unique therapeutic profile, distinct from the current CETP drugs being evaluated in late-stage clinical trials.

3.2.4. Fourth Part of RCT

SR-BI Activators

SR-BI, the HDL receptor, is expressed on hepatocytes and facilitates selective absorption of cholesterol ester from HDL. The discovery and development of traditional drugs that can modulate SR-BI expression and/or activity are being investigated through high-throughput screening of chemical compound libraries. Endogenous or exogenous agents (such as natural products) and the detailed high-resolution molecular structure of SR-BI protein, the regulators of SR-BI activity, should provide new insights for the progress of non-genetic therapies to modulate HDL metabolism *in vivo*.

As an alternative to traditional drugs, gene therapeutics are being extensively explored. In general, miRNA-125a and miRNA-455 can bind to specific sites in the 3' UTR of SR-BI mRNA and act as endogenous attenuators of SR-BI protein expression [137]. It is clear that activation of miRNA-125a and miRNA-455 shows a negative relationship with SR BI-mediated selective HDL uptake and SR-BI-supported steroid hormone synthesis. Therefore, inhibition of miRNA-125a and miRNA-455 may enhance SR-BI expression to alter the course of the atherogenic sequence by increasing plasma HDL-C flux. Furthermore, in a recent report, the level of SR-BI expression was repressed by miR-185, miR-96, and miR-223, individually, in HepG2 cells [138]. Inhibitions of these miRNAs were associated with increased SR-BI expression and reduced AS by facilitating RCT and cholesterol removal from the body.

3.3. Natural Drugs Associated with HDL at the Future Stage

Nature is an irrefutable source of inspiration for the modern man in many aspects. The observation and understanding of nature have allowed the development of new materials, new sources of energies, new drugs, *etc.* Specifically, natural products provide a great contribution to the development of new agents for the treatment of hyperlipidemic diseases. Compared with chemical drugs or other synthetically created products, natural products could more closely mimic physiological processes and may be more effective in treatment of cardiovascular diseases. There are many natural drugs for the treatment of AS associated with HDL, such as polysaccharide, sesamin, anthocyanins, 24(S)-Saringosterol and many others. Chitosan and its related products, which are polysaccharides, are used to enhance natural products and may represent promising strategies in the near future.

3.3.1. Chitosan

Chitosan (CTS), the only positive alkaline polysaccharide extracted from shrimp or crab shells and exhibiting biocompatibility and a nontoxic nature, has the potential for hypolipidemic and weight loss activities. In 1980, the first article demonstrating that proper supplementation of chitosan to the diet seemed to be effective in lowering plasma cholesterol in rats was published [139]. And the meta-analysis by Baker *et al.*, based on six randomized placebo-controlled clinical trials in hypercholesterolemic patients has showed that chitosan only induced a decrease in total cholesterol level but without any significant changes in LDL-cholesterol, HDL-cholesterol or triglyceride concentrations [140]. Since then, the research of CTS in treatment of hyperlipemia has been extensively undertaken. It is reported that because CTS is a biodegradable carbohydrate polymer, it has been prepared in a variety of dosages for use in delivery systems in previous studies [141–143], and these new preparations were found to have a more effective capability of improving hyperlipidemia in rats [144,145].

3.3.2. Chitosan Oligosaccharides

Chitosan oligosaccharides (COS) are depolymerized products of chitosan by either chemical or enzymatic hydrolysis. COS is a polymer of glucosamine with a number of bioactive properties. Recent studies have suggested that COS inhibits adipogenesis and promotes RCT through altered expression of a number of key regulators of lipid metabolism, including leptin [146], SR-BI and CYP7A1. It is reported that COS plays a positive role in the RCT pathway *in vivo* and stimulates hepatic LDL-r expression, inducing the LDL cholesterol lowering. Furthermore, chitosan oligosaccharides have anti-inflammatory functions similar to that of HDL, which downregulates the expression of E-selectin, ICAM-1 and IL-8 induced by LPS in endothelial cells through blockade of p38 MAPK and PI3K/Akt signaling pathways [147,148].

4. Discussion

HDL particles have various effects *in vitro* and *in vivo* that may protect arteries from chemical or biological hazards or facilitate repair of injuries. Nevertheless, HDL has not yet been successfully exploited for therapy. One possible reason may be the complexity of HDL particles, resulting in the physiological heterogeneity that contributes to the antiatherogenic functions of HDL. Moreover, for more than 50 years, HDL-C has been known as an independent clinical biomarker of cardiovascular risk. However, the failures of drugs to increase HDL-C drive scientists to search for new biomarkers to replace it, such as HDL functions, HDL size, and HDL-P. Among these, HDL functions will be a reliable diagnostic biomarker for the identification, personalized treatment stratification, and monitoring of patients at increased cardiovascular risk. The functionality of HDLs has two important roles. First, it promotes reverse cholesterol transport; second, it modulates inflammation and oxidation. HDL-based interventions in promoting the RCT process may be more promising. Meanwhile, some natural products with functions similar to that of HDL also play unique roles in the RCT process and will enter a new era in treatment of CVD in the near future (Table 2).

Table 2. Overview of Classes of HDL-based therapies. HDL-based therapies are an innovative approach against atherosclerosis. In this review, they can be summarized as the following three categories: strategies increasing HDL, strategies of RCT in four steps and natural drugs. ●: primary; ◆: secondary.

Strategies Increasing HDL		Strategies of RCT in Four Steps			Natural Drugs	
●Infusions of special HDL	◆ rHDL: CSL-111 CER-001 CSL-112	●First part of RCT		●Second part of RCT	●Polysaccharide:	Chitosan; Chitosan oligosaccharides
		ApoA-I mimetic peptides; ApoA-I upregulator		LCAT Agonists; ◆ rLCAT: ACP-501		
		LXR agonists; Mir-33; PPAR modulators			●Anthocyanins	
		●Third part of RCT		●Fourth part of RCT		
●Autologous delipidated HDL	◆ CETP inhibitor:	Anacetrapib; Evacetrapib; BAY 60-5521; TA-8995; CETP ASO	◆ SR-BI activators:	Traditional drugs; Gene therapeutics	●Sesamin	
					●24(S)-Saringosterol	
					●Others	

Acknowledgments: This project was financially supported by the National Science Foundation of China (no. 81173107), the Science and Technology Planning Project of Guangdong, China (2013B021100018, 2013B090600050, 2015A010101318).

References

1. Roger, V.L.; Go, A.S.; Lloyd-Jones, D.M.; Benjamin, E.J.; Berry, J.D.; Borden, W.B.; Bravata, D.M.; Dai, S.; Ford, E.S.; Fox, C.S.; *et al.* Executive summary: Heart disease and stroke statistics-2012 update: A report from the American heart association. *Circulation* **2012**, *125*, 188–197. [PubMed]

2. Gordon, T.; Castelli, W.P.; Hjortland, M.C.; Kannel, W.B.; Dawber, T.R. High density lipoprotein as a protective factor against coronary heart disease. The framingham study. *Am. J. Med.* **1977**, *62*, 707–714. [CrossRef]

3. Baigent, C.; Blackwell, L.; Emberson, J.; Holland, L.E.; Reith, C.; Bhala, N.; Peto, R.; Barnes, E.H.; Keech, A.; Simes, J.; *et al.* Efficacy and safety of more intensive lowering of LDL cholesterol: A meta-analysis of data from 170,000 participants in 26 randomised trials. *Lancet* **2010**, *376*, 1670–1681. [PubMed]

4. Barter, P.; Gotto, A.M.; LaRosa, J.C.; Maroni, J.; Szarek, M.; Grundy, S.M.; Kastelein, J.J.; Bittner, V.; Fruchart, J.C. HDL cholesterol, very low levels of LDL cholesterol, and cardiovascular events. *N. Engl. J. Med.* **2007**, *357*, 1301–1310. [CrossRef] [PubMed]

5. Dumitrescu, L.; Goodloe, R.; Bradford, Y.; Farber-Eger, E.; Boston, J.; Crawford, D.C. The effects of electronic medical record phenotyping details on genetic association studies: HDL-C as a case study. *Biodata Min.* **2015**, *8*, 15. [CrossRef] [PubMed]

6. Remaley, A.T.; Norata, G.D.; Catapano, A.L. Novel concepts in HDL pharmacology. *Cardiovasc. Res.* **2014**, *103*, 423–428. [CrossRef] [PubMed]

7. Schwartz, G.G.; Olsson, A.G.; Abt, M.; Ballantyne, C.M.; Barter, P.J.; Brumm, J.; Chaitman, B.R.; Holme, I.M.; Kallend, D.; Leiter, L.A.; *et al.* Effects of dalcetrapib in patients with a recent acute coronary syndrome. *N. Engl. J. Med.* **2012**, *367*, 2089–2099. [CrossRef] [PubMed]

8. Barter, P.J.; Caulfield, M.; Eriksson, M.; Grundy, S.M.; Kastelein, J.J.; Komajda, M.; Lopez-Sendon, J.; Mosca, L.; Tardif, J.C.; Waters, D.D.; *et al.* Effects of torcetrapib in patients at high risk for coronary events. *N. Engl. J. Med.* **2007**, *357*, 2109–2122. [CrossRef] [PubMed]

9. Marsche, G.; Saemann, M.D.; Heinemann, A.; Holzer, M. Inflammation alters HDL composition and function: Implications for HDL-raising therapies. *Pharmacol. Ther.* **2013**, *137*, 341–351. [CrossRef] [PubMed]

10. Shah, P.K. Atherosclerosis: Targeting endogenous apo AI—A new approach for raising HDL. *Nat. Rev. Cardiol.* **2011**, *8*, 187–188. [CrossRef] [PubMed]

11. Holleboom, A.G.; Jakulj, L.; Franssen, R.; Decaris, J.; Vergeer, M.; Koetsveld, J.; Luchoomun, J.; Glass, A.; Hellerstein, M.K.; Kastelein, J.J.; *et al. In vivo* tissue cholesterol efflux is reduced in carriers of a mutation in APOA1. *J. Lipid Res.* **2013**, *54*, 1964–1971. [CrossRef] [PubMed]

12. Umemoto, T.; Han, C.Y.; Mitra, P.; Averill, M.M.; Tang, C.; Goodspeed, L.; Omer, M.; Subramanian, S.; Wang, S.; den Hartigh, L.J.; *et al.* Apolipoprotein AI and high-density lipoprotein have anti-inflammatory effects on adipocytes via cholesterol transporters: ATP-binding cassette A-1, ATP-binding cassette G-1, and scavenger receptor B-1. *Circ. Res.* **2013**, *112*, 1345–1354. [CrossRef] [PubMed]

13. Navab, M.; Reddy, S.T.; van Lenten, B.J.; Fogelman, A.M. HDL and cardiovascular disease: Atherogenic and atheroprotective mechanisms. *Nat. Rev. Cardiol.* **2011**, *8*, 222–232. [CrossRef] [PubMed]

14. Hewing, B.; Parathath, S.; Barrett, T.; Chung, W.K.; Astudillo, Y.M.; Hamada, T.; Ramkhelawon, B.; Tallant, T.C.; Yusufishaq, M.S.; Didonato, J.A.; *et al.* Effects of native and myeloperoxidase-modified apolipoprotein A-I on reverse cholesterol transport and atherosclerosis in mice. *Arterioscler. Thromb. Vasc. Biol.* **2014**, *34*, 779–789. [CrossRef] [PubMed]

15. Rader, D.J.; Alexander, E.T.; Weibel, G.L.; Billheimer, J.; Rothblat, G.H. The role of reverse cholesterol transport in animals and humans and relationship to atherosclerosis. *J. Lipid Res.* **2009**, *50*, S189–S194. [CrossRef] [PubMed]

16. Hartman, J.; Frishman, W.H. Inflammation and atherosclerosis: A review of the role of interleukin-6 in the development of atherosclerosis and the potential for targeted drug therapy. *Cardiol. Rev.* **2014**, *22*, 147–151. [CrossRef] [PubMed]

17. Glass, C.K.; Witztum, J.L. Atherosclerosis. The road ahead. *Cell* **2001**, *104*, 503–516. [CrossRef]

18. Libby, P. Inflammation in atherosclerosis. *Nature* **2002**, *420*, 868–874. [CrossRef] [PubMed]

19. Prasad, V.; Bonow, R.O. The cardiovascular biomarker conundrum: Challenges and solutions. *JAMA* **2011**, *306*, 2151–2152. [CrossRef] [PubMed]

20. The AIM-HIGH Investigators. The role of niacin in raising high-density lipoprotein cholesterol to reduce cardiovascular events in patients with atherosclerotic cardiovascular disease and optimally treated low-density lipoprotein cholesterol: baseline characteristics of study participants. The Atherothrombosis Intervention in Metabolic syndrome with low HDL/high triglycerides: Impact on Global Health outcomes (AIM-HIGH) trial. *Am. Heart J.* **2011**, *161*, 538–543.

21. Boden, W.E.; Probstfield, J.L.; Anderson, T.; Chaitman, B.R.; Desvignes-Nickens, P.; Koprowicz, K.; McBride, R.; Teo, K.; Weintraub, W. Niacin in patients with low HDL cholesterol levels receiving intensive statin therapy. *N. Engl. J. Med.* **2011**, *365*, 2255–2267. [PubMed]

22. Li, C.; Zhang, W.; Zhou, F.; Chen, C.; Zhou, L.; Li, Y.; Liu, L.; Pei, F.; Luo, H.; Hu, Z.; *et al.* Cholesteryl ester transfer protein inhibitors in the treatment of dyslipidemia: A systematic review and meta-analysis. *PLoS ONE* **2013**, *8*, e77049. [CrossRef] [PubMed]

23. Boekholdt, S.M.; Arsenault, B.J.; Hovingh, G.K.; Mora, S.; Pedersen, T.R.; Larosa, J.C.; Welch, K.M.; Amarenco, P.; Demicco, D.A.; Tonkin, A.M.; *et al.* Levels and changes of HDL cholesterol and apolipoprotein A-I in relation to risk of cardiovascular events among statin-treated patients: A meta-analysis. *Circulation* **2013**, *128*, 1504–1512. [CrossRef] [PubMed]

24. Keene, D.; Price, C.; Shun-Shin, M.J.; Francis, D.P. Effect on cardiovascular risk of high density lipoprotein targeted drug treatments niacin, fibrates, and CETP inhibitors: Meta-analysis of randomised controlled trials including 117,411 patients. *BMJ* **2014**, *349*, g4379. [CrossRef] [PubMed]

25. Voight, B.F.; Peloso, G.M.; Orho-Melander, M.; Frikke-Schmidt, R.; Barbalic, M.; Jensen, M.K.; Hindy, G.; Holm, H.; Ding, E.L.; Johnson, T.; *et al.* Plasma HDL cholesterol and risk of myocardial infarction: a mendelian randomisation study. *Lancet* **2012**, *380*, 572–580. [CrossRef]

26. Saely, C.H.; Vonbank, A.; Drexel, H. HDL cholesterol and residual risk of first cardiovascular events. *Lancet* **2010**, *376*, 1738–1739. [CrossRef]

27. Mora, S.; Glynn, R.J.; Boekholdt, S.M.; Nordestgaard, B.G.; Kastelein, J.J.; Ridker, P.M. On-treatment non-high-density lipoprotein cholesterol, apolipoprotein B, triglycerides, and lipid ratios in relation to residual vascular risk after treatment with potent statin therapy: JUPITER (justification for the use of statins in prevention: An intervention trial evaluating rosuvastatin). *J. Am. Coll. Cardiol.* **2012**, *59*, 1521–1528. [PubMed]

28. Rye, K.A.; Bursill, C.A.; Lambert, G.; Tabet, F.; Barter, P.J. The metabolism and anti-atherogenic properties of HDL. *J. Lipid Res.* **2009**, *50*, S195–S200. [CrossRef] [PubMed]

29. Barter, P.; Kastelein, J.; Nunn, A.; Hobbs, R. High density lipoproteins (HDLs) and atherosclerosis: The unanswered questions. *Atherosclerosis* **2003**, *168*, 195–211. [CrossRef]

30. Arsenault, B.J.; Lemieux, I.; Despres, J.P.; Gagnon, P.; Wareham, N.J.; Stroes, E.S.; Kastelein, J.J.; Khaw, K.T.; Boekholdt, S.M. HDL particle size and the risk of coronary heart disease in apparently healthy men and women: the EPIC-Norfolk prospective population study. *Atherosclerosis* **2009**, *206*, 276–281. [CrossRef] [PubMed]

31. Azevedo, C.H.; Wajngarten, M.; Prete, A.C.; Diament, J.; Maranhao, R.C. Simultaneous transfer of cholesterol, triglycerides, and phospholipids to high-density lipoprotein in aging subjects with or without coronary artery disease. *Clinics* **2011**, *66*, 1543–1548. [PubMed]

32. Pascot, A.; Lemieux, I.; Prud'Homme, D.; Tremblay, A.; Nadeau, A.; Couillard, C.; Bergeron, J.; Lamarche, B.; Despres, J.P. Reduced HDL particle size as an additional feature of the atherogenic dyslipidemia of abdominal obesity. *J. Lipid Res.* **2001**, *42*, 2007–2014. [PubMed]

33. Du, X.M.; Kim, M.J.; Hou, L.; le Goff, W.; Chapman, M.J.; van Eck, M.; Curtiss, L.K.; Burnett, J.R.; Cartland, S.P.; Quinn, C.M.; *et al.* HDL particle size is a critical determinant of ABCA1-mediated macrophage cellular cholesterol export. *Circ. Res.* **2015**, *116*, 1133–1142. [PubMed]

34. Kim, D.S.; Burt, A.A.; Rosenthal, E.A.; Ranchalis, J.E.; Eintracht, J.F.; Hatsukami, T.S.; Furlong, C.E.; Marcovina, S.; Albers, J.J.; Jarvik, G.P. HDL-3 is a superior predictor of carotid artery disease in a case-control cohort of 1725 participants. *J. Am. Heart Assoc.* **2014**, *3*, e902. [CrossRef] [PubMed]

35. Ridker, P.M.; Genest, J.; Boekholdt, S.M.; Libby, P.; Gotto, A.M.; Nordestgaard, B.G.; Mora, S.; MacFadyen, J.G.; Glynn, R.J.; Kastelein, J.J. HDL cholesterol and residual risk of first cardiovascular events after treatment with potent statin therapy: An analysis from the JUPITER trial. *Lancet* **2010**, *376*, 333–339. [CrossRef]

36. Mora, S.; Glynn, R.J.; Ridker, P.M. High-density lipoprotein cholesterol, size, particle number, and residual vascular risk after potent statin therapy. *Circulation* **2013**, *128*, 1189–1197. [CrossRef] [PubMed]

37. El, H.K.; Arsenault, B.J.; Franssen, R.; Despres, J.P.; Hovingh, G.K.; Stroes, E.S.; Otvos, J.D.; Wareham, N.J.; Kastelein, J.J.; Khaw, K.T.; *et al.* High-density lipoprotein particle size and concentration and coronary risk. *Ann. Intern. Med.* **2009**, *150*, 84–93.

38. Mora, S.; Otvos, J.D.; Rifai, N.; Rosenson, R.S.; Buring, J.E.; Ridker, P.M. Lipoprotein particle profiles by nuclear magnetic resonance compared with standard lipids and apolipoproteins in predicting incident cardiovascular disease in women. *Circulation* **2009**, *119*, 931–939. [CrossRef] [PubMed]

39. Ala-Korpela, M.; Soininen, P.; Savolainen, M.J. Letter by Ala-Korpela et al regarding article, "Lipoprotein particle profiles by nuclear magnetic resonance compared with standard lipids and apolipoproteins in predicting incident cardiovascular disease in women". *Circulation* **2009**, *120*, e149–e150. [CrossRef] [PubMed]

40. Hutchins, P.M.; Ronsein, G.E.; Monette, J.S.; Pamir, N.; Wimberger, J.; He, Y.; Anantharamaiah, G.M.; Kim, D.S.; Ranchalis, J.E.; Jarvik, G.P.; *et al.* Quantification of HDL particle concentration by calibrated ion mobility analysis. *Clin. Chem.* **2014**, *60*, 1393–1401. [CrossRef] [PubMed]

41. Dahlback, B.; Nielsen, L.B. Apolipoprotein M—A novel player in high-density lipoprotein metabolism and atherosclerosis. *Curr. Opin. Lipidol.* **2006**, *17*, 291–295. [CrossRef] [PubMed]

42. Elsoe, S.; Christoffersen, C.; Luchoomun, J.; Turner, S.; Nielsen, L.B. Apolipoprotein M promotes mobilization of cellular cholesterol *in vivo*. *Biochim. Biophys. Acta* **2013**, *1831*, 1287–1292. [CrossRef] [PubMed]

43. Wolfrum, C.; Poy, M.N.; Stoffel, M. Apolipoprotein M is required for prebeta-HDL formation and cholesterol efflux to HDL and protects against atherosclerosis. *Nat. Med.* **2005**, *11*, 418–422. [CrossRef] [PubMed]

44. Su, W.; Jiao, G.; Yang, C.; Ye, Y. Evaluation of apolipoprotein M as a biomarker of coronary artery disease. *Clin. Biochem.* **2009**, *42*, 365–370. [CrossRef] [PubMed]

45. Borup, A.; Christensen, P.M.; Nielsen, L.B.; Christoffersen, C. Apolipoprotein M in lipid metabolism and cardiometabolic diseases. *Curr. Opin. Lipidol.* **2015**, *26*, 48–55. [CrossRef] [PubMed]

46. Brea, D.; Sobrino, T.; Blanco, M.; Fraga, M.; Agulla, J.; Rodriguez-Yanez, M.; Rodriguez-Gonzalez, R.; Perez, D.L.O.N.; Leira, R.; Forteza, J.; *et al.* Usefulness of haptoglobin and serum amyloid A proteins as biomarkers for atherothrombotic ischemic stroke diagnosis confirmation. *Atherosclerosis* **2009**, *205*, 561–567. [CrossRef] [PubMed]

47. King, V.L.; Thompson, J.; Tannock, L.R. Serum amyloid A in atherosclerosis. *Curr. Opin. Lipidol.* **2011**, *22*, 302–307. [CrossRef] [PubMed]

48. Liuzzo, G.; Biasucci, L.M.; Gallimore, J.R.; Grillo, R.L.; Rebuzzi, A.G.; Pepys, M.B.; Maseri, A. The prognostic value of C-reactive protein and serum amyloid a protein in severe unstable angina. *N. Engl. J. Med.* **1994**, *331*, 417–424. [CrossRef] [PubMed]

49. Delanghe, J.R.; Langlois, M.R.; de Bacquer, D.; Mak, R.; Capel, P.; van Renterghem, L.; de Backer, G. Discriminative value of serum amyloid A and other acute-phase proteins for coronary heart disease. *Atherosclerosis* **2002**, *160*, 471–476. [CrossRef]

50. Lepedda, A.J.; Nieddu, G.; Zinellu, E.; de Muro, P.; Piredda, F.; Guarino, A.; Spirito, R.; Carta, F.; Turrini, F.; Formato, M. Proteomic analysis of plasma-purified VLDL, LDL, and HDL fractions from atherosclerotic patients undergoing carotid endarterectomy: Identification of serum amyloid A as a potential marker. *Oxid. Med. Cell. Longev.* **2013**, *2013*, 385214. [CrossRef] [PubMed]

51. McMahon, M.; Grossman, J.; FitzGerald, J.; Dahlin-Lee, E.; Wallace, D.J.; Thong, B.Y.; Badsha, H.; Kalunian, K.; Charles, C.; Navab, M.; *et al.* Proinflammatory high-density lipoprotein as a biomarker for atherosclerosis in patients with systemic lupus erythematosus and rheumatoid arthritis. *Arthritis Rheum.* **2006**, *54*, 2541–2549. [CrossRef] [PubMed]

52. Fung, E.T.; Thulasiraman, V.; Weinberger, S.R.; Dalmasso, E.A. Protein biochips for differential profiling. *Curr. Opin. Biotechnol.* **2001**, *12*, 65–69. [CrossRef]

53. Issaq, H.J.; Veenstra, T.D.; Conrads, T.P.; Felschow, D. The SELDI-TOF MS approach to proteomics: Protein profiling and biomarker identification. *Biochem. Biophys. Res. Commun.* **2002**, *292*, 587–592. [CrossRef] [PubMed]

54. Watanabe, J.; Chou, K.J.; Liao, J.C.; Miao, Y.; Meng, H.H.; Ge, H.; Grijalva, V.; Hama, S.; Kozak, K.; Buga, G.; *et al.* Differential association of hemoglobin with proinflammatory high density lipoproteins in atherogenic/hyperlipidemic mice. A novel biomarker of atherosclerosis. *J. Biol. Chem.* **2007**, *282*, 23698–23707. [CrossRef] [PubMed]

55. Frohlich, J.; Al-Sarraf, A. Cholesterol efflux capacity and atherosclerosis. *N. Engl. J. Med.* **2011**, *364*, 1474–1475. [PubMed]

56. Uto-Kondo, H.; Ayaori, M.; Ogura, M.; Nakaya, K.; Ito, M.; Suzuki, A.; Takiguchi, S.; Yakushiji, E.; Terao, Y.; Ozasa, H.; *et al.* Coffee consumption enhances high-density lipoprotein-mediated cholesterol efflux in macrophages. *Circ. Res.* **2010**, *106*, 779–787. [CrossRef] [PubMed]

57. Oram, J.F.; Lawn, R.M.; Garvin, M.R.; Wade, D.P. ABCA1 is the cAMP-inducible apolipoprotein receptor that mediates cholesterol secretion from macrophages. *J. Biol. Chem.* **2000**, *275*, 34508–34511. [CrossRef] [PubMed]

58. Santamarina-Fojo, S.; Peterson, K.; Knapper, C.; Qiu, Y.; Freeman, L.; Cheng, J.F.; Osorio, J.; Remaley, A.; Yang, X.P.; Haudenschild, C.; *et al.* Complete genomic sequence of the human ABCA1 gene: analysis of the human and mouse ATP-binding cassette A promoter. *Proc. Natl. Acad. Sci. USA* **2000**, *97*, 7987–7992. [CrossRef] [PubMed]

59. Wang, N.; Lan, D.; Chen, W.; Matsuura, F.; Tall, A.R. ATP-binding cassette transporters G1 and G4 mediate cellular cholesterol efflux to high-density lipoproteins. *Proc. Natl. Acad. Sci. USA* **2004**, *101*, 9774–9779. [CrossRef] [PubMed]

60. Nakamura, K.; Kennedy, M.A.; Baldan, A.; Bojanic, D.D.; Lyons, K.; Edwards, P.A. Expression and regulation of multiple murine ATP-binding cassette transporter G1 mRNAs/isoforms that stimulate cellular cholesterol efflux to high density lipoprotein. *J. Biol. Chem.* **2004**, *279*, 45980–45989. [CrossRef] [PubMed]

61. Yancey, P.G.; Bortnick, A.E.; Kellner-Weibel, G.; de la Llera-Moya, M.; Phillips, M.C.; Rothblat, G.H. Importance of different pathways of cellular cholesterol efflux. *Arterioscler. Thromb. Vasc. Biol.* **2003**, *23*, 712–719. [CrossRef] [PubMed]

62. Dikkers, A.; Freak, D.B.J.; Annema, W.; Groen, A.K.; Tietge, U.J. Scavenger receptor BI and ABCG5/G8 differentially impact biliary sterol secretion and reverse cholesterol transport in mice. *Hepatology* **2013**, *58*, 293–303. [CrossRef] [PubMed]

63. Von Eckardstein, A.; Nofer, J.R.; Assmann, G. High density lipoproteins and arteriosclerosis. Role of cholesterol efflux and reverse cholesterol transport. *Arterioscler. Thromb. Vasc. Biol.* **2001**, *21*, 13–27. [CrossRef] [PubMed]

64. Rosenson, R.S.; Brewer, H.J.; Davidson, W.S.; Fayad, Z.A.; Fuster, V.; Goldstein, J.; Hellerstein, M.; Jiang, X.C.; Phillips, M.C.; Rader, D.J.; *et al.* Cholesterol efflux and atheroprotection: Advancing the concept of reverse cholesterol transport. *Circulation* **2012**, *125*, 1905–1919. [CrossRef] [PubMed]

65. Joy, T.; Hegele, R.A. The end of the road for CETP inhibitors after torcetrapib? *Curr. Opin. Cardiol.* **2009**, *24*, 364–371. [CrossRef] [PubMed]

66. Wang, N.; Tall, A.R. Regulation and mechanisms of ATP-binding cassette transporter A1-mediated cellular cholesterol efflux. *Arterioscler. Thromb. Vasc. Biol.* **2003**, *23*, 1178–1184. [CrossRef] [PubMed]

67. Curtiss, L.K.; Valenta, D.T.; Hime, N.J.; Rye, K.A. What is so special about apolipoprotein AI in reverse cholesterol transport? *Arterioscler. Thromb. Vasc. Biol.* **2006**, *26*, 12–19. [CrossRef] [PubMed]

68. Kontush, A.; Chapman, M.J. Functionally defective high-density lipoprotein: A new therapeutic target at the crossroads of dyslipidemia, inflammation, and atherosclerosis. *Pharmacol. Rev.* **2006**, *58*, 342–374. [CrossRef] [PubMed]

69. Freeman, S.R.; Jin, X.; Anzinger, J.J.; Xu, Q.; Purushothaman, S.; Fessler, M.B.; Addadi, L.; Kruth, H.S. ABCG1-mediated generation of extracellular cholesterol microdomains. *J. Lipid Res.* **2014**, *55*, 115–127. [CrossRef] [PubMed]

70. Song, G.J.; Kim, S.M.; Park, K.H.; Kim, J.; Choi, I.; Cho, K.H. SR-BI mediates high density lipoprotein (HDL)-induced anti-inflammatory effect in macrophages. *Biochem. Biophys. Res. Commun.* **2015**, *457*, 112–118. [CrossRef] [PubMed]

71. Wang, X.; Collins, H.L.; Ranalletta, M.; Fuki, I.V.; Billheimer, J.T.; Rothblat, G.H.; Tall, A.R.; Rader, D.J. Macrophage ABCA1 and ABCG1, but not SR-BI, promote macrophage reverse cholesterol transport *in vivo*. *J. Clin. Investig.* **2007**, *117*, 2216–2224. [CrossRef] [PubMed]

72. Daniil, G.; Zannis, V.I.; Chroni, A. Effect of apoA-I Mutations in the capacity of reconstituted HDL to promote ABCG1-mediated cholesterol efflux. *PLoS ONE* **2013**, *8*, e67993. [CrossRef] [PubMed]

73. Westerterp, M.; Murphy, A.J.; Wang, M.; Pagler, T.A.; Vengrenyuk, Y.; Kappus, M.S.; Gorman, D.J.; Nagareddy, P.R.; Zhu, X.; Abramowicz, S.; *et al.* Deficiency of ATP-binding cassette transporters A1 and G1 in macrophages increases inflammation and accelerates atherosclerosis in mice. *Circ. Res.* **2013**, *112*, 1456–1465. [CrossRef] [PubMed]

74. Bultel, S.; Helin, L.; Clavey, V.; Chinetti-Gbaguidi, G.; Rigamonti, E.; Colin, M.; Fruchart, J.C.; Staels, B.; Lestavel, S. Liver X receptor activation induces the uptake of cholesteryl esters from high density lipoproteins in primary human macrophages. *Arterioscler. Thromb. Vasc. Biol.* **2008**, *28*, 2288–2295. [CrossRef] [PubMed]

75. Hanf, R.; Millatt, L.J.; Cariou, B.; Noel, B.; Rigou, G.; Delataille, P.; Daix, V.; Hum, D.W.; Staels, B. The dual peroxisome proliferator-activated receptor α/δ agonist GFT505 exerts anti-diabetic effects in db/db mice without peroxisome proliferator-activated receptor gamma-associated adverse cardiac effects. *Diabetes Vasc. Dis. Res.* **2014**, *11*, 440–447. [CrossRef] [PubMed]

76. Colin, S.; Briand, O.; Touche, V.; Wouters, K.; Baron, M.; Pattou, F.; Hanf, R.; Tailleux, A.; Chinetti, G.; Staels, B.; et al. Activation of intestinal peroxisome proliferator-activated receptor-α increases high-density lipoprotein production. *Eur. Heart J.* **2013**, *34*, 2566–2574. [CrossRef] [PubMed]

77. Sahebkar, A.; Chew, G.T.; Watts, G.F. New peroxisome proliferator-activated receptor agonists: Potential treatments for atherogenic dyslipidemia and non-alcoholic fatty liver disease. *Expert Opin. Pharmacother.* **2014**, *15*, 493–503. [CrossRef] [PubMed]

78. Rousset, X.; Shamburek, R.; Vaisman, B.; Amar, M.; Remaley, A.T. Lecithin cholesterol acyltransferase: An anti- or pro-atherogenic factor? *Curr. Atheroscler. Rep.* **2011**, *13*, 249–256. [CrossRef] [PubMed]

79. Soran, H.; Hama, S.; Yadav, R.; Durrington, P.N. HDL functionality. *Curr. Opin. Lipidol.* **2012**, *23*, 353–366. [CrossRef] [PubMed]

80. Olivecrona, G.; Olivecrona, T. Triglyceride lipases and atherosclerosis. *Curr. Opin. Lipidol.* **2010**, *21*, 409–415. [CrossRef] [PubMed]

81. Chatterjee, C.; Sparks, D.L. Hepatic lipase, high density lipoproteins, and hypertriglyceridemia. *Am. J. Pathol.* **2011**, *178*, 1429–1433. [CrossRef] [PubMed]

82. Yasuda, T.; Ishida, T.; Rader, D.J. Update on the role of endothelial lipase in high-density lipoprotein metabolism, reverse cholesterol transport, and atherosclerosis. *Circ. J.* **2010**, *74*, 2263–2270. [CrossRef] [PubMed]

83. Annema, W.; Tietge, U.J. Role of hepatic lipase and endothelial lipase in high-density lipoprotein-mediated reverse cholesterol transport. *Curr. Atheroscler. Rep.* **2011**, *13*, 257–265. [CrossRef] [PubMed]

84. Ishida, T.; Choi, S.; Kundu, R.K.; Hirata, K.; Rubin, E.M.; Cooper, A.D.; Quertermous, T. Endothelial lipase is a major determinant of HDL level. *J. Clin. Investig.* **2003**, *111*, 347–355. [CrossRef] [PubMed]

85. Ruel, I.L.; Couture, P.; Cohn, J.S.; Bensadoun, A.; Marcil, M.; Lamarche, B. Evidence that hepatic lipase deficiency in humans is not associated with proatherogenic changes in HDL composition and metabolism. *J. Lipid Res.* **2004**, *45*, 1528–1537. [CrossRef] [PubMed]

86. Lambert, G.; Amar, M.J.; Martin, P.; Fruchart-Najib, J.; Foger, B.; Shamburek, R.D.; Brewer, H.J.; Santamarina-Fojo, S. Hepatic lipase deficiency decreases the selective uptake of HDL-cholesteryl esters *in vivo*. *J. Lipid Res.* **2000**, *41*, 667–672. [PubMed]

87. Jaye, M.; Lynch, K.J.; Krawiec, J.; Marchadier, D.; Maugeais, C.; Doan, K.; South, V.; Amin, D.; Perrone, M.; Rader, D.J. A novel endothelial-derived lipase that modulates HDL metabolism. *Nat. Genet.* **1999**, *21*, 424–428. [PubMed]

88. Escola-Gil, J.C.; Chen, X.; Julve, J.; Quesada, H.; Santos, D.; Metso, J.; Tous, M.; Jauhiainen, M.; Blanco-Vaca, F. Hepatic lipase- and endothelial lipase-deficiency in mice promotes macrophage-to-feces RCT and HDL antioxidant properties. *Biochim. Biophys. Acta* **2013**, *1831*, 691–697. [CrossRef] [PubMed]

89. Zhang, L.; Yan, F.; Zhang, S.; Lei, D.; Charles, M.A.; Cavigiolio, G.; Oda, M.; Krauss, R.M.; Weisgraber, K.H.; Rye, K.A.; et al. Structural basis of transfer between lipoproteins by cholesteryl ester transfer protein. *Nat. Chem. Biol.* **2012**, *8*, 342–349. [CrossRef] [PubMed]

90. Chapman, M.J.; le Goff, W.; Guerin, M.; Kontush, A. Cholesteryl ester transfer protein: At the heart of the action of lipid-modulating therapy with statins, fibrates, niacin, and cholesteryl ester transfer protein inhibitors. *Eur. Heart J.* **2010**, *31*, 149–164. [CrossRef] [PubMed]

91. Rao, R.; Albers, J.J.; Wolfbauer, G.; Pownall, H.J. Molecular and macromolecular specificity of human plasma phospholipid transfer protein. *Biochemistry* **1997**, *36*, 3645–3653. [CrossRef] [PubMed]

92. Yu, Y.; Guo, S.; Feng, Y.; Feng, L.; Cui, Y.; Song, G.; Luo, T.; Zhang, K.; Wang, Y.; Jiang, X.C.; et al. Phospholipid transfer protein deficiency decreases the content of S1P in HDL via the loss of its transfer capability. *Lipids* **2014**, *49*, 183–190. [CrossRef] [PubMed]

93. Albers, J.J.; Vuletic, S.; Cheung, M.C. Role of plasma phospholipid transfer protein in lipid and lipoprotein metabolism. *Biochim. Biophys. Acta* **2012**, *1821*, 345–357. [CrossRef] [PubMed]

94. Jiang, X.C.; Bruce, C.; Mar, J.; Lin, M.; Ji, Y.; Francone, O.L.; Tall, A.R. Targeted mutation of plasma phospholipid transfer protein gene markedly reduces high-density lipoprotein levels. *J. Clin. Investig.* **1999**, *103*, 907–914. [CrossRef] [PubMed]

95. Yazdanyar, A.; Quan, W.; Jin, W.; Jiang, X.C. Liver-specific phospholipid transfer protein deficiency reduces high-density lipoprotein and non-high-density lipoprotein production in mice. *Arterioscler. Thromb. Vasc. Biol.* **2013**, *33*, 2058–2064. [CrossRef] [PubMed]

96. Jiang, X.C.; Qin, S.; Qiao, C.; Kawano, K.; Lin, M.; Skold, A.; Xiao, X.; Tall, A.R. Apolipoprotein B secretion and atherosclerosis are decreased in mice with phospholipid-transfer protein deficiency. *Nat. Med.* **2001**, *7*, 847–852. [CrossRef] [PubMed]

97. Luo, Y.; Shelly, L.; Sand, T.; Reidich, B.; Chang, G.; Macdougall, M.; Peakman, M.C.; Jiang, X.C. Pharmacologic inhibition of phospholipid transfer protein activity reduces apolipoprotein-B secretion from hepatocytes. *J. Pharmacol. Exp. Ther.* **2010**, *332*, 1100–1106. [CrossRef] [PubMed]

98. Rinninger, F.; Heine, M.; Singaraja, R.; Hayden, M.; Brundert, M.; Ramakrishnan, R.; Heeren, J. High density lipoprotein metabolism in low density lipoprotein receptor-deficient mice. *J. Lipid Res.* **2014**, *55*, 1914–1924. [CrossRef] [PubMed]

99. Van der Velde, A.E.; Vrins, C.L.; van den Oever, K.; Kunne, C.; Oude, E.R.; Kuipers, F.; Groen, A.K. Direct intestinal cholesterol secretion contributes significantly to total fecal neutral sterol excretion in mice. *Gastroenterology* **2007**, *133*, 967–975. [CrossRef] [PubMed]

100. Van der Velde, A.E.; Brufau, G.; Groen, A.K. Transintestinal cholesterol efflux. *Curr. Opin. Lipidol.* **2010**, *21*, 167–171. [CrossRef] [PubMed]

101. Blanchard, C.; Moreau, F.; Cariou, B.; Le May, C. Trans-intestinal cholesterol excretion (TICE): A new route for cholesterol excretion. *Med. Sci.* **2014**, *30*, 896–901.

102. Vrins, C.L.; van der Velde, A.E.; van den Oever, K.; Levels, J.H.; Huet, S.; Oude, E.R.; Kuipers, F.; Groen, A.K. Peroxisome proliferator-activated receptor delta activation leads to increased transintestinal cholesterol efflux. *J. Lipid Res.* **2009**, *50*, 2046–2054. [CrossRef] [PubMed]

103. Vrins, C.L.; Ottenhoff, R.; van den Oever, K.; de Waart, D.R.; Kruyt, J.K.; Zhao, Y.; van Berkel, T.J.; Havekes, L.M.; Aerts, J.M.; van Eck, M.; *et al.* Trans-intestinal cholesterol efflux is not mediated through high density lipoprotein. *J. Lipid Res.* **2012**, *53*, 2017–2023. [CrossRef] [PubMed]

104. Kontush, A.; Chantepie, S.; Chapman, M.J. Small, dense HDL particles exert potent protection of atherogenic LDL against oxidative stress. *Arterioscler. Thromb. Vasc. Biol.* **2003**, *23*, 1881–1888. [CrossRef] [PubMed]

105. Kontush, A.; Chapman, M.J. Antiatherogenic function of HDL particle subpopulations: Focus on antioxidative activities. *Curr. Opin. Lipidol.* **2010**, *21*, 312–318. [CrossRef] [PubMed]

106. Mackness, B.; Mackness, M. The antioxidant properties of high-density lipoproteins in atherosclerosis. *Panminerva Med.* **2012**, *54*, 83–90. [PubMed]

107. Vohl, M.C.; Neville, T.A.; Kumarathasan, R.; Braschi, S.; Sparks, D.L. A novel lecithin-cholesterol acyltransferase antioxidant activity prevents the formation of oxidized lipids during lipoprotein oxidation. *Biochemistry* **1999**, *38*, 5976–5981. [CrossRef] [PubMed]

108. Navab, M.; Hama, S.Y.; Anantharamaiah, G.M.; Hassan, K.; Hough, G.P.; Watson, A.D.; Reddy, S.T.; Sevanian, A.; Fonarow, G.C.; Fogelman, A.M. Normal high density lipoprotein inhibits three steps in the formation of mildly oxidized low density lipoprotein: Steps 2 and 3. *J. Lipid Res.* **2000**, *41*, 1495–1508. [PubMed]

109. Turunen, P.; Jalkanen, J.; Heikura, T.; Puhakka, H.; Karppi, J.; Nyyssonen, K.; Yla-Herttuala, S. Adenovirus-mediated gene transfer of Lp-PLA2 reduces LDL degradation and foam cell formation *in vitro*. *J. Lipid Res.* **2004**, *45*, 1633–1639. [CrossRef] [PubMed]

110. Chen, N.; Liu, Y.; Greiner, C.D.; Holtzman, J.L. Physiologic concentrations of homocysteine inhibit the human plasma GSH peroxidase that reduces organic hydroperoxides. *J. Lab. Clin. Med.* **2000**, *136*, 58–65. [CrossRef] [PubMed]

111. Besler, C.; Heinrich, K.; Rohrer, L.; Doerries, C.; Riwanto, M.; Shih, D.M.; Chroni, A.; Yonekawa, K.; Stein, S.; Schaefer, N.; *et al.* Mechanisms underlying adverse effects of HDL on eNOS-activating pathways in patients with coronary artery disease. *J. Clin. Investig.* **2011**, *121*, 2693–2708. [CrossRef] [PubMed]

112. Sorrentino, S.A.; Besler, C.; Rohrer, L.; Meyer, M.; Heinrich, K.; Bahlmann, F.H.; Mueller, M.; Horvath, T.; Doerries, C.; Heinemann, M.; *et al.* Endothelial-vasoprotective effects of high-density lipoprotein are impaired in patients with type 2 diabetes mellitus but are improved after extended-release niacin therapy. *Circulation* **2010**, *121*, 110–122. [CrossRef] [PubMed]

113. Levine, D.M.; Parker, T.S.; Donnelly, T.M.; Walsh, A.; Rubin, A.L. *In vivo* protection against endotoxin by plasma high density lipoprotein. *Proc. Natl. Acad. Sci. USA* **1993**, *90*, 12040–12044. [CrossRef] [PubMed]

114. Nissen, S.E.; Tsunoda, T.; Tuzcu, E.M.; Schoenhagen, P.; Cooper, C.J.; Yasin, M.; Eaton, G.M.; Lauer, M.A.; Sheldon, W.S.; Grines, C.L.; *et al.* Effect of recombinant ApoA-I Milano on coronary atherosclerosis in patients with acute coronary syndromes: A randomized controlled trial. *JAMA* **2003**, *290*, 2292–2300. [CrossRef] [PubMed]

115. Ibanez, B.; Giannarelli, C.; Cimmino, G.; Santos-Gallego, C.G.; Alique, M.; Pinero, A.; Vilahur, G.; Fuster, V.; Badimon, L.; Badimon, J.J. Recombinant HDL(Milano) exerts greater anti-inflammatory and plaque stabilizing properties than HDL(wild-type). *Atherosclerosis* **2012**, *220*, 72–77. [CrossRef] [PubMed]

116. Tardy, C.; Goffinet, M.; Boubekeur, N.; Ackermann, R.; Sy, G.; Bluteau, A.; Cholez, G.; Keyserling, C.; Lalwani, N.; Paolini, J.F.; *et al.* CER-001, a HDL-mimetic, stimulates the reverse lipid transport and atherosclerosis regression in high cholesterol diet-fed LDL-receptor deficient mice. *Atherosclerosis* **2014**, *232*, 110–118. [CrossRef] [PubMed]

117. Tardif, J.C.; Ballantyne, C.M.; Barter, P.; Dasseux, J.L.; Fayad, Z.A.; Guertin, M.C.; Kastelein, J.J.; Keyserling, C.; Klepp, H.; Koenig, W.; *et al.* Effects of the high-density lipoprotein mimetic agent CER-001 on coronary atherosclerosis in patients with acute coronary syndromes: A randomized trial. *Eur. Heart J.* **2014**, *35*, 3277–3286. [CrossRef] [PubMed]

118. Murphy, A.J.; Funt, S.; Gorman, D.; Tall, A.R.; Wang, N. Pegylation of high-density lipoprotein decreases plasma clearance and enhances antiatherogenic activity. *Circ. Res.* **2013**, *113*, e1–e9. [CrossRef] [PubMed]

119. Waksman, R.; Torguson, R.; Kent, K.M.; Pichard, A.D.; Suddath, W.O.; Satler, L.F.; Martin, B.D.; Perlman, T.J.; Maltais, J.A.; Weissman, N.J.; *et al.* A first-in-man, randomized, placebo-controlled study to evaluate the safety and feasibility of autologous delipidated high-density lipoprotein plasma infusions in patients with acute coronary syndrome. *J. Am. Coll. Cardiol.* **2010**, *55*, 2727–2735. [CrossRef] [PubMed]

120. Sacks, F.M.; Rudel, L.L.; Conner, A.; Akeefe, H.; Kostner, G.; Baki, T.; Rothblat, G.; de la Llera-Moya, M.; Asztalos, B.; Perlman, T.; *et al.* Selective delipidation of plasma HDL enhances reverse cholesterol transport *in vivo*. *J. Lipid Res.* **2009**, *50*, 894–907. [CrossRef] [PubMed]

121. Van Capelleveen, J.C.; Brewer, H.B.; Kastelein, J.J.; Hovingh, G.K. Novel therapies focused on the high-density lipoprotein particle. *Circ. Res.* **2014**, *114*, 193–204. [CrossRef] [PubMed]

122. Zhao, Y.; Imura, T.; Leman, L.J.; Curtiss, L.K.; Maryanoff, B.E.; Ghadiri, M.R. Mimicry of high-density lipoprotein: Functional peptide-lipid nanoparticles based on multivalent peptide constructs. *J. Am. Chem. Soc.* **2013**, *135*, 13414–13424. [CrossRef] [PubMed]

123. Joseph, S.B.; Castrillo, A.; Laffitte, B.A.; Mangelsdorf, D.J.; Tontonoz, P. Reciprocal regulation of inflammation and lipid metabolism by liver X receptors. *Nat. Med.* **2003**, *9*, 213–219. [CrossRef] [PubMed]

124. Lo, S.G.; Murzilli, S.; Salvatore, L.; D'Errico, I.; Petruzzelli, M.; Conca, P.; Jiang, Z.Y.; Calabresi, L.; Parini, P.; Moschetta, A. Intestinal specific LXR activation stimulates reverse cholesterol transport and protects from atherosclerosis. *Cell Metab.* **2010**, *12*, 187–193.

125. Bartel, D.P. MicroRNAs: Genomics, biogenesis, mechanism, and function. *Cell* **2004**, *116*, 281–297. [CrossRef]

126. Rayner, K.J.; Esau, C.C.; Hussain, F.N.; McDaniel, A.L.; Marshall, S.M.; van Gils, J.M.; Ray, T.D.; Sheedy, F.J.; Goedeke, L.; Liu, X.; *et al.* Inhibition of miR-33a/b in non-human primates raises plasma HDL and lowers VLDL triglycerides. *Nature* **2011**, *478*, 404–407. [CrossRef] [PubMed]

127. Zhao, R.; Feng, J.; He, G. miR-613 regulates cholesterol efflux by targeting LXRα and ABCA1 in PPARβ activated THP-1 macrophages. *Biochem. Biophys. Res. Commun.* **2014**, *448*, 329–334. [CrossRef] [PubMed]

128. Simonelli, S.; Tinti, C.; Salvini, L.; Tinti, L.; Ossoli, A.; Vitali, C.; Sousa, V.; Orsini, G.; Nolli, M.L.; Franceschini, G.; *et al.* Recombinant human LCAT normalizes plasma lipoprotein profile in LCAT deficiency. *Biologicals* **2013**, *41*, 446–449. [CrossRef] [PubMed]

129. Aguilar-Espinosa, S.L.; Mendoza-Espinosa, P.; Delgado-Coello, B.; Mas-Oliva, J. Lecithin cholesterol acyltransferase (LCAT) activity in the presence of Apo-AI-derived peptides exposed to disorder-order conformational transitions. *Biochem. Biophys. Res. Commun.* **2013**, *441*, 469–475. [CrossRef] [PubMed]

130. Barylski, M.; Toth, P.P.; Nikolic, D.; Banach, M.; Rizzo, M.; Montalto, G. Emerging therapies for raising high-density lipoprotein cholesterol (HDL-C) and augmenting HDL particle functionality. *Best Pract. Res. Clin. Endocrinol. Metab.* **2014**, *28*, 453–461. [CrossRef] [PubMed]

131. Barter, P.J.; Rye, K.A. Cholesteryl ester transfer protein inhibition as a strategy to reduce cardiovascular risk. *J. Lipid Res.* **2012**, *53*, 1755–1766. [CrossRef] [PubMed]

132. Mohammadpour, A.H.; Akhlaghi, F. Future of cholesteryl ester transfer protein (CETP) inhibitors: A pharmacological perspective. *Clin. Pharmacokinet.* **2013**, *52*, 615–626. [CrossRef] [PubMed]

133. Cao, G.; Beyer, T.P.; Zhang, Y.; Schmidt, R.J.; Chen, Y.Q.; Cockerham, S.L.; Zimmerman, K.M.; Karathanasis, S.K.; Cannady, E.A.; Fields, T.; *et al.* Evacetrapib is a novel, potent, and selective inhibitor of cholesteryl ester transfer protein that elevates HDL cholesterol without inducing aldosterone or increasing blood pressure. *J. Lipid Res.* **2011**, *52*, 2169–2176. [CrossRef] [PubMed]

134. Ford, J.; Lawson, M.; Fowler, D.; Maruyama, N.; Mito, S.; Tomiyasu, K.; Kinoshita, S.; Suzuki, C.; Kawaguchi, A.; Round, P.; *et al.* Tolerability, pharmacokinetics and pharmacodynamics of TA-8995, a selective cholesteryl ester transfer protein (CETP) inhibitor, in healthy subjects. *Br. J. Clin. Pharmacol.* **2014**, *78*, 498–508. [CrossRef] [PubMed]

135. Boettcher, M.F.; Heinig, R.; Schmeck, C.; Kohlsdorfer, C.; Ludwig, M.; Schaefer, A.; Gelfert-Peukert, S.; Wensing, G.; Weber, O. Single dose pharmacokinetics, pharmacodynamics, tolerability and safety of BAY 60–5521, a potent inhibitor of cholesteryl ester transfer protein. *Br. J. Clin. Pharmacol.* **2012**, *73*, 210–218. [CrossRef] [PubMed]

136. Bell, T.R.; Graham, M.J.; Lee, R.G.; Mullick, A.E.; Fu, W.; Norris, D.; Crooke, R.M. Antisense oligonucleotide inhibition of cholesteryl ester transfer protein enhances RCT in hyperlipidemic, CETP transgenic, LDLr$^{-/-}$ mice. *J. Lipid Res.* **2013**, *54*, 2647–2657. [CrossRef] [PubMed]

137. Hu, Z.; Shen, W.J.; Kraemer, F.B.; Azhar, S. MicroRNAs 125a and 455 repress lipoprotein-supported steroidogenesis by targeting scavenger receptor class B type I in steroidogenic cells. *Mol. Cell. Biol.* **2012**, *32*, 5035–5045. [CrossRef] [PubMed]

138. Wang, L.; Jia, X.J.; Jiang, H.J.; Du, Y.; Yang, F.; Si, S.Y.; Hong, B. MicroRNAs 185, 96, and 223 repress selective high-density lipoprotein cholesterol uptake through posttranscriptional inhibition. *Mol. Cell. Biol.* **2013**, *33*, 1956–1964. [CrossRef] [PubMed]

139. Sugano, M.; Fujikawa, T.; Hiratsuji, Y.; Nakashima, K.; Fukuda, N.; Hasegawa, Y. A novel use of chitosan as a hypocholesterolemic agent in rats. *Am. J. Clin. Nutr.* **1980**, *33*, 787–793. [PubMed]

140. Baker, W.L.; Tercius, A.; Anglade, M.; White, C.M.; Coleman, C.I. A meta-analysis evaluating the impact of chitosan on serum lipids in hypercholesterolemic patients. *Ann. Nutr. Metab.* **2009**, *55*, 368–374. [CrossRef] [PubMed]

141. Su, Z.Q.; Wu, S.H.; Zhang, H.L.; Feng, Y.F. Development and validation of an improved Bradford method for determination of insulin from chitosan nanoparticulate systems. *Pharm. Biol.* **2010**, *48*, 966–973. [CrossRef] [PubMed]

142. Tan, S.; Gao, B.; Tao, Y.; Guo, J.; Su, Z.Q. Antiobese effects of capsaicin-chitosan microsphere (CCMS) in obese rats induced by high fat diet. *J. Agric. Food Chem.* **2014**, *62*, 1866–1874. [CrossRef] [PubMed]

143. Chen, J.; Huang, G.D.; Tan, S.R.; Guo, J.; Su, Z.Q. The preparation of capsaicin-chitosan microspheres (CCMS) enteric coated tablets. *Int. J. Mol. Sci.* **2013**, *14*, 24305–24319. [CrossRef] [PubMed]

144. Tao, Y.; Zhang, H.L.; Hu, Y.M.; Wan, S.; Su, Z.Q. Preparation of chitosan and water-soluble chitosan microspheres via spray-drying method to lower blood lipids in rats fed with high-fat diets. *Int. J. Mol. Sci.* **2013**, *14*, 4174–4184. [CrossRef] [PubMed]

145. Pan, H.; Guo, J.; Su, Z. Advances in understanding the interrelations between leptin resistance and obesity. *Physiol. Behav.* **2014**, *130*, 157–169. [CrossRef] [PubMed]

146. Zhang, H.L.; Tao, Y.; Guo, J.; Hu, Y.M.; Su, Z.Q. Hypolipidemic effects of chitosan nanoparticles in hyperlipidemia rats induced by high fat diet. *Int. Immunopharmacol.* **2011**, *11*, 457–461. [CrossRef] [PubMed]

147. Li, Y.; Xu, Q.; Wei, P.; Cheng, L.; Peng, Q.; Li, S.; Yin, H.; Du, Y. Chitosan oligosaccharides downregulate the expression of E-selectin and ICAM-1 induced by LPS in endothelial cells by inhibiting MAP kinase signaling. *Int. J. Mol. Med.* **2014**, *33*, 392–400. [PubMed]

148. Liu, H.T.; Huang, P.; Ma, P.; Liu, Q.S.; Yu, C.; Du, Y.G. Chitosan oligosaccharides suppress LPS-induced IL-8 expression in human umbilical vein endothelial cells through blockade of p38 and Akt protein kinases. *Acta Pharmacol. Sin.* **2011**, *32*, 478–486. [CrossRef] [PubMed]

6

Intracranial Thrombus Morphology and Composition Undergoes Time-Dependent Changes in Acute Ischemic Stroke

Slaven Pikija [1], Jozef Magdic [2], Vladimir Trkulja [3], Peter Unterkreuter [4],
Johannes Sebastian Mutzenbach [1], Helmut F. Novak [1], Friedrich Weymayr [5], Larissa Hauer [6,†]
and Johann Sellner [1,7,8,*,†]

[1] Department of Neurology, Christian Doppler Medical Center, Paracelsus Medical University, 5020 Salzburg,
    Austria; s.pikija@salk.at (S.P.); j.mutzenbach@salk.at (J.S.M.); h.novak@salk.at (H.F.N.)
[2] Department of Neurology, Univerzitetni Klinični Center, 2000 Maribor, Slovenia; jozef_magdic@yahoo.com
[3] Department for Pharmacology, School of Medicine, University of Zagreb, 10000 Zagreb, Croatia;
    vtrkulja@mef.hr
[4] Department of Neurology, Bezirkskrankenhaus Lienz, 9900 Lienz, Austria; p.unterkreuter@kh-lienz.at
[5] Division of Neuroradiology, Christian Doppler Medical Center, Paracelsus Medical University,
    5020 Salzburg, Austria; f.weymayr@salk.at
[6] Department of Psychiatry, Christian Doppler Medical Center, Paracelsus Medical University, 5020 Salzburg,
    Austria; l.hauer@salk.at
[7] Department of Neurology, Klinikum rechts der Isar, Technische Universität, 81675 München, Germany
[8] Institute of Linguistics, University of Salzburg, 5020 Salzburg, Austria
*   Correspondence: j.sellner@salk.at;
†   These authors contributed equally to this work.

Academic Editor: Michael Henein

Abstract: The aim of our study was to assess whether cerebral artery clots undergo time-dependent morphological and compositional changes in acute ischemic stroke. We performed a retrospective chart review of patients admitted within 5 h from symptom onset to three European stroke centers and evaluated non-contrast-enhanced CT (NECT) for hyperdense artery signs (HAS) in 2565 scans. The occlusion site, density of HAS expressed in Hounsfield units (HU), area of HAS, and relative density (rHU) (HU clot/HU non-affected artery) were studied and related to time from symptom onset, clinical severity, stroke etiology, and laboratory parameters. A HAS was present in the middle cerebral artery (MCA) in 185 (7.2%) and further explored. The mean time from symptom onset to CT was 100 min (range 17–300). We found a time-dependent loss of density in the occluded M1 segment within the first 5 h ($N = 118$, 95% CI $[-15, -2]$, $p = 0.01$). Further, the thrombus area in the M2 segment decreased with time (cubic trend $N = 67$, 95% CI $[-63, -8]$, $p = 0.02$). Overall, and especially in the M2 segment, a lower clot area was associated with higher fibrinogen (-21.7%, 95% CI $[-34.8, -5.8]$, $p = 0.009$). In conclusion, our results disclosed time-dependent changes of intracranial thrombi with regard to occlusion site, density and area.

Keywords: acute ischemic stroke; intracranial clot; vascular disease; atherosclerosis; neuroimaging; hyperdense artery sign; biomarker

1. Introduction

Acute occlusion of intracranial vessels is responsible for up to 80% of ischemic strokes [1,2]. The susceptibility of clot material to reperfusion therapy is being actively researched; however, more data is needed to fill the knowledge gap [3–6]. The composition of clots is thought to be dependent on the embolic source. Hence, fibrin-rich "white" thrombi are presumed to originate from high-flow larger arteries and thrombi with a predominant red blood cell (RBC) composition are more likely to stem from low-flow cardiac sources [3]. The clots composed predominantly of RBC are considered to be fresh, less compact and more hyperdense than fibrin-rich clots. After local plaque rupture in coronary vessels, the development of proximal and distal of fibrin-/thrombocyte-rich nidus have been reported [7]. A similar mechanism could take place for embolized clots in acute ischemic stroke (AIS). Indeed, interspersed formations of fibrin-platelet-rich deposits with linear collections of nucleated cells and erythrocytes have also been reported in AIS [4]. Several later studies, however, disclosed that the thrombi from these two locations do not differ in composition, being heterogeneous with both fibrin- and RBC-rich layers interspersed, probably reflecting time-dependent changes [4,8]. A recent CT densitometry study hypothesized that the clot loses its density by acquiring fibrin, since more hypodense clots were found in patients with lower fibrinogen values [9]. The RBC count, on the other hand, showed no correlation with clot density. In addition, the fibrinogen serum levels were lower in patients with larger intracranial clots.

In AIS, the hyperdense artery sign (HAS) on non-contrast-enhanced computed tomography (NECT) is thought to represent the intraluminal thrombus and subsequent arterial obstruction. A recent meta-analysis found a sensitivity and specificity of HAS for arterial obstruction on angiography of 52% and 95%, respectively [10]. Of note, thrombus characteristics can be evaluated reliably on non-contrast-enhanced CT by further characterizing the HAS [11,12]. In this regard, thrombi with lower Hounsfield units (HU) on NECT appear to be more resistant to pharmacological lysis and mechanical thrombectomy [11,13–15]. Given the varied choice of catheters and techniques currently available, pre-therapeutic thrombus characterization may help in the selection of the most effective method [16]. Here, we present the results of the retrospective three-center study on the time-dependent thrombus dynamics seen as HAS on NECT in patients with AIS.

2. Results

2.1. Patient Eligibility and Characteristics

Of the 2562 patients with NECT scans, a HAS was present in 270 cases. Of those, 250 patients had the time between symptom onset and NECT scan exactly recorded: in 41 patients the elapsed time was >300 min (up to 960) (Figure 1). To avoid a potential bias arising from a lower number of patients beyond 300 min, only the patients with NECT performance within 300 min were selected for detailed analysis. Among the remaining 209, an occlusion of the middle cerebral artery (MCA) was by far prevailing (Figure 1).

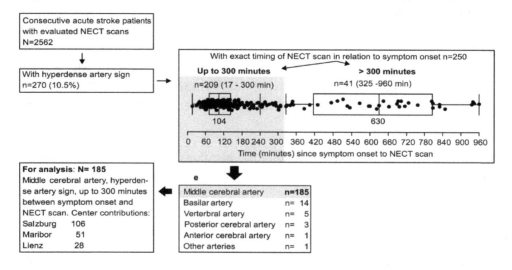

Figure 1. Flow of the patient selection process.

To avoid a further bias due to low patient numbers for other occluded vessels, the present analysis was restricted to 185 patients with MCA involvement (Figure 1). Clinical details are depicted in Table 1 and give insight to characteristics of the entire cohort and in subgroups stratified for the affected MCA segment (proximal or distal). Patient subsets by MCA segment were fairly comparable in all aspects, except that thrombectomy was, by far, more frequently performed when proximal MCA was affected (Table 1).

Table 1. Patient characteristics, overall and by the affected medial cerebral artery (MCA) segment. Data are median (range) or count (percent), unless otherwise stated.

Variables	All Patients		Proximal MCA		Distal MCA	
	N	Values	N	Values	N	Values
Age (years)	185	75 (19–98)	118	75 (41–97)	67	75 (19–98)
Men	185	82 (44.3)	118	52 (44.1)	67	30 (44.8)
Symptom onset to NECT (min)	185	100 (17–300) (Q1–Q3 = 71–136)	118	104 (31–286) (Q1–Q3 = 71–133)	67	94 (17–300) (Q1–Q3 = 70–147)
Side affected (left/right)	185	92 (49.7)/93	118	62 (52.5)/56	67	30 (44.8)/37
Average clot density (HU)	185	46.3 (36.1–56.1)	118	46.5 (36.9–56.1)	67	45.9 (36.1–55.3)
Non-affected side density (HU)	185	35.8 (18.6–45.7)	118	35.7 (24.4–45.7)	67	33.9 (18.6–45.7)
Ratio clot/non-affected rHU	185	1.30 (0.86–2.75)	118	1.30 (1.02–2.18)	67	1.32 (0.86–2.75)
Hyperdense area (mm^2)	176	30.2 (2.5–211.4)	115	31.7 (2.9–211.4)	61	28.2 (2.5–119.0)
Admission NIHSS	185	16 (0–32)	118	17 (0–32)	67	13 (0–32)
TOAST class	185		118		67	
Cardioembolic		93 (50.3)		59 (50.0)		34 (50.8)
Large artery atherosclerosis		23 (12.4)		20 (16.9)		3 (4.5)
Other (all arterial dissections)		6 (3.2)		4 (3.4)		2 (3.0)
Undetermined		9 (4.9)		3 (2.5)		6 (8.9)
Unknown		54 (29.1)		32 (27.1)		22 (32.8)
Angiography performed *	185	118 (63.8)	118	89 (75.4)	67	29 (43.3)
Thrombolysis	185	139 (75.1)	118	90 (76.3)	67	49 (73.1)
Thrombectomy	185	52 (28.1)	118	48 (40.7)	67	4 (6.0)
Thrombolysis + thrombectomy	185	44 (23.8)	118	40 (33.9)	67	4 (6.0)
Usage of antiplatelets	185	55 (29.7)	118	33 (28.0)	67	22 (32.8)
Usage of anticoagulants	185	19 (10.3)	118	12 (10.2)	67	7 (10.5)
History of stroke or TIA	185	25 (13.5)	118	14 (11.9)	67	11 (16.4)
Peripheral arterial disease	185	14 (7.6)	118	9 (7.6)	67	5 (7.5)
Atrial fibrillation	185	91 (49.5)	118	56 (47.5)	67	35 (53.0)
Diabetes mellitus	185	31 (16.8)	118	19 (16.1)	67	12 (17.9)
Arterial hypertension	185	127 (68.6)	118	84 (71.2)	67	43 (64.2)
Carotid stenosis >50%	185	24 (13.0)	118	16 (13.6)	67	8 (11.9)
Chronic heart failure	185	30 (16.2)	118	21 (17.8)	67	9 (13.4)
Blood glucose (mg/dL)	184	119 (76–351)	118	119 (76–254)	66	120 (77–351)
Total cholesterol (mg/dL)	160	181 (78–300)	102	185 (78–300)	58	175 (99–275)
Serum fibrinogen (mg/dL)	170	346 (55–785)	111	350 (166–785)	59	335 (55–685)

* Computed tomography or/and magnetic resonance or/and digital subtraction angiography. HU—Hounsfield units; NECT—non-contrast enhanced computed tomography; NIHSS—National Institutes of Health Stroke Scale score; TIA—transitory ischemic attack; TOAST—trial of Org 10172 in acute stroke treatment criteria.

2.2. Univariate Association between Timing of NECT (Non-Contrast-Enhanced CT) Relative to Symptom Onset and Ratio of Density (rHU) or Hyperdense Area

Initial exploration of the relationship between the timing of NECT relative to symptom onset (time-lag) and the ratio of the density (rHU) or hyperdense area indicated that these relationships were apparently different at the proximal and distal MCA (Figure 2). In detail, rHU tended to decrease with a longer time-lag at the proximal MCA but not at the distal MCA, and the difference between the slopes of the two regression lines of ln(rHU) vs. time was significant ($p = 0.019$). In contrast, the hyperdense area tended to decrease with a longer time-lag at the distal MCA, but not at the proximal MCA. The difference between the slopes of the two regression lines of ln(hyperdense area) vs. time was significant ($p = 0.018$).

106   Cardiovascular Imaging: From Techniques to Clinical Interpretation

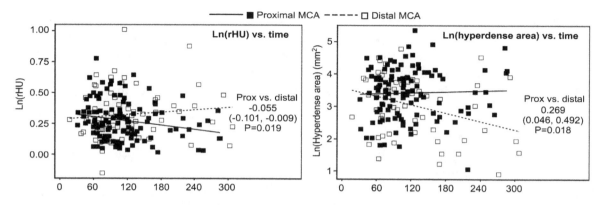

Figure 2. Exploration of the relationship between timing of NECT relative to symptom onset and ratio of density (rHU) (**left**) or hyperdense area (**right**). A separate linear mixed model (center as a cluster) was fitted to ln-transformed rHU and hyperdense area (to achieve normality of residuals) with time, MCA segment and time × MCA segment interaction term as independent variables. In the analysis of ln(rHU), there was no overall effect of time ($F = 0.05$, $p = 0.824$) and no overall difference between the MCA segments ($F = 1.21$, $p = 0.274$), but the interaction term was significant ($F = 5.61$, $p = 0.019$). Difference in slopes of ln(rHU) vs. time (per 60 min) at the two MCA segments is depicted numerically. Similarly, in the analysis of ln(hyperdense area), there was no overall effect of time ($F = 1.27$, $p = 0.261$) and no overall difference between the two MCA segments ($F = 0.00$, $p = 0.964$), but the interaction term was significant ($F = 5.68$, $p = 0.018$). Difference in slopes of ln(hyperdense area) vs. time (per 60 min) at the two MCA segments is depicted numerically.

Since the sample was limited, and particularly for the MCA subset groups with inadequate power for an analysis based on an interaction term (MCA segment × time), we assessed the relationships of interest separately at the proximal MCA and the distal MCA. Moreover, we treated time as a categorical variable (by quartiles, see Table 1 for limit values) since cases for the later time-lag were relatively sparse and variable. The relationship between the rHU and hyperdense area vs. quartiles of time-lag is shown in Figure 3. The key findings were:

(a)   rHU decreased linearly across quartiles of time (linear trend $p = 0.025$) at the proximal MCA and values at Q4 were 9% lower than at Q1 ($p = 0.010$) (Figure 1A); at the distal MCA, an apparent cubic trend ($p = 0.016$) was observed since rHU values declined from Q1 to Q2 and then increased at Q3 and Q4, and hence values at Q4 were actually no different than the values at Q1 (Figure 3A);

(b)   At the proximal MCA, there was no apparent difference regarding the hyperdense area across quartiles of time (Figure 3B), whereas at distal MCA there was a significant cubic trend ($p = 0.017$)—the values slightly increased from Q1 to Q3, and then declined at Q4, so that the values at Q4 were 42% lower than at Q1 ($p = 0.020$) (Figure 3B).

2.3. Multivariate (Independent) Association between Timing of NECT Relative to Symptom Onset and Ratio of Density (rHU) or Hyperdense Area

With adjustment for age, we analyzed the clinical severity of disease at presentation (represented by the NIHSS score) and stroke etiology (TOAST criteria) categorized as "cardioembolic", "large artery atherosclerosis" (two readily identifiable categories with specific, distinct pathophysiology) and "other" (unknown or undetermined) with different readouts of clot characteristics. The relationship between the timing of NECT relative to the symptom onset and rHU and hyperdense area remained practically unchanged (Table 2). Further findings were:

(a)   At the proximal MCA, the rHU linearly decreased across quartiles of the time-lag (linear trend $p = 0.019$) and values at the fourth quartile were 10% lower than at the first quartile ($p = 0.008$); at the distal MCA, the cubic trend remained significant and there was no difference in rHU at the fourth vs. first quartile of the time-lag; and

(b)   At the proximal MCA there was no apparent change in the hyperdense area across quartiles of the time-lag, whereas at the distal MCA the cubic trend remained significant and values at the fourth quartile were 39% lower than at the first quartile (Table 2).

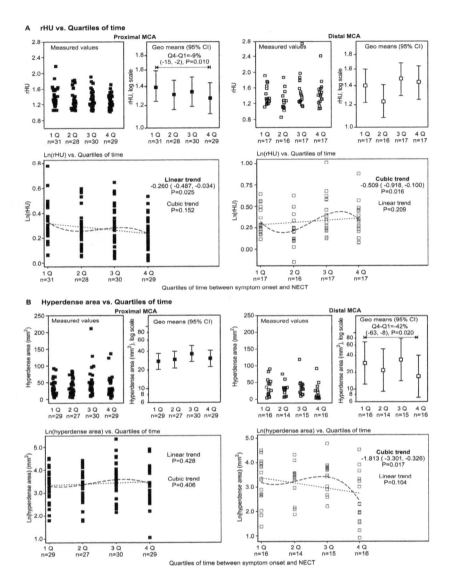

Figure 3. Univariate relationship between timing of NECT relative to symptom onset (as quartiles of time-lag) and ratio of density (rHU) (**A**) or hyperdense area (**B**) by segment of medial cerebral artery (MCA). (**A**) A mixed model (center as a cluster) was fitted to ln-transformed rHU (to achieve normality of residuals) with time-lag as the only independent variable. The relationship was tested for a linear, quadratic and cubic trend. At the proximal MCA, a significant linear decreasing trend was observed (depicted numerically) across quartiles of time-lag and values at the fourth quartile of elapsed time were by 9% lower than at the first quartile. At the distal MCA, values at the second quartile were lower than at the first quartile of the time-lag, and then increased to the third and fourth quartile, yielding a significant cubic trend (depicted numerically); however values at the fourth quartile of the time-lag were closely similar to the values at the first quartile; (**B**) The same analysis was repeated for the ln-transformed hyperdense area. At the proximal MCA, no apparent trend across quartiles of time was observed and values at the fourth quartile were closely similar to the values at the first quartile. At the distal MCA, values slightly increased towards the third quartile and then decreased to the fourth quartile of the time-lag, yielding a significant cubic trend (depicted numerically), and values at the fourth quartile were 42% lower than at the first quartile. Percentage difference between the fourth and the first quartile of time-lag = $(1 - e^{\text{coeff}}) \times 100$.

Table 2. Independent association between timing of NECT relative to the symptoms onset and ratio of density (rHU) or hyperdense area: summary of adjusted effects.

Associations	At Proximal MCA		At Distal MCA	
	Estimate (95% CI)	p	Estimate (95% CI)	p
Dependent: rHU				
Linear trend across time-lag quartiles	−0.280 (−0.513, −0.046)	0.019	0.230 (−0.224, 0.684)	0.315
Cubic trend across time-lag quartiles	−0.169 (−0.404, 0.066)	0.158	−0.480 (−0.914, −0.046)	0.031
Difference in fourth to first quartile (%)	−10 (−16, −3)	0.008	2 (−11, 17)	0.761
Dependent: hyperdense area				
Linear trend across time-lag quartiles	0.652 (−0.543, 1.848)	0.282	−0.976 (−2.586, 0.671)	0.243
Cubic trend across time-lag quartiles	−0.906 (−2.104, 0.292)	0.137	−2.092 (−3.672, −0.512)	0.011
Difference in fourth to first quartile (%)	11 (−24, 62)	0.581	−39 (−63, −1)	0.046

A separate mixed model (center as a cluster) was fitted to the ln-transformed rHU and hyperdense area (to achieve normality of residuals) with quartiles of time-lag, age, NIHSS score at admission and stroke etiology by TOAST criteria (categorized as "cardioembolic", "large artery atherosclerosis" or "other") as independents, and the linear, quadratic and cubic relationships between time and dependent variables were tested. Depicted are adjusted effects. Percentage difference between the fourth and the first quartile of time-lag = $(1 - e^{\text{coeff}}) \times 100$.

2.4. Exploration of the Relationship between Serum Fibrinogen Levels and rHU or Hyperdense Area

On-admission serum fibrinogen levels were available for 170/185 patients (91.9%). Among these patients there were 111/118 (94.1%) with proximal MCA and 59/67 (88.1%) with distal MCA pathology. A separate mixed model (center as a cluster) was fitted to ln(rHU) and ln(hyperdense area) with the MCA segment, serum fibrinogen, stroke type (by TOAST criteria) and MCA segment × fibrinogen interaction term. Figure 4 depicts adjusted regressions of either dependent variable on the serum fibrinogen and adjusted estimates are shown in Table 3. In detail, we found:

(a) there was an overall trend of association between higher serum fibrinogen and higher rHU (2.3% higher with 100 mg/dL increase in fibrinogen). However, there was no association between fibrinogen and rHU in patients with an affected proximal MCA, whereas the association was stronger and statistically significant in patients with an affected distal MCA (4.2% higher rHU by 100 mg/dL increase in fibrinogen);

(b) for the entire cohort, higher fibrinogen was associated with a smaller hyperdense area (15% by 100 mg/dL increase in fibrinogen) ($p = 0.005$). However, this association was much weaker and not statistically significant in patients with an affected proximal MCA, whereas it was stronger and significant in patients with an affected distal MCA (Table 3). Due to incompleteness, data should be viewed with caution, but suggest that at proximal MCA, rHU apparently declines over the first 300 min after the stroke onset, though the hyperdense area does not appear to change. Further, neither of these two radiological outcomes seems to be associated with serum fibrinogen levels. Moreover, at the distal MCA, rHU does not appear to change while the hyperdense area tends to diminish over the first 300 min after the stroke onset. At the same time, a higher rHU and lower hyperdense area appear to be associated with higher serum fibrinogen.

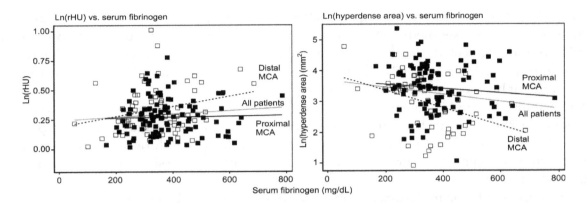

Figure 4. Adjusted regression lines of ln-transformed rHU (**left**) and hyperdense area (**right**) vs. serum fibrinogen, overall and by the segment of medial cerebral artery (MCA). Regressions are from the model depicted in Table 3.

Table 3. Association between serum fibrinogen and ratio of density (rHU) or hyperdense area: summary of adjusted effects expressed as % change in dependent variable by 100 mg/dL increase in serum fibrinogen.

Affected Artery	rHU		Hyperdense Area (mm^2)	
	Estimate (95% CI)	p	Estimate (95% CI)	p
Proximal and distal MCA	2.27% (−0.10, 4.67)	0.059	−15.2% (−24.3, −5.0)	0.005
Proximal MCA	0.41% (−2.23, 3.17)	0.769	−8.2% (−29.3, 4.5)	0.191
Distal MCA	4.16% (0.39, 8.08)	0.031	−21.7% (−34.8, −5.8)	0.009

A separate mixed model (center as a cluster) was fitted to the ln-transformed rHU and hyperdense area (to achieve normality of residuals) with quartiles of time-lag, stroke etiology by TOAST criteria (categorized as "cardioembolic", "large artery atherosclerosis" or "other"), serum fibrinogen levels, MCA segment and fibrinogen × MCA segment interaction as independent variables. Percentage change in rHU or hyperdense area = $(1 - e^{coeff}) \times 100$.

3. Discussion

The efficacy of recanalization efforts in AIS is variable and biomarkers for stratifying patients with a lower probability of success are eagerly awaited. The anatomical site, composition and spread of clot in various arteries are potential parameters which could assist decision-making processes in order to individually optimize treatment [17,18]. NECT is a fast, widely available and readily used method in acute stroke and it enables non-invasive thrombus characterization. Importantly, thrombus characterization by NECT could provide additional useful information regarding clot susceptibility to thrombolysis and mechanical recanalization. Clot characteristics, however, could undergo dynamic changes over time as a multitude of biochemical pathways are activated when a vessel is occluded and the clot is exposed to hemodynamic and humoral changes of the local milieu [19–21]. These include a combination of proximal and distal apposition of new thrombotic material as well as proteolytic processes, which dissolve less compact thrombus material and leave a place for further fibrin meshwork propagation.

Here, we found indirect evidence of changes in clot composition and morphology within the first 5 h of AIS. Our study disclosed that MCA M1 clots, but not MCA M2 loses its density within the first 5 h. Moreover, we report a decline of the clot plane over time for the M2 segment. The area reduction was also associated with higher fibrinogen blood levels, which corroborates our previous observation [9]. The clots situated in the M1 segment did not change with regard to area and time, and thrombus characteristics did not correlate with fibrinogen levels.

Why is there a difference between the proximal and distal MCA occlusion with regard to time-dependent changes? This observation could, on one hand, be related to differences of embolic material, and indeed, large artery atherosclerosis was a more frequent etiology in M1 segment occlusion

(16.9% vs. 4.5%). The other factor playing a possible role could be the availability of collateral perfusion regarding the occluded segment. This issue was not assessed in our study. Although there are conflicting reports, Kim et al. found higher proportions of RBCs and a lower proportion of fibrin in clots arising from cardioembolic (CE) than in those with large artery arteriosclerosis (LAA) etiology. The predominant histology of distal clots is not reported in published studies. Accordingly, we could speculate that distal thrombi, having originally more fibrin content that is more resistant to endogenous lysis, shield the RBC-rich part from degradation and accordingly these clots do not change in density with time. However, the later the patient arrives, the area of the distal thrombi seems to be somewhat smaller, possibly reflecting the degradation of RBC content later in time since the change is not obvious until the last quartile of time.

A time-dependent drop in clot density (absolute HU) was previously reported by Topcuoglu et al. [22]. In contrast to our findings, one study with 106 patients showed no changes in the relative HU density of the hyperdense artery within the first 4.5 h [23]. The reason for this discrepancy remains unclear. The density of the clot as seen on NECT is augmented by RBC content. Loss of density after embolism in MCA M1 occlusion is probably due to the preferential degradation of the erythrocyte-rich part of the clot [7]. Reports from a murine ischemic model provide evidence that the urokinase plasminogen activator is activated in the first 1 to 2 h following acute MCA occlusion, with gradual weakening of activity thereafter, which could explain our observation [19].

The second largest group concerning stroke pathogenesis consisted of patients with unknown etiology, accounting for 29%. Although we have not specifically reassessed details of the diagnostic stroke workup, the usual standard of care in stroke units includes blood analysis, 24 h electrocardiography (ECG), heart ultrasound and vessel imaging in every patient. Accordingly, it is unlikely that a lack of workup is responsible for this unexpectedly high number of cryptogenic strokes. With the presence of the intracranial clot, many of these patients could be classified as embolic stroke of undetermined source (ESUS) as the underlying etiology [24]. The prevalence of cryptogenic or ESUS strokes in cohorts with evaluation of the HAS is rarely reported. A pilot study identified nine patients with HAS of the MCA, which accounted for 20% of all stroke cases. Cryptogenic and ESUS stroke made up 26% of stroke cases in a larger study [25]. One study revealed that patients without detectable stroke etiology may have better clinical outcomes [26]. Further studies are required to prove whether hints for stroke etiology could be determined by analysis of clot morphology on NECT in cases where the causality remains unclear from ancillary investigations.

Limitations of our study are the usage of different scanning parameters and non-uniform slice thickness. This influences the detection rate of HA which is known to be dependent on slice thickness, and studies confirmed that thinner NECT slices have a greater sensitivity [12]. In addition, the rather low detection rate of HA in nearly 10% of all consecutive strokes could be interpreted as low sensitivity of our study. However, the prevalence of the HA sign among non-selected stroke patients and larger cohorts has not been reported so far. Selected populations, i.e., patients chosen for thrombolysis or with specific stroke syndromes such as posterior cerebral artery stroke, have higher detection rates, but this varies widely (5%–75%) [27]. In our study, some form of angiography (CT, magnetic resonance imaging (MRI) or digital subtraction angiography (DSA)) was performed in 63.8% patients with a correlation of vessel occlusion. For other patients, the clinical stroke syndrome was taken for the verification of vessel obstruction and this always corresponded to the side of the artery occlusion. Of note, we acknowledge the difficulty of discerning the hyperdense artery on plain CT without additional angiography but we presume that the combination of hematocrit correction and correlation with the clinical syndrome suffices for the identification of the occluded artery. Naturally, the presumption that time-dependent changes can be approximated from various patients is subjected to biases. Ideally, each patient should be re-examined with NECT at fixed time points. Such an approach, however, is not feasible due to ethical constraints and patient safety. Nevertheless, in our population, on follow up CT scans in 45 patients, HA was still visible (29%); of them 32 (71%) showed no change or had a drop in rHU values, thus further confirming our findings. Eventually, our observation needs to be confirmed in a larger cohort. Moreover, the characterization of thrombus dynamics beyond 5 h from symptom onset should follow as well.

4. Materials and Methods

We performed a retrospective study of consecutive patients with AIS who presented to the emergency department in three stroke centers. These were Christian-Doppler-Klinik Salzburg, Austria (CDK), University Clinical Center Maribor, Slovenia (MB) and Bezirkskrankenhaus Lienz, Austria (LZ). The study periods for CDK and MB were 2013–2015, and for LZ 2011–2014.

The inclusion criteria were age ≥18 years, presentation within 16 h from stroke onset and available head NECT. We excluded those cases were brain hemorrhage, brain tumor or non-stroke pathology was seen. In addition to usual laboratory examinations we recorded HbA1c and acute fibrinogen values. Stroke subtypes were classified according to the modified Trial of Org 10172 in Acute Treatment (TOAST) criteria [28]. NECT was performed before treatment with rt-PA in all patients.

CT scans were acquired in LZ and CDK with the multidetector CT scanner Sensation 64 (Siemens, Erlangen, Germany) and in MB with the multidetector CT scanner (Aquilion 64, Toshiba Medical Systems, Tochigi, Japan). The CT scans were reconstructed into 4, 2.4 and 3 mm (for CDK, LZ and MB, respectively) thick adjacent slices through the whole brain with the specifications of 120 kV (all centers) and 250, 440 and 150–350 mAs (for CDK, LZ and MB respectively) (mean value, using automatic exposure control) and matrix size of 512 × 512. The mean equivalent dose was 1.2 mSv for CDK and LZ and 1.9 mSv for MB.

The evaluation of CT-scans were performed by two experienced stroke physicians who were blinded to the clinical data. When in doubt of presence of hyperdense vessel sign, consensus was reached. HAS was recognized as the area of hyperattenuating artery on NECT. The hyperdense area was manually delineated in IMPAX software (Impax Laboratories Inc., Hayward, CA, USA), the vessel location and the side (when applicable) were recorded. Areas with calcifications (HU > 90) were not delineated. Measurements of hyperdense artery were made as previously described [11]. In short, the region of interest (ROI) was manually placed on the margins of the clot. Average HU was then obtained from all voxels within the ROI, summed across all slices (if present on more than one) producing HU sum. The final HU value was calculated by dividing the HU sum with number of slices. We recorded area in mm^2 of manually circumscribed hyperdensity. The area was summed across slices (when present in more than one). Analyses depending on variables including time, disease severity and location of the HAS were performed with respective cohorts.

In order to correct for the impact of hematocrit values we measured the density of the vessel contralateral to affected one, in the case of basilar artery hyperdensity the measurement was in posterior cerebral artery. From measured final HU value, relative HU ratio (rHU) (final HU value divided by average HU of contralateral/appropriate non-affected artery) was derived. After hyperdense artery detection, the medical records were checked to ensure correspondence with clinical symptoms.

Data Analysis

In line with the study objective, data analysis was conceived to explore the relationship, univariate and independent (adjusted), between time (defined as time elapsed between symptom onset and NECT scan, i.e., time-lag) and the two radiological outcomes—rHU and size of the hyperdense area. For all analyses, center was treated as a random effect to account for potential correlation of data coming from one site. In randomized trials, this approach was shown to improve power and maintain nominal coverage rates [29]. Univariate models contained "time" as the only fixed effect. Selection of covariates (additional fixed effects) in multivariate models was based on rationale that adjustments should account for biologically plausible potential confounders and/or moderators. We did not intend to detect "all possible effects" or to define the best set of explanatory variables of variability of rHU or hyperdense area. Finally, in an attempt to explore a potential biological background for the observed time effects on rHU and hyperdense area, we investigated the relationship between these outcomes and serum fibrinogen levels at admission. All mixed models were fitted using SAS for Windows 9.4 software (SAS Inc., Cary, NC, USA).

5. Conclusions

There are time-dependent changes in MCA thrombus morphology and composition within the first 5 h from symptom onset in patients with AIS. Moreover, we found that proximal and distal MCA clots differ with regard to these dynamics. Further studies, ideally with the evaluation of mechanically retrieved intracranial clots, are required to understand the complex pathophysiological processes determining the intrinsic and extrinsic post-processing of an intracranial thrombus.

Acknowledgments: The preparation of the manuscript was supported by Teva-Ratiopharm, open access publishing was covered by the University of Salzburg.

Author Contributions: Slaven Pikija, Larissa Hauer and Johann Sellner conceived and designed the experiments; Slaven Pikija, Jozef Magdic and Peter Unterkreuter performed the experiments; Slaven Pikija, Vladimir Trkulja, Johannes Sebastian Mutzenbach, Helmut F. Novak, Friedrich Weymayr, Larissa Hauer and Johann Sellner analyzed the data; Slaven Pikija, Larissa Hauer and Johann Sellner wrote the paper; all authors contributed to the revision.

Abbreviations

AIS	Acute ischemic stroke
LAA	Large artery atherosclerosis
HAS	Hyperdense artery sign
NECT	Non-enhanced CT
TOAST	Trial of Org 10172 in Acute Treatment criteria
HU	Hounsfield units
rHU	Average HU of hyperdense artery/average HU of non-affected artery
DSA	Digital subtraction angiography
MRI	Magnetic resonance imaging
CT	Computertomography
ESUS	Embolic stroke of unknown source
CE	Cardioembolic

References

1. Williams, G.R.; Jiang, J.G.; Matchar, D.B.; Samsa, G.P. Incidence and occurrence of total (first-ever and recurrent) stroke. *Stroke* **1999**, *30*, 2523–2528. [CrossRef] [PubMed]
2. Pikija, S.; Trkulja, V.; Malojcic, B.; Mutzenbach, J.S.; Sellner, J. A High Burden of Ischemic Stroke in Regions of Eastern/Central Europe is Largely Due to Modifiable Risk Factors. *Curr. Neurovasc. Res.* **2015**, *12*, 341–352. [CrossRef] [PubMed]
3. Goldmakher, G.V.; Camargo, E.C.; Furie, K.L.; Singhal, A.B.; Roccatagliata, L.; Halpern, E.F.; Chou, M.J.; Biagini, T.; Smith, W.S.; Harris, G.J.; et al. Hyperdense basilar artery sign on unenhanced CT predicts thrombus and outcome in acute posterior circulation stroke. *Stroke* **2009**, *40*, 134–139. [CrossRef] [PubMed]
4. Marder, V.J.; Chute, D.J.; Starkman, S.; Abolian, A.M.; Kidwell, C.; Liebeskind, D.; Ovbiagele, B.; Vinuela, F.; Duckwiler, G.; Jahan, R.; et al. Analysis of thrombi retrieved from cerebral arteries of patients with acute ischemic stroke. *Stroke* **2006**, *37*, 2086–2093. [CrossRef] [PubMed]
5. Mattle, H.P.; Arnold, M.; Georgiadis, D.; Baumann, C.; Nedeltchev, K.; Benninger, D.; Remonda, L.; von Budingen, C.; Diana, A.; Pangalu, A.; et al. Comparison of intraarterial and intravenous thrombolysis for ischemic stroke with hyperdense middle cerebral artery sign. *Stroke* **2008**, *39*, 379–383. [CrossRef] [PubMed]
6. Niesten, J.M.; van der Schaaf, I.C.; Biessels, G.J.; van Otterloo, A.E.; van Seeters, T.; Horsch, A.D.; Luitse, M.J.; van der Graaf, Y.; Kappelle, L.J.; Mali, W.P.; et al. Relationship between thrombus attenuation and different stroke subtypes. *Neuroradiology* **2013**, *55*, 1071–1079. [CrossRef] [PubMed]

7.   Jang, I.K.; Gold, H.K.; Ziskind, A.A.; Fallon, J.T.; Holt, R.E.; Leinbach, R.C.; May, J.W.; Collen, D. Differential sensitivity of erythrocyte-rich and platelet-rich arterial thrombi to lysis with recombinant tissue-type plasminogen activator. A possible explanation for resistance to coronary thrombolysis. *Circulation* **1989**, *79*, 920–928. [CrossRef] [PubMed]

8.   Liebeskind, D.S.; Sanossian, N.; Yong, W.H.; Starkman, S.; Tsang, M.P.; Moya, A.L.; Zheng, D.D.; Abolian, A.M.; Kim, D.; Ali, L.K.; et al. CT and MRI early vessel signs reflect clot composition in acute stroke. *Stroke* **2011**, *42*, 1237–1243. [CrossRef] [PubMed]

9.   Pikija, S.; Trkulja, V.; Mutzenbach, J.S.; McCoy, M.R.; Ganger, P.; Sellner, J. Fibrinogen consumption is related to intracranial clot burden in acute ischemic stroke: A retrospective hyperdense artery study. *J. Transl. Med.* **2016**, *14*, 250. [CrossRef] [PubMed]

10. Mair, G.; Boyd, E.V.; Chappell, F.M.; von Kummer, R.; Lindley, R.I.; Sandercock, P.; Wardlaw, J.M.; Group, I.S.T.C. Sensitivity and specificity of the hyperdense artery sign for arterial obstruction in acute ischemic stroke. *Stroke* **2015**, *46*, 102–107. [CrossRef] [PubMed]

11. Puig, J.; Pedraza, S.; Demchuk, A.; Daunis, I.E.J.; Termes, H.; Blasco, G.; Soria, G.; Boada, I.; Remollo, S.; Banos, J.; et al. Quantification of thrombus hounsfield units on noncontrast CT predicts stroke subtype and early recanalization after intravenous recombinant tissue plasminogen activator. *Am. J. Neuroradiol.* **2012**, *33*, 90–96. [CrossRef] [PubMed]

12. Riedel, C.H.; Jensen, U.; Rohr, A.; Tietke, M.; Alfke, K.; Ulmer, S.; Jansen, O. Assessment of thrombus in acute middle cerebral artery occlusion using thin-slice nonenhanced Computed Tomography reconstructions. *Stroke* **2010**, *41*, 1659–1664. [CrossRef] [PubMed]

13. Moftakhar, P.; English, J.D.; Cooke, D.L.; Kim, W.T.; Stout, C.; Smith, W.S.; Dowd, C.F.; Higashida, R.T.; Halbach, V.V.; Hetts, S.W. Density of thrombus on admission CT predicts revascularization efficacy in large vessel occlusion acute ischemic stroke. *Stroke* **2013**, *44*, 243–245. [CrossRef] [PubMed]

14. Niesten, J.M.; van der Schaaf, I.C.; van der Graaf, Y.; Kappelle, L.J.; Biessels, G.J.; Horsch, A.D.; Dankbaar, J.W.; Luitse, M.J.; van Seeters, T.; Smit, E.J.; et al. Predictive value of thrombus attenuation on thin-slice non-contrast CT for persistent occlusion after intravenous thrombolysis. *Cerebrovasc. Dis.* **2014**, *37*, 116–122. [CrossRef] [PubMed]

15. Mokin, M.; Morr, S.; Natarajan, S.K.; Lin, N.; Snyder, K.V.; Hopkins, L.N.; Siddiqui, A.H.; Levy, E.I. Thrombus density predicts successful recanalization with Solitaire stent retriever thrombectomy in acute ischemic stroke. *J. Neurointerv. Surg.* **2015**, *7*, 104–107. [CrossRef] [PubMed]

16. Bouchez, L.; Lovblad, K.O.; Kulcsar, Z. Pretherapeutic characterization of the clot in acute stroke. *J. Neuroradiol.* **2016**, *43*, 163–166. [CrossRef] [PubMed]

17. Riedel, C.H.; Zimmermann, P.; Jensen-Kondering, U.; Stingele, R.; Deuschl, G.; Jansen, O. The importance of size: Successful recanalization by intravenous thrombolysis in acute anterior stroke depends on thrombus length. *Stroke* **2011**, *42*, 1775–1777. [CrossRef] [PubMed]

18. Molina, C.A. Imaging the clot: Does clot appearance predict the efficacy of thrombolysis? *Stroke* **2005**, *36*, 2333–2334. [CrossRef] [PubMed]

19. Hosomi, N.; Lucero, J.; Heo, J.H.; Koziol, J.A.; Copeland, B.R.; del Zoppo, G.J. Rapid differential endogenous plasminogen activator expression after acute middle cerebral artery occlusion. *Stroke* **2001**, *32*, 1341–1348. [CrossRef] [PubMed]

20. Alvarez-Perez, F.J.; Castelo-Branco, M.; Alvarez-Sabin, J. Usefulness of measurement of fibrinogen, D-dimer, D-dimer/fibrinogen ratio, C reactive protein and erythrocyte sedimentation rate to assess the pathophysiology and mechanism of ischaemic stroke. *J. Neurol. Neurosurg. Psychiatry* **2011**, *82*, 986–992. [CrossRef] [PubMed]

21. De Meyer, S.F.; Denorme, F.; Langhauser, F.; Geuss, E.; Fluri, F.; Kleinschnitz, C. Thromboinflammation in Stroke Brain Damage. *Stroke* **2016**, *47*, 1165–1172. [CrossRef] [PubMed]

22. Topcuoglu, M.A.; Arsava, E.M.; Akpinar, E. Clot Characteristics on Computed Tomography and Response to Thrombolysis in Acute Middle Cerebral Artery Stroke. *J. Stroke Cerebrovasc. Dis.* **2015**, *24*, 1363–1372. [CrossRef] [PubMed]

23. Haridy, J.; Churilov, L.; Mitchell, P.; Dowling, R.; Yan, B. Is there association between hyperdense middle cerebral artery sign on CT scan and time from stroke onset within the first 24-hours? *BMC Neurol.* **2015**, *15*, 101. [CrossRef] [PubMed]

24. Hart, R.G.; Diener, H.C.; Connolly, S.J. Embolic strokes of undetermined source: Support for a new clinical construct—Authors' reply. *Lancet Neurol.* **2014**, *13*, 967. [CrossRef]

25. Fonseca, A.C.; Ferro, J.M. Cryptogenic stroke. *Eur. J. Neurol.* **2015**, *22*, 618–623. [CrossRef] [PubMed]

26. Scullen, T.A.; Monlezun, D.J.; Siegler, J.E.; George, A.J.; Schwickrath, M.; El Khoury, R.; Cho, M.C.; Martin-Schild, S. Cryptogenic stroke: Clinical consideration of a heterogeneous ischemic subtype. *J. Stroke Cerebrovasc. Dis.* **2015**, *24*, 993–999. [CrossRef] [PubMed]

27. Krings, T.; Noelchen, D.; Mull, M.; Willmes, K.; Meister, I.G.; Reinacher, P.; Toepper, R.; Thron, A.K. The hyperdense posterior cerebral artery sign: A computed tomography marker of acute ischemia in the posterior cerebral artery territory. *Stroke* **2006**, *37*, 399–403. [CrossRef] [PubMed]

28. Kolominsky-Rabas, P.L.; Weber, M.; Gefeller, O.; Neundoerfer, B.; Heuschmann, P.U. Epidemiology of ischemic stroke subtypes according to TOAST criteria: Incidence, recurrence, and long-term survival in ischemic stroke subtypes: A population-based study. *Stroke* **2001**, *32*, 2735–2740. [CrossRef] [PubMed]

29. Kahan, B.C.; Morris, T.P. Adjusting for multiple prognostic factors in the analysis of randomised trials. *BMC Med. Res. Methodol.* **2013**, *13*, 99. [CrossRef] [PubMed]

7

Ultrasound Tissue Characterization of Vulnerable Atherosclerotic Plaque

Eugenio Picano [1,*] **and Marco Paterni** [2]

[1] Biomedicine Department, NU School of Medicine, Astana 010000, Kazakistan

[2] CNR (Consiglio Nazionale Ricerche), Institute of Clinical Physiology, 56124 Pisa, Italy; marco.paterni@ifc.cnr.it

* Correspondence: picano@ifc.cnr.it;

Academic Editor: Michael Henein

Abstract: A thrombotic occlusion of the vessel fed by ruptured coronary atherosclerotic plaque may result in unstable angina, myocardial infarction or death, whereas embolization from a plaque in carotid arteries may result in transient ischemic attack or stroke. The atherosclerotic plaque prone to such clinical events is termed high-risk or vulnerable plaque, and its identification in humans before it becomes symptomatic has been elusive to date. Ultrasonic tissue characterization of the atherosclerotic plaque is possible with different techniques—such as vascular, transesophageal, and intravascular ultrasound—on a variety of arterial segments, including carotid, aorta, and coronary districts. The image analysis can be based on visual, video-densitometric or radiofrequency methods and identifies three distinct textural patterns: hypo-echoic (corresponding to lipid- and hemorrhage-rich plaque), iso- or moderately hyper-echoic (fibrotic or fibro-fatty plaque), and markedly hyperechoic with shadowing (calcific plaque). Hypoechoic or dishomogeneous plaques, with spotty microcalcification and large plaque burden, with plaque neovascularization and surface irregularities by contrast-enhanced ultrasound, are more prone to clinical complications than hyperechoic, extensively calcified, homogeneous plaques with limited plaque burden, smooth luminal plaque surface and absence of neovascularization. Plaque ultrasound morphology is important, along with plaque geometry, in determining the atherosclerotic prognostic burden in the individual patient. New quantitative methods beyond backscatter (to include speed of sound, attenuation, strain, temperature, and high order statistics) are under development to evaluate vascular tissues. Although not yet ready for widespread clinical use, tissue characterization is listed by the American Society of Echocardiography roadmap to 2020 as one of the most promising fields of application in cardiovascular ultrasound imaging, offering unique opportunities for the early detection and treatment of atherosclerotic disease.

Keywords: atherosclerosis; plaque; tissue characterization; ultrasound

1. Tissue Characterization of Vulnerable Plaque: From Histology to Ultrasound

The underlying hypothesis in tissue characterization studies is that a different biochemical structure, internal architectural arrangement or physiologic state of normal *vs.* diseased tissue can affect the physical properties of the tissue and can therefore be detected by ultrasound. Tissue characterization can be performed using three main approaches with increasing degrees of complexity and accuracy: visual eyeballing, software-assisted videodensitometry of standard digitized images, and backscatter analysis of native radiofrequency signal (Figure 1). Visual eyeballing is the "first generation" approach (arising in the 1980s) and is still the only clinically viable option for large-scale use, but it can only detect the most obvious changes in tissue structure such as a hypoechoic, hyperechoic, or calcified carotid plaque. Videodensitometry is the "second-generation" approach, implemented since the mid-1990s, more objective than visual assessment and based on quantitative analysis of digitized video images. It samples the commercial video signal downstream to the processing chain distorting the linear relationship between received signal and displayed image. Radiofrequency analysis is a more technologically demanding "third generation" approach, commercially developed over the last 15 years and theoretically the most accurate, since the native ultrasonic signal is sampled upstream to the video display, and is not distorted by the post-processing function of the imaging chain. According to recent recommendations, "The long history of the ultrasound tissue characterization technique compared with its rare clinical use tells its own story in relation to its difficulty" [1]. This procedure is complex, subject to artifacts related to image settings, and the exact location of the sample volume. Calibrated backscatter has a value as a marker of fibrosis and calcification, but—the guidelines conclude—this methodology remains more of a research instrument than a clinical tool in echocardiography.

In spite of these recognized difficulties, the clinical yield of ultrasonic tissue characterization remains especially attractive in atherosclerosis, especially for the acoustic identification of vulnerable or high-risk plaques, a challenging but achievable target—as recently outlined by National Heart Lung and Blood Institute (NHLBI) Working Group [2]—for future research in the field. The carotid plaque is defined as "a focal structure that encroaches into the arterial lumen of at least 0.5 mm or 50% of the surrounding intima-media thickness or demonstrated a thickness of greater than or equal to 1.5 mm" [3]. For the clinician, there is a need to characterize "vulnerable plaque", i.e., the plaque susceptible to rupture, which can give rise to clinical complications, from embolization to thrombosis leading to symptoms, myocardial infarction, stroke and death. The vulnerability features are only weakly related to plaque size and stenosis and are also related to plaque morphology and histologic content: plaque size matters, but shape and content of the plaque also matter. Vulnerable, high-risk plaque is histologically different from stable, benign, clinically asymptomatic plaque—not only regarding its larger plaque burden but also for its higher content of lipids, with necrotic cores due to invasion of lipid pools by macrophages and other inflammatory cells with speckled micro-calcification (Table 1). The necrotic core can show hemorrhages due to extravasation of erythrocytes from the intimal neo-vascularization originating from the adventitia. The fibrous cap is usually thin, and the luminal contours may be irregular rather than smooth. All these histologic features can leave their readout on a variety of acoustic parameters, based on acoustic backscatter, attenuation, spatial texture, angular variability, plaque neo-vascularization detected through contrast administration, and acoustic internal homogeneity of spatial gray-level distribution. In order to have a comprehensive evaluation of plaque prognostic potential we need the assessment of plaque hemodynamic severity—as can be optimally provided by Duplex scan including Doppler and conventional B-mode—but also better insight into plaque content and morphology, as potentially provided by the tissue characterization approach [4].

Table 1. The vulnerable plaque read-out: from histology to ultrasound.

Histology	Ultrasound
Outward remodeling	Stenosis > 70%
Decreased Fibrous Tissue	Hypoechoic core
Increased Lipid-Hemorrhages	Hypoechoic core
More necrotic core	Dishomogeneous texture
Macrophages—inflammation	Dishomogeneous texture
Micro-calcification	Spotty hyper-dense foci
Endothelial rupture	Irregular border by CEUS
Intimal neovessel formation	Vascularization by CEUS

CEUS, contrast-enhanced ultrasound.

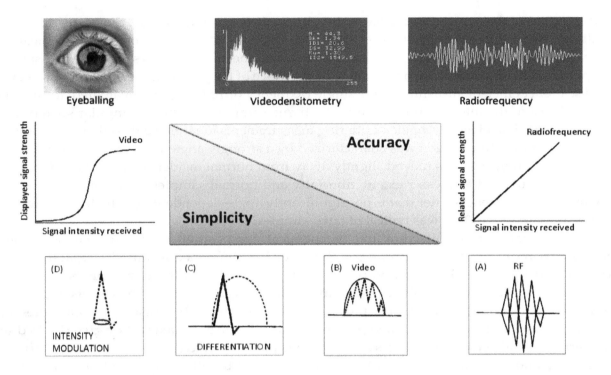

Figure 1. Approaches to tissue characterization: visual eyeballing analysis; videodensitometric analysis of digitized image by descriptors of image brightness and gray level spatial distribution; backscatter based sampling of received signal. The latter method is the most technically demanding, available in some but not all commercially available instruments, but it works on a linear relationship between received and displayed signal. This relationship is non-linear for visual and videodensitometric methods, working downstream to the electronic chain of signal processing, shown in the bottom panel, from right (panel **A**, original radiofrequency) to left (panels **B–D**, video, distorted, signal).

2. Tissue Characterization of the Atherosclerotic Plaque: *Ex Vivo* Studies

In the 1984 edition of Braunwald's classic Textbook of Cardiology, Wissler stated that "at our present stage of technology and knowledge, it is virtually impossible to evaluate the quantities of the major components in any given plaque in the human subject at any specific time, short of surgical removal or examination at autopsy" [5]. Since then, there has been growing interest in characterization of the acoustic properties of the vascular wall to identify and define the composition of atherosclerotic plaque non-invasively, and several *in vitro* studies have established a solid experimental foundation of ultrasonic tissue characterization of the atherosclerotic plaque. These studies aimed (1) to clarify the biological determinants of vascular acoustic properties; (2) to test, under controlled conditions, ultrasonic parameters of potential diagnostic use; (3) to propose an anatomic-geometrical model of arterial scatterers in different stages of normality and disease; and (4) to orient the technological efforts necessary to translate the most meaningful laboratory information into a clinically feasible tool.

The normal wall can be distinguished from atherosclerotic plaque by a variety of acoustic parameters. The peak amplitude value of reflected signal is low in normal walls and fatty plaques, intermediate in fibrous plaques, and highest in calcific plaques. This index is strongly phase-sensitive and angle-dependent, but also very simple [6]. Plaques can also be identified with parameters based on acoustic attenuation [7]. In particular, calcific plaques show an attenuation 700% greater than that found in normal wall, and 300% greater than that found in atherosclerotic non-calcific plaques. This finding is the experimental counterpart of the clinical echo finding of acoustic shadowing associated with focal calcification. A third parameter of interest for characterizing atherosclerotic plaque as well as in the elaboration of an anatomic-geometrical model of arterial scatterers is the backscatter angular dependence [8]. In contrast to the echoes arising from the myocardium, which are relatively independent of the angle of incidence of the ultrasonic beam to the tissue, those arising from arterial walls are generally said to be of a specular type. This is a major limitation to any application based on a quantitative diagnostic approach *in vivo* because specular reflectors give rise to a signal whose amplitude is highly dependent on the angle of incidence of the ultrasonic beam to the tissue target. The backscatter coefficient, measured at the single frequency of 10 MHz, was evaluated at a normal angle of incidence of the interrogating beam to the tissue sample and over an angular span of 60° ($\pm$30° around normal incidence). Angular scattering measurements identified a directive and a non-directive pattern. The directive pattern was characterized by a strongly angle-dependent backscatter that falls abruptly when the beam is moved slightly away from normal incidence. This pattern was typical of calcific, fibrous, and to a lesser extent, fibrofatty and normal samples. The non-directive pattern is characterized by a backscatter that is not significantly angle-dependent and fluctuates throughout the entire angular range. This was typical of fatty samples.

The histological architecture and biochemical composition of the arterial wall might be a reasonable morphological substrate for the recorded difference in angular scattering, which is determined by size and orientation of the scatterers relative to the ultrasonic beam. A directive angular response may be attributable to simple planar organization of the targets within the tissue. Scatterers in the normal wall might be physically identified in the thin elastic membrane present within the normal media layer and oriented perpendicularly to the beam axis. They give rise to directional scattering typical of that in structures in which large plane interfaces exist within the scattering volume. In fibrous and calcified specimens, the scatterers might be physically identified in thick collagen bundles and calcium laminae, which like elastic membranes are oriented perpendicularly to the beam. This might explain the very high directivity of these plaques. In fatty plaques, lipids accumulate in the intima, mainly in the amorphous state but also as cholesterol crystals. Such crystals are comparable in size to the wavelength of the beam, and are spatially arranged in a random fashion. The absence of a spatial orientation and the small size of the scatterers both contribute to the nondirective type of angular scattering in the plaques. In the fibrofatty plaque, the markedly directive response is probably attributable to the fibrous cap; however, the coexistence within the scattering volume of a nondirective structure (the fatty core, absent in the purely fibrous plaques) partially blunts the directivity of the angular response, which is substantially less than in the fibrous samples.

Another potentially useful parameter is the spatial distribution of echo density in an arterial region of interest. In this approach, the information is less dependent on the absolute value of echodensity, and more related to the relative value of different pixels within a region of interest [9]. The shape of the integrated backscatter amplitude distribution is more spread out and flat in the atherosclerotic region.

Another approach is the analysis of the echo signal in time domain (across the depth wall), conceptually similar to the old A-mode representation of ultrasound [10]. If one measures only the first interface aqueous-intimal echo, there is a variable amplitude value for all plaque subsets except for lipidic plaque, which shows a consistently low amplitude value.

These findings were confirmed by different laboratories using qualitative assessment of B-mode images [11] or more quantitative backscatter analysis [12–14] and the overall conclusion is that the atherosclerotic plaque composition leaves several ultrasonic fingerprints which can be fruitfully used for tissue characterization of the vulnerable plaque (Table 1, right side). Even under ideal imaging conditions (*in vitro*, no interposed tissue, controlled angle of insonation, quantitative analysis of reflected signal) lipids and hemorrhages cannot be distinguished by ultrasound, and both appear as low echogenic ("soft") tissue.

3. *In Vivo* Ultrasonic Tissue Characterization

Clinical studies have confirmed that the vulnerable, lipid-rich plaque can be identified in the carotid with all three approaches of tissue characterization: visual eyeballing [15–19], videodensitometry [20–22] and backscatter [23–25] (Table 2). Whatever the method, plaque morphology assessment is critically dependent on image quality and the echogenicity is usually normalized for an internal standard, such as—for visual assessment—the flowing blood (black) or far wall media-adventitia surface (white). Eyeballing characterization of plaque texture is subjective and operator-dependent, polluted by technological speckle, but it remains an attractive option since it is simple, straightforward, and still capable of detecting quickly and simply any obvious changes in plaque composition [15–18] with an acceptable reproducibility in controlled conditions when compared to more complex methods [19]. Videodensitometry is quantitative, and still widely applicable in the current era, with most instruments generating a picture describing the image texture through mean gray level and higher order statistics (such as entropy) for spatial distribution of texture.

Table 2. Ultrasonic tissue characterization: tools.

Parameter	B-Mode Ultrasound Imaging		
	Vascular	**Transesophageal**	**Intravascular**
Ultrasound frequency	5–15	5–10	15–20
Signal-to-noise ratio	++	++	+++
Accuracy	++	++	+++
Prognostic value	++	++	+++
Applicability	Bedside	Echo lab	Cath lab
Invasiveness	Non-invasive	Semi-invasive	Invasive
Main target artery	Carotid (femoral)	Thoracic Aorta	Coronary

− = poor; ± = fair; + = good; ++ = very good; +++ = excellent.

Videodensitometry is quantitative, and still widely applicable in the current era, with most instruments generating a picture describing the image texture through mean gray level and higher order statistics (such as entropy) for spatial distribution of texture. The vulnerable plaque is more often hypoechoic, with lower mean gray level and higher entropy values (an index of spatial heterogeneity of gray level distribution) in the region of interest [19–22]. Calibrating the system in a 256 gray level scale with blood equal to 0 (=black), perfect white = 255 and the far wall, strongly reflective adventitial interface = 190, the lipid-hemorrhagic plaques (with blood-like backscatter) remain below 30, with stable plaques showing higher mean gray levels and—with texture analysis—higher entropy values associated with less homogeneous spatial pattern. Radiofrequency analysis is more technologically demanding, and theoretically more accurate, since the "native" ultrasonic signal is sampled, which is not distorted by the post-processing function of the imaging chain [23–25]. It can be applied in the carotid and in the coronary [24,26] districts, with similar findings. Calibrating the system with blood equal to 0 decibels (dB) and the perfect artificial reflector equal to 50 dB, the lipid-hemorrhagic plaques (with blood-like backscatter) remain below 14, fibrous and fibro-fatty plaques in between 14 and 26, and calcific plaques above 27. Although the radiofrequency approach is the most quantitative, the other, simpler approaches can also provide clinically valuable information for *in vivo* characterization of the ultrasonic plaque. The echogenicity is usually expressed with a qualitative score with visual assessment (from black = 1 to white = 4), in grey level units with videodensitometry (from black = 0 to white = 255), in absolute decibel values in radiofrequency analysis (Table 3). Additional echographic features of plaque instability are the neovascularization of the plaque and the irregular contour of plaque surface which are best detected by contrast-enhanced ultrasound (CEUS) [27–29].

4. Ultrasound Plaque Morphology as an Index of Clinical Instability

Although the field suffers from lack of standardization, steady changes in image technology, and lack of prospective randomized trials, over the last 30 years a series of observational studies has built up respectable evidence that an unstable plaque morphology by ultrasound identifies a higher risk subset when evaluated by different approaches (visual, videodensitometry, backscatter, CEUS) in different districts (carotid, aorta, coronary arteries) with different methods (vascular, transesophageal, intravascular ultrasound), on different populations (from acute and stable coronary patients to stable and unstable cerebrovascular or peripheral artery disease patients to asymptomatic persons at risk).

Subjects with echo-lucent and/or heterogeneous and/or neovascularized (by CEUS) atherosclerotic plaques in carotid arteries have increased risk of ischemic cerebrovascular and cardiovascular events independently of both degree of stenosis and cardiovascular risk factors [30–37].

The link between echo plaque structure and prognosis do not appear to be limited to the carotid arteries but may apply to virtually all vascular districts where atherosclerotic plaques can be imaged by ultrasound technology including femoral artery [38]. In the ascending thoracic aorta, non-calcified aortic plaques detected by TEE in brain infarction have been associated with a tenfold increased risk of subsequent events when compared to calcified plaque [39].

In coronary arteries evaluated by intracoronary ultrasound, a meta-analysis of 16 studies totaling 1693 patients who underwent PCI showed that the necrotic core (hypoechoic) component derived from virtual histology—IVUS at the minimum lumen sizes were significantly greater in the embolization (no-reflow) group compared with the no-embolization group [40]. Necrotic core was identified in the color-coded analysis as "red" (different from green, fibrotic, yellow-green, fibrofatty, and white, dense calcium). The larger the amount of attenuated coronary plaque by intracoronary ultrasound, the greater the likelihood of no-reflow [41].

Recent studies support the concept that plaque instability is not merely a local vascular incident but rather that plaque instability exists simultaneously at multiple sites of the vascular bed [42]. Similar features can be recognized in unstable patients not only in the symptomatic carotid plaque but also in the contralateral asymptomatic side, suggesting that the vulnerable plaque is also a part of the systemic inflammatory process of the vulnerable patient [43]. Ultrasonic features of instability are potentially a biomarker not only of the vulnerable plaque but—in a certain sense—of the vulnerable patient.

5. Clinical Implications

Information on plaque characterization can be obtained by ultrasound and is clinically important for several reasons. First, ultrasonically heterogeneous or soft plaques are associated with lipids and hemorrhages and have a greater tendency to ulceration, embolization, and development of symptoms. Second, anti-atherosclerotic statin treatment may induce a biochemical remodeling of the atherosclerotic plaque, with greater effect on lipidic components than on overall plaque size, which appear more echo-dense (and therefore less vulnerable) after therapy both in the coronary [44,45] and the carotid [46–51] arteries.

Table 3. Plaque imaging by ultrasound: criteria of instability.

Type of Plaque	Unstable	Stable
Visual assessment	Hypo-, Anechoic Heterogeneous Irregular surface	Iso-, Hyper-echoic Homogeneous Regular surface
Videodensitometry	Low median gray level High entropy	High median gray level Low entropy
Radiofrequency	<13 dB	14–33 dB
CEUS	Neovessel Present	Neovessel Absent

Higher values correspond to higher echodensity. Visual assessment of echogenicity refers black as blood and white as far-wall adventitia interface (Gray-Weale, 1988 [16]). Homogeneity is defined according to Joakimsen, 1997 [17] and surface regularity as in Ibrahimi, 2014 [43]. Videodensitometry values are expressed in median grey levels (MGL, 0 black–255 white), with 0 = black as blood and 190 = bright as far-wall adventitia (Ibrahimi, 2014 [43]). Backscatter values are expressed in decibels (dB, calibrated with 0 dB = blood and 50 dB = stainless steel specular interface), according to Kawasaky, 2001 [24]. CEUS binary criteria for intimal neovascularization were proposed by Coli, 2008 [27].

Whatever the method available (visual, videodensitometry or backscatter-based), a simple description of plaque morphology can be helpful to the clinician as a clue to separate stable and unstable plaques (Table 4). Conventional echography and ultrasonic tissue characterization are not mutually exclusive, and any commercial device has—or will soon have—both conventional imaging and quantitative tissue characterization imaging built into the same hybrid basic hardware. Information on tissue characterization of the atherosclerotic plaque can be obtained with other imaging techniques, including MRI, CCTA, PET with FDG and—invasively—by OCT [4].

Table 4. Ultrasound appearance and plaque risk.

Risk	Low-Risk	High-Risk
Plaque border profile	Smooth	Irregular
Echo-density	Iso-, Hyper-echoic	Hypo-, Anechoic
Plaque luminal border *	Regular	Irregular
Plaque neovascularization *	Absent	Present
Spotty calcification	Rare	Frequent
Massive calcification	Frequent	Rare
Plaque burden	Low (<40% stenosis)	High (>70% stenosis)

* By CEUS, contrast-enhanced ultrasound. Carotid plaques are imaged by Duplex scan, coronary plaques by invasive intracoronary ultrasound.

The ultrasound approach has clear advantages over other clinically viable imaging approaches used to detect the vulnerable plaque: non-invasive (differently from OCT—although intracoronary ultrasound can be used, with higher frequencies and better signal-to-noise ratio than vascular ultrasound), radiation-free (differently from CCTA and PET), low cost and high spatial and temporal resolution [4]. Carotid duplex imaging is suitable for evaluation of extracranial cerebral vessels, but cannot image intracranial portion of the carotid artery and is less accurate in presence of dense calcification [3].

6. Conclusions

Ultrasonic tissue characterization of atherosclerotic plaque began 30 years ago, and while not yet ready for clinical use it is today regarded as one of the most promising fields of application in cardiovascular ultrasound imaging. In particular, it has the potential to identify—for any given stenosis—vulnerable, lipid-rich, unstable plaques more prone to complications such as embolization and rupture, and also receiving the greatest benefit from pharmacological and mechanical intervention strategies to prevent such events. Although fascinating, the imaging approach has inherent limitations, since not all ruptured plaques have histologic features of vulnerability (and 20% have none of them), and not all vulnerable plaques by histology criteria do eventually rupture in their natural history [3]. With these caveats, the imaging of plaque vulnerability remains a reasonable approach to bridging the current gap in understanding clinical manifestations of atherosclerotic disease, especially regarding the striking clinical mismatch between atherosclerosis extent and severity and its clinical manifestations, and the therapeutic mismatch between reductions of clinical events obtained with statins and the limited—if any—reduction in atheroma size. New quantitative methods beyond backscatter (to include speed of sound, attenuation, strain, temperature, and high order statistics) will be developed to evaluate vascular tissues. These image methods may offer opportunities for the early detection and treatment of the disease [52]. Once the methodology and analysis have been standardized, the stage will be set for future prospective randomized trials to evaluate whether quantitative tissue characterization-based information on plaque vulnerability can be used to tailor risk and treatment in patients with clinically symptomatic and high-risk asymptomatic atherosclerosis.

Acknowledgments: The authors thank Letizia Morelli for secretarial assistance.

References

1. Mor-Avi, V.; Lang, R.M.; Badano, L.P.; Belohlavek, M.; Cardim, N.M.; Derumeaux, G.; Galderisi, M.; Marwick, T.; Nagueh, S.F.; Sengupta, P.P.; *et al.* Current and evolving echocardiographic techniques for the quantitative evaluation of cardiac mechanics: ASE/EAE consensus statement on methodology and indications endorsed by the Japanese Society of Echocardiography. *Eur. J. Echocardiogr.* **2011**, *12*, 167–205. [CrossRef] [PubMed]

2. Fleg, J.L.; Stone, G.W.; Fayad, Z.A.; Granada, J.F.; Hatsukami, T.S.; Kolodgie, F.D.; Ohayon, J.; Pettigrew, R.; Sabatine, M.S.; Tearney, G.J.; *et al.* Detection of high-risk atherosclerotic plaque: Report of the NHLBI Working Group on current status and future directions. *JACC Cardiovasc. Imaging* **2012**, *5*, 941–955. [CrossRef] [PubMed]

3. Stein, J.H.; Korcarz, C.E.; Hurst, R.T.; Lonn, E.; Kendall, C.B.; Mohler, E.R.; Najjar, S.S.; Rembold, C.M.; Post, W.S.; American Society of Echocardiography Carotid Intima-Media Thickness Task Force. Use of carotid ultrasound to identify subclinical cardiovascular disease risk: Consensus statement from the American society of echocardiography. *J. Am. Soc. Echocardiogr.* **2008**, *21*, 93–111. [CrossRef] [PubMed]

4. Gallino, A.; Stuber, M.; Crea, F.; Falk, E.; Corti, R.; Lekakis, J.; Schwitter, J.; Camici, P.; Gaemperli, O.; di Valentino, M.; *et al. In vivo* imaging of atherosclerosis. *Atherosclerosis* **2012**, *224*, 25–36. [CrossRef] [PubMed]

5. Wissler, R.W. Principles of the pathogenesis of atherosclerosis. In *Heart Disease: A Textbook of Cardiovascular Medicine*; Braunwald, E., Ed.; Saunders: Philadelphia, PA, USA, 1984; pp. 1183–1194.

6. Picano, E.; Landini, L.; Distante, A.; Sarnelli, R.; Benassi, A.; L'Abbate, A. Different degrees of atherosclerosis detected by backscattered ultrasound: An *in vitro* study on fixed human aortic walls. *J. Clin. Ultrasound* **1983**, *11*, 375–379. [CrossRef] [PubMed]

7. Picano, E.; Landini, L.; Distante, A.; Benassi, A.; Sarnelli, R.; L'Abbate, A. Fibrosis, lipids, and calcium in human atherosclerotic plaque. *In vitro* differentiation from normal aortic walls by ultrasonic attenuation. *Circ. Res.* **1985**, *56*, 556–562.

8. Picano, E.; Landini, L.; Distante, A.; Salvadori, M.; Lattanzi, F.; Masini, M.; L'Abbate, A. Angle dependence of ultrasonic backscatter in arterial tissues: A study *in vitro. Circulation* **1985**, *72*, 572–576. [CrossRef] [PubMed]

9. Picano, E.; Landini, L.; Lattanzi, F.; Mazzarisi, A.; Sarnelli, R.; Distante, A.; Benassi, A.; L'Abbate, A. The use of frequency histograms of ultrasonic backscatter amplitudes for detection of atherosclerosis *in vitro. Circulation* **1986**, *74*, 1093–1098. [CrossRef] [PubMed]

10. Picano, E.; Landini, L.; Lattanzi, F.; Salvadori, M.; Benassi, A.; L'Abbate, A. Time domain echo pattern evaluations from normal and atherosclerotic arterial walls: A study *in vitro. Circulation* **1988**, *77*, 654–659. [CrossRef] [PubMed]

11. Wolverson, M.K.; Bashiti, H.M.; Peterson, G.J. Ultrasonic tissue characterization of atheromatous plaques using a high resolution real time scanner. *Ultrasound Med. Biol.* **1983**, *9*, 599–609. [CrossRef] [PubMed]

12. Barzilai, B.; Saffitz, J.E.; Miller, J.G.; Sobel, B.E. Quantitative ultrasonic characterization of the nature of atherosclerotic plaques in human aorta. *Circ. Res.* **1987**, *60*, 459–463. [CrossRef] [PubMed]

13. Hiro, T.; Leung, C.Y.; Karimi, H.; Farvid, A.R.; Tobis, J.M. Angle dependence of intravascular ultrasound imaging and its feasibility in tissue characterization of human atherosclerotic tissue. *Am. Heart J.* **1999**, *137*, 476–481. [CrossRef] [PubMed]

14. Komiyama, N.; Berry, G.J.; Kolz, M.L.; Oshima, A.; Metz, J.A.; Preuss, P.; Brisken, A.F.; Pauliina Moore, M.; Yock, P.G.; Fitzgerald, P.J. Tissue characterization of atherosclerotic plaques by intravascular radiofrequency signal analysis: An *in vitro* study of human coronary artery. *Am. Heart J.* **2000**, *140*, 565–574. [CrossRef] [PubMed]

15. Reilly, L.M.; Lusby, R.J.; Hughes, L.; Ferrell, L.D.; Stoney, R.J.; Ehrenfeld, W.K. Carotid plaque histology using real time ultrasonography. Clinical and therapeutic implications. *Am. J. Surg.* **1983**, *146*, 188–193. [CrossRef] [PubMed]

16. Gray-Weale, A.C.; Graham, J.C.; Burnett, J.R.; Byrne, K.; Lusby, R.J. Carotid artery atheroma: Comparison of preoperative B-mode ultrasound appearance with carotid endarterectomy specimen pathology. *J. Cardiovasc. Surg.* **1988**, *29*, 676–681.

17. European Carotid Plaque Study Group. Carotid artery composition—Relation to clinical presentation and ultrasound B-mode imaging. *Eur. J. Endovasc. Surg.* **1995**, *10*, 23–32.

18. Joakimsen, O.; Bıııona, K.H.; Stensland-Bugge, E. Reproducibility of ultrasound assessment of carotid plaque occurrence, thickness, and morphology. The Tromsø study. *Stroke* **1997**, *28*, 2201–2207. [CrossRef] [PubMed]

19. Grønholdt, M.L.; Wiebe, B.M.; Laursen, H.; Nielsen, T.G.; Schroeder, T.V.; Sillesen, H. Lipid-rich carotid artery plaques appear echolucent on ultrasound B-mode images and may be associated with intraplaque hemorrhage. *Eur. J. Vasc. Endovasc. Surg.* **1997**, *14*, 439–445. [CrossRef] [PubMed]

20. Mazzone, A.M.; Urbani, M.P.; Picano, E.; Paterni, M.; Borgatti, E.; de Fabritiis, A.; Landini, L. *In vivo* ultrasonic parametric imaging of carotid atherosclerotic plaque by videodensitometric technique. *Angiology* **1995**, *46*, 663–672. [CrossRef] [PubMed]

21. El-Barghouty, N.M.; Levine, T.; Ladva, S.; Flanagan, A.; Nicolaides, A. Histological verification of computerized carotid plaque characterization. *Eur. J. Vasc. Endovasc. Surg.* **1996**, *11*, 414–416. [CrossRef] [PubMed]

22. Baroncini, L.A.V.; Pazin Filho, A.; Murta, O., Jr.; Martins, A.R.; Ramos, S.O.; Cherri, J.; Piccinato, C.E. Ultrasonic tissue characterization of vulnerable carotid plaque: Correlation between videodensitometric method and histological exam. *Cardiov. Ultrasound* **2006**, *4*. [CrossRef]

23. Urbani, M.P.; Picano, E.; Parenti, G.; Mazzarisi, A.; Fiori, L.; Paterni, M.; Pelosi, G.; Landini, L. *In vivo* radiofrequency-based ultrasonic tissue characterization of the atherosclerotic plaque. *Stroke* **1993**, *24*, 1507–1512. [CrossRef] [PubMed]

24. Kawasaki, M.; Takatsu, H.; Noda, T.; Ito, Y.; Kunishima, A.; Arai, M.; Nishigaki, K.; Takemura, G.; Morita, N.; Minatoguchi, S.; *et al.* Noninvasive quantitative tissue characterization and two-dimensional color-coded map of human atherosclerotic lesions using ultrasound integrated backscatter. Comparison between histology and integrated backscatter images before and after death. *J. Am. Coll. Cardiol.* **2001**, *38*, 486–492. [CrossRef] [PubMed]

25. Waki, H.; Masuyama, T.; Mori, H.; Maeda, T.; Kitade, K.; Moriyasu, K.; Tsujimoto, M.; Fujimoto, K.; Koshimae, N.; Matsuura, N. Ultrasonic tissue characterization of the atherosclerotic carotid plaque: Histologic correlates of carotid integrated backscatter. *Circ. J.* **2003**, *67*, 1013–1016. [CrossRef] [PubMed]

26. Gussenhoven, W.J.; Essed, C.E.; Frietman, P.; Mastik, F.; Lancee, C.; Slager, C.; Serruys, P.; Gerritsen, P.; Pieterman, H.; Bom, N. Intravascular echographic assessment of vessel wall characteristics: A correlation with histology. *Int. J. Cardiovasc. Imaging* **1989**, *4*, 105–116. [CrossRef]

27. Coli, S.; Magnoni, M.; Sangiorgi, G.; Marrocco-Trischitta, M.M.; Melisurgo, G.; Mauriello, A.; Spagnoli, L.; Chiesa, R.; Cianflone, D.; Maseri, A. Contrast-enhanced ultrasound imaging of intraplaque neovascularization in carotid arteries: Correlation with histology and plaque echogenicity. *J. Am. Coll. Cardiol.* **2008**, *52*, 223–230. [CrossRef] [PubMed]

28. Faggioli, G.L.; Pini, R.; Mauro, R.; Pasquinelli, G.; Fittipaldi, S.; Freyrie, A.; Serra, C.; Stella, A. Identification of carotid vulnerable plaque in contrast-enhanced ultrasound: Correlation with plaque histology, symptoms and cerebral computed tomography. *Eur. J. Vasc. Endovasc. Surg.* **2011**, *41*, 238–248. [CrossRef] [PubMed]

29. Partovi, S.; Loebe, M.; Aschwanden, M.; Baldi, T.; Jäger, K.A.; Feinstein, S.B.; Staub, D. Contrast-enhanced ultrasound for assessing carotid atherosclerosis plaque lesions. *Am. J. Radiol.* **2012**, *198*, W13–W19.

30. Gronholdt, M.L.; Nordestgaard, B.G.; Schroeder, T.V.; Vorstrup, S.; Sillesen, H. Ultrasound echolucent carotid plaques predict future strokes. *Circulation* **2001**, *104*, 68–73. [CrossRef] [PubMed]

31. Mathiesen, E.B.; Bonaa, K.H.; Joakimsen, O. Echo-lucent plaques are associated with high risk of ischemic cerebrovascular events in carotid stenosis. *Circulation* **2001**, *103*, 2171–2175. [CrossRef] [PubMed]

32. Honda, O.; Sugiyama, S.; Kugiyama, K.; Fukushima, H.; Nakamura, S.; Koide, S.; Kojima, S.; Hirai, N.; Kawano, H.; Soejima, H.; *et al.* Echolucent carotid plaques predict future coronary events in patients with coronary artery disease. *J. Am. Coll. Cardiol.* **2004**, *43*, 1177–1184. [CrossRef] [PubMed]

33. Biasi, G.M.; Froio, A.F.; Diethrich, E.B.; Deleo, G.; Galimberti, S.; Mingazzini, P.; Nicolaides, A.N.; Griffin, M.; Raithel, D.; Reid, D.B.; *et al.* Carotid plaque echolucency increases the risk of stroke in carotid stenting. The Imaging in Carotid Angioplasty and Risk of Stroke (ICAROS) study. *Circulation* **2004**, *110*, 756–762. [CrossRef] [PubMed]

34. Petersen, C.; Peçanha, P.B.; Venneri, L.; Pasanisi, E.; Pratali, L.; Picano, E. The impact of carotid plaque presence and morphology on mortality outcome in cardiological patients. *Cardiovasc. Ultrasound* **2006**, *4*. [CrossRef]

35. Yamada, K.; Kawasaki, M.; Yoshima, S.; Enomoto, Y.; Asano, T.; Minatocuchi, S.; Iwana, T. Prediction of silent ischemic lesions after carotid stenting using integrated backscatter ultrasouns and magnetic resonance imaging. *Atherosclerosis* **2010**, *208*, 161–166. [CrossRef] [PubMed]

36. Irie, Y.; Katakami, N.; Kaneto, H.; Takahara, M.; Nishio, M.; Kasami, R.; Sakamoto, K.; Umayahara, Y.; Sumitsuji, S.; Ueda, Y.; *et al.* The utility of ultrasound tissue characterization in the prediction of cardiovascular events in diabetic patients. *Atherosclerosis* **2013**, *230*, 399–403. [CrossRef] [PubMed]

37. Zhu, Y.; Deng, Y.B.; Liu, Y.N.; Bi, X.J.; Sun, J.; Tang, Q.Y.; Deng, Q. Use of carotid plaque neovascularization of contrast-enhanced ultrasound to predict coronary events in patients with coronary artery disease. *Radiology* **2013**, *268*, 54–61. [CrossRef] [PubMed]

38. Schmidt, C.; Fagerberg, B.; Hulthe, J. Non-stenotic echolucent ultrasound-assessed femoral artery plaques are predictive for future cardiovascular events in middle-aged men. *Atherosclerosis* **2005**, *181*, 125–130. [CrossRef] [PubMed]

39. Cohen, A.; Tzourio, C.; Bertrand, B.; Chauvel, C.; Bousser, M.G.; Amarenco, P. Aortic plaque morphology and vascular events: A follow-up study in patients with ischemic stroke. FAPS Investigators. French Study of Aortic Plaques in Stroke. *Circulation* **1997**, *96*, 3838–3841. [CrossRef] [PubMed]

40. Jang, J.S.; Jin, H.Y.; Seo, J.S.; Yang, T.H.; Kim, D.K.; Park, Y.A.; Cho, K.I.; Park, Y.H.; Kim, D.S. Meta-analysis of plaque composition by intravascular ultrasound and its relation to distal emboli after percutaneous coronary interventions. *Am. J. Cardiol.* **2013**, *111*, 968–972. [CrossRef] [PubMed]

41. Xu, Y.; Mintz, G.S.; Tam, A.; McPherson, J.A.; Iñiguez, A.; Fajadet, J.; Fahy, M.; Weisz, G.; de Bruyne, B.; Serruys, P.W.; *et al.* Prevalence, distribution, predictors and outcomes of patients with calcified nodules in native coronary arteries: A 3-vessel intravascular ultrasound anaysis from Providing Regional Observations to Study predictors of Events in the Coronary Tree (PROSPECT). *Circulation* **2012**, *126*, 537–545. [CrossRef] [PubMed]

42. Lombardo, A.; Biasucci, L.M.; Lanza, G.A.; Coli, S.; Silvestri, P.; Cianflone, D.; Liuzzo, G.; Burzotta, F.; Crea, F.; Maseri, A. Inflammation as a possible link between coronary and carotid plaque instability. *Circulation* **2004**, *109*, 3158–3163. [CrossRef] [PubMed]

43. Ibrahimi, P.; Jashari, F.; Johansson, E.; Gronlund, C.; Bajraktari, G.; Wester, P.; Henein, M.Y. Vulnerable plaques in the contralateral carotid arteries in symptomatic patients: A detailed ultrasonic analysis. *Atherosclerosis* **2014**, *235*, 526–531. [CrossRef] [PubMed]

44. Kawasaki, M.; Sano, K.; Okubo, M.; Yokoyama, H.; Ito, Y.; Murata, I.; Tsuchiya, K.; Minatoguchi, S.; Zhou, X.; Fujita, H.; *et al.* Volumetric quantitative analysis of tissue characteristics of coronary plaques after statin therapy using three-dimensional integrated backscatter intravascular ultrasound. *J. Am. Coll. Cardiol.* **2005**, *45*, 1946–1953. [CrossRef] [PubMed]

45. Yokoyama, M.; Komiyama, N.; Courtney, B.K.; Nakayama, T.; Namikawa, S.; Kuriyama, N.; Koizumi, T.; Nameki, M.; Fitzgerald, P.J.; Komuro, I. Plasma low-density lipoprotein reduction and structural effects on coronary atherosclerotic plaques by atorvastatin as clinically assessed with intravascular ultrasound radio-frequency signal analysis: A randomized prospective study. *Am. Heart J.* **2005**, *150*, 287. [CrossRef] [PubMed]

46. Yamada, K.; Yoshimura, S.; Kawasaki, M.; Enomoto, Y.; Asano, T.; Minatoguchi, S.; Iwama, T. Effects of atorvastatin on carotid atherosclerotic plaques: A randomized trial with quantitative tissue characterization of carotid atherosclerotic plaques with integrated backscatter. *Cerebrovasc. Dis.* **2009**, *28*, 417–424. [CrossRef] [PubMed]

47. Watanabe, K.; Sugiyama, S.; Kugiyama, K.; Honda, O.; Fukushima, H.; Koga, H.; Horibata, Y.; Hirai, T.; Sakamoto, T.; Yoshimura, M.; *et al.* Stabilization of carotid atheroma assessed by quantitative ultrasound analysis in non-hypercholesterolemic patients with coronary artery disease. *J. Am. Coll. Cardiol.* **2005**, *46*, 2022–2030. [CrossRef] [PubMed]

48. Kadoglou, N.P.; Gerasimidis, T.; Moumtzouoglou, A.; Kapelouzou, A.; Sailer, N.; Fotiadis, G.; Vitta, I.; Katinios, A.; Kougias, P.; Bandios, S.; *et al.* Intensive lipid-lowering therapy ameliorates novel calcification markers and GSM score in patients with carotid stenosis. *Eur. J. Vasc. Endovasc. Surg.* **2008**, *35*, 661–668. [CrossRef] [PubMed]

49. Yamagami, H.; Sakaguchi, M.; Furukado, S.; Hoshi, T.; Abe, Y.; Hougaku, H.; Hori, M.; Kitagawa, K. Statin therapy increases carotid plaque echogenicity in hypercholesterolemic patients. *Ultrasound Med. Biol.* **2008**, *34*, 1353–1359. [CrossRef] [PubMed]

50. Della-Morte, D.; Moussa, I.; Elkind, M.S.; Sacco, R.L.; Rundek, T. The short-term effects of atorvastatin on carotid plaque morphology assessed by computer-assisted gray scale densitometry: A pilot study. *Neurol. Res.* **2011**, *33*, 991–994. [CrossRef] [PubMed]

51. Ostling, G.; Gonçalves, I.; Wikstrand, J.; Berglund, G.; Nilsson, J.; Hedblad, B. Long-term treatment with low dose metoprolol is associated with increased plaque echogenicity: The β-blocker cholesterol lowering asymptomatic plaque study. *Atherosclerosis* **2011**, *215*, 440–445. [CrossRef] [PubMed]

52. Pellikka, P.A.; Douglas, P.S.; Miller, J.G.; Abraham, T.P.; Baumann, R.; Buxton, D.B.; Byrd, B.F., III; Chen, P.; Cook, N.L.; Gardin, J.M.; *et al.* American Society of Echocardiography Cardiovascular technology and research summit: A roadmap for 2020. *J. Am. Soc. Echocardiogr.* **2013**, *26*, 325–338. [CrossRef] [PubMed]

8

Asymmetric Dimethylarginine *versus* Proton Pump Inhibitors Usage in Patients with Stable Coronary Artery Disease

Olga Kruszelnicka [1,*], **Jolanta Świerszcz** [2], **Jacek Bednarek** [3], **Bernadeta Chyrchel** [2], **Andrzej Surdacki** [2,†] **and Jadwiga Nessler** [1,†]

[1] Department of Coronary Artery Disease and Heart Failure, Jagiellonian University Medical College and John Paul II Hospital, 80 Prądnicka, 31-202 Cracow, Poland; jnessler@interia.pl

[2] Second Department of Cardiology, Jagiellonian University Medical College and University Hospital, 17 Kopernika, 31-501 Cracow, Poland; grasshoppers@interia.eu (J.Ś.); chyrchelb@gmail.com (B.C.); surdacki.andreas@gmx.net (A.S.)

[3] Department of Electrocardiology, John Paul II Hospital, 80 Prądnicka, 31-202 Cracow, Poland; bednareks@op.pl

* Correspondence: olga.kruszelnicka@onet.pl;

† Joint senior authors on this work.

Academic Editor: Michael Henein

Abstract: A recent experimental study suggested that proton pump inhibitors (PPI), widely used to prevent gastroduodenal complications of dual antiplatelet therapy, may increase the accumulation of the endogenous nitric oxide synthesis antagonist asymmetric dimethylarginine (ADMA), an adverse outcome predictor. Our aim was to assess the effect of PPI usage on circulating ADMA in coronary artery disease (CAD). Plasma ADMA levels were compared according to PPI use for ≥ 1 month prior to admission in 128 previously described non-diabetic men with stable CAD who were free of heart failure or other coexistent diseases. Patients on PPI tended to be older and with insignificantly lower estimated glomerular filtration rate (GFR). PPI use was not associated with any effect on plasma ADMA (0.51 ± 0.11 (SD) *vs.* 0.50 ± 0.10 μmol/L for those with PPI ($n = 53$) and without PPI ($n = 75$), respectively; $p = 0.7$). Additionally, plasma ADMA did not differ between PPI users and non-users stratified by a history of current smoking, CAD severity or extent. The adjustment for patients' age and GFR did not substantially change the results. Thus, PPI usage does not appear to affect circulating ADMA in non-diabetic men with stable CAD. Whether novel mechanisms of adverse PPI effects on the vasculature can be translated into clinical conditions, requires further studies.

Keywords: asymmetric dimethylarginine; coronary artery disease; proton pump inhibitors

1. Introduction

Proton pump inhibitors (PPI)—widely used to prevent gastroduodenal complications of dual antiplatelet therapy—have recently been demonstrated to raise intracellular levels of asymmetric dimethylargininie (ADMA), an endogenous inhibitor of nitric oxide (NO) synthesis, which was accompanied by a lower NO formation, depressed endothelium-mediated vasorelaxation *in vitro* and increased circulating ADMA by about 20% in mice. These effects were ascribed to a PPI-dependent direct inhibition of the activity of the major ADMA-degrading enzyme type 1 dimethylarginine dimethylaminohydrolase (DDAH-1) [1].

Because ADMA is a recognized adverse outcome predictor in coronary artery disease (CAD) patients [2–4], the PPI-ADMA interaction might contribute to an excessive cardiovascular risk in patients on PPI irrespective of the use of antiplatelet agents including clopidogrel, or a prior history of myocardial infarction [5–11]. Importantly, an elevated risk of myocardial infarction was associated with the usage of PPI but not H_2-receptor antagonists also in the general population subjects, mainly without aspirin or clopidogrel, which may suggest an underlying mechanism not directly involving either platelet aggregation or changed drug absorption due to a rise in gastric pH [11,12]. Admittedly, potential negative clinical impacts of PPI on the risk of adverse cardiovascular events are still controversial [13] with conflicting results between randomized trials and observational studies [10,14]. Nevertheless, the proposed mechanistic concept [1] was not confirmed in a recent placebo-controlled, open-label, cross-over study where PPI administration for four weeks was not associated with significant effects on plasma ADMA or flow-dependent vasodilation in adults [15].

Therefore, our aim was to estimate the effect of PPI usage on circulating ADMA in stable CAD.

2. Results

Clinical and angiographic characteristics according to PPI use are shown in Table 1. Patients taking a PPI prior to admission (mainly omeprazole 20 mg o.i.d. or pantoprazole 20 mg o.i.d.) tended to be older and with lower estimated glomerular filtration rate (GFR).

Table 1. Characteristics of CAD patients according to PPI use prior to admission on a background of concomitant low-dose aspirin, ACEI and statin.

Characteristic	Patients on PPI ($n = 53$)	Patients without PPI ($n = 75$)	p-Value
Age (years)	59 ± 11	56 ± 10	0.12
Body-mass index (kg/m^2)	27.7 ± 3.6	27.4 ± 3.5	0.6
History of current smoking, n (%)	16 (30%)	20 (27%)	0.8
Multivessel CAD, n (%)	41 (77%)	54 (72%)	0.6
CAD extent score	31 (21–44)	28 (19–40)	0.5
Left ventricular ejection fraction (%)	70 ± 7	68 ± 6	0.2
Hypertension, n (%)	43 (80%)	56 (75%)	0.4
Mean blood pressure (mm Hg)	96 ± 11	95 ± 10	0.7
Estimated GFR (mL/min per 1.73 m^2)	69 ± 9	72 ± 11	0.09
LDL cholesterol (mmol/L)	2.8 ± 0.7	2.8 ± 0.6	0.8
HDL cholesterol (mmol/L)	0.9 ± 0.3	1.0 ± 0.3	0.2
Triglycerides (mmol/L)	1.4 ± 0.6	1.5 ± 0.7	0.3
Glucose (mmol/L)	5.8 ± 0.9	5.7 ± 0.8	0.5
High-sensitivity C-reactive protein (mg/L)	1.9 (1.1–4.0)	1.8 (1.0–3.8)	0.8

Data are shown as mean $\pm$ SD, median (interquartile range) or n (%); p-values by 2-tailed Student's t-test or Mann-Whitney U test, and chi-squared test for proportions. CAD: coronary artery disease; ADMA: asymmetric dimethylarginine; ACEI: angiotensin-converting enzyme inhibitors; GFR: glomerular filtration rate calculated according to the Modification of Diet in Renal Disease study formula; HDL: high-density lipoproteins; LDL: low-density lipoproteins; PPI: proton pump inhibitors.

The use of PPI was not associated with any effect on plasma ADMA (Table 2). In addition, there were no interactions between PPI use and the categorized potential confounders, *i.e.*, current smoking, angiographic CAD severity or extent in terms of plasma ADMA ($p > 0.3$), so that ADMA levels did not differ between PPI users and PPI non-users stratified by a history of current smoking, the presence of multivessel CAD or an over-median Sullivan score of angiographic CAD extent (Table 2). Adjustment for patients' age and GFR by means of ANCOVA did not substantially change the results.

Table 2. Plasma ADMA levels according to PPI use prior to admission.

	ADMA before Admission (μmol/L)		p-Value
	PPI Users ($n = 53$)	PPI Non-Users ($n = 75$)	
All CAD subjects, $n = 128$	0.51 ± 0.11	0.50 ± 0.10	0.7
History of current smoking			
Yes, $n = 36$	0.51 ± 0.11	0.50 ± 0.10	0.4
No, $n = 92$	0.51 ± 0.10	0.51 ± 0.11	0.8
Severity of angiographic CAD			
One-vessel disease, $n = 33$	0.48 ± 0.10	0.49 ± 0.10	0.7
Multivessel disease, $n = 95$	0.52 ± 0.11	0.51 ± 0.11	0.9
Extent of angiographic CAD			
Sullivan extent score $\leqslant 29$, $n = 65$	0.48 ± 0.09	0.49 ± 0.10	0.6
Sullivan extent score > 29, $n = 63$	0.54 ± 0.11	0.52 ± 0.10	0.3

Data are shown as mean $\pm$ SD; p-values by 2-tailed Student's t-test. Abbreviations as in Table 1.

3. Discussion

Our salient finding was a similar plasma level of ADMA in PPI users and non-users. This observation appears inconsistent with the previously reported ability of PPI to augment ADMA accumulation *in vitro* and in an animal model through a direct inhibition of DDAH-1 [1], an enzyme influencing circulating ADMA [16–19]. On the other hand, in subjects with a history of vascular disease, Ghebremariam *et al.* [15] observed a more pronounced trend towards higher ADMA while on PPI compared to placebo in an interventional cross-over study, nevertheless the differences did not reach the statistical significance, which is in agreement with our cross-sectional retrospective analysis. To the best of our knowledge, our study is the second clinical report on ADMA levels in relation to PPI use.

3.1. Mechanistic Considerations

There are several potential explanations of these apparent discrepancies. First, all the patients were receiving angiotensin-converting enzyme inhibitors (ACEI), aspirin and statins, all of which had been previously shown to lower ADMA levels [20–22], thereby obscuring the putative influence of PPI on ADMA. On the other hand, ADMA concentrations in our patients were only slightly lower than ADMA levels measured by the same enzyme-linked immunosorbent assay (ELISA) in control groups of largely untreated subjects of similar age from European populations and without evidence of atherosclerotic vascular disease [23–25], which argues against the proposed explanation and strengthens our findings.

Second, even if the PPI-DDAH-1 interaction took place *in vivo*, its effects on plasma ADMA could be attenuated or nullified by an effective counter-regulatory mechanism. This hypothetical mechanism might involve any of the recognized determinants of circulating ADMA levels including DDAH-mediated ADMA degradation, urinary ADMA excretion, the activity of type I protein-arginine N-methyltransferases (PRMTs-I), proteolysis rate of proteins with dimethylated arginine residues, and interorgan ADMA transport [26]. Of note, Becker *et al.* [27] described depressed nicotinamide adenine dinucleotide phosphate (NADPH)-dependent superoxide release and augmented expression of the antioxidant defense enzyme type 1 heme oxygenase (HO-1) in human endothelial cells exposed for 8–24 h to lansoprazole at final concentrations as low as 30 μmol/L, *i.e.*, similar to PPI levels (20 μmol/L) that increased intracellular ADMA concentrations by about 30% via DDAH-1 inhibition as shown by Ghebremariam *et al.* [1]. The PPI-dependent HO-1 induction occurred at the level of transcription [27], in contrast to PPI direct effects on DDAH-1 activity [1], which can probably further potentiate the former effect in subjects on chronic PPI therapy. Accordingly, because oxidative stress stimulates PRMTs-I expression [28] and inhibits DDAH activity [29,30], the PPI-mediated decrease in endothelial superoxide formation [27] could possibly indirectly downregulate ADMA formation and enhance ADMA degradation, thus counteracting the ADMA-increasing effect of the direct DDAH-1 inhibition by PPI [1].

Third, findings from animal experiments cannot be simply extrapolated to clinical conditions because the presence of atherosclerotic cardiovascular disease and risk factors may interfere with ADMA-regulating pathways. Nevertheless, in our hands, there were no significant interactions between PPI use and angiographic CAD extent or severity in terms of plasma ADMA and the results did not substantially change upon exclusion of current smokers from the analysis.

3.2. Study Limitations

First, a retrospective study design constrains conclusions drawn from our data. Second, our findings would be strengthened if we also assessed characteristics previously linked to adverse cardiovascular effects of PPI, *i.e.*, magnesium or homocysteine (due to a putative PPI-induced vitamin B_{12} deficiency), and platelet response to aspirin (attributable to reduced aspirin absorption at a higher intragastric pH). Nevertheless, chronic PPI therapy is unlikely to induce clinically relevant changes in serum magnesium [31], vitamin B_{12} or homocysteine [32]. With regard to aspirin antiplatelet effect, contradictory results were reported in patients on a low-dose aspirin treated with concomitant PPI [33,34] and no involvement of ADMA in this interaction [33] has been demonstrated so far. Third, coexistent diseases could affect our results, although we applied a wide range of exclusion criteria to limit the heterogeneity of the study population. Finally, PPI pharmacokinetics is profoundly modulated by genetic loss-of-function polymorphisms of cytochrome P450 (CYP) 2C19 isoform. Compared to so-called extensive metabolizers with both wild-type CYP2C19 alleles, poor mobilizers (those with both mutated CYP2C19 alleles) exhibit elevated circulating PPI levels, e.g., after oral omeprazole its peak plasma level was about 5-fold higher and the area under the concentration-time curve approximately 9-fold higher [35]. Admittedly, we did not perform either genetic or epigenetic testing. However, our aim was to compare ADMA in relation to PPI use in real-world clinical practice irrespective of genotype status. Additionally, the frequency of CYP2C19 poor metabolizers in Caucasian populations averages only about 2%–3% [36,37].

4. Materials and Methods

4.1. Patients

We performed an additional analysis of the dataset including ADMA levels and clinical and angiographic characteristics of stable CAD men who had previously been described [38]. The study subjects were free of heart failure or diabetes and exhibited the presence of $\geqslant 1$ significant epicardial coronary stenosis on elective coronary angiography in our tertiary-care center [38]. All the patients were receiving a low-dose aspirin, ACEI and statin for at least 3 months prior to the hospitalization. As described previously [38], a wide set of exclusion criteria had been applied, including significant valvular heart disease, infections within previous 2 months, relevant coexistent diseases (e.g., severe renal insufficiency) and chronic non-cardiovascular medication with non-selective non-steroidal anti-inflammatory drugs or coxibs. Out of 151 CAD patients 23 were excluded from the current analysis due to missing data with regard to PPI use for $\geqslant 1$ month before the index hospitalization.

In line with the Declaration of Helsinki, the study protocol was approved by the Bioethics Committee of the Jagiellonian University (Approval numbers: KBET/63/B/2006 dated 27 April 2006 and KBET/364/B/2012 dated 20 December 2012) and informed consent was obtained from the patients, as mentioned previously [38].

4.2. Procedure

A sample of peripheral venous blood was collected into ethylenediaminetetraacetic acid tubes in the fasting state in the morning prior to coronary angiography and plasma was kept frozen at $-70\,^\circ\mathrm{C}$ for subsequent biochemical analyses.

ADMA levels were measured by a commercially available ELISA (DLD Diagnostika GmbH., Hamburg, Germany)—as reported in detail [38]—and compared between 2 subgroups of the study subjects divided on the basis of a history of PPI use for ≥ 1 month before blood sampling on admission for ADMA assay. In addition, we compared ADMA levels in PPI users and non-users according to a history of current smoking, angiographic CAD severity (multivessel *vs.* one-vessel CAD) [39] and CAD extent quantified by means of the Sullivan score representing a percentage of the vessels with vascular wall irregularities on coronary angiography [40].

4.3. Statistical Analysis

Data have been presented as means $\pm$ SD (standard deviation) or medians (interquartile range) for continuous characteristics with normal and non-normal distribution, respectively. The concordance with a Gaussian distribution was checked by the Lilliefors' test. The patients were compared according to PPI use by 2-tailed Student's *t*-test or Mann-Whitney U test, and chi-squared test for continuous and categorical characteristics, respectively. According to a *post hoc* power calculation for the study group as a whole, the study design allowed to detect a difference in plasma ADMA between PPI users ($n = 53$) and non-users ($n = 75$) of 0.05 µmol/L (0.5 SD) with a power of 80% at a type I error rate of 0.05.

In order to test whether an effect of PPI use on circulating ADMA levels was modified by selected categorized covariates, a two-way analysis of variance (ANOVA) was performed to assess these potential interactions with plasma ADMA as a dependent variable and 2 independent factors: PPI use on the one hand and—on the other hand—a history of self-reported current smoking or angiographic CAD severity (multivessel *vs.* one-vessel CAD) or dichotomized CAD extent (an over-median (>29) *vs.* below-median (≤ 29) Sullivan score) as a coexistent factor; then an interaction between these factors was estimated. In addition, analysis of covariance (ANCOVA) was used to adjust for continuous clinical characteristics, for which the *p*-value in a univariate comparison between patients with and without PPI did not exceed 0.15. A *p*-value below 0.05 was inferred significant.

5. Conclusions

Thus, our preliminary cross-sectional findings suggest that PPI use does not appear to considerably affect circulating ADMA in non-diabetic men with stable CAD. Whether novel mechanisms of adverse PPI effects on the vasculature can be translated into clinical conditions, requires validation in large well-designed studies.

Acknowledgments: This work was supported in part by a research grant (No. K/ZDS/003761) from the Jagiellonian University Medical College, Cracow, Poland. The publication of this paper was supported by the Faculty of Medicine, Jagiellonian University Medical College, Leading National Research Center (KNOW) 2012–2017.

Author Contributions: Olga Kruszelnicka conceived and designed the study, analyzed and interpreted data, and wrote the manuscript. Jolanta Świerszcz, Jacek Bednarek and Bernadeta Chyrchel contributed to data collection and analysis. Jadwiga Nessler and Andrzej Surdacki contributed to study design and discussion, and supervised the study. All authors read, critically revised and approved the final manuscript.

Abbreviations

ACEI	angiotensin-converting enzyme inhibitors
ADMA	asymmetric dimethylarginine
ANCOVA	analysis of covariance
ANOVA	analysis of variance
CAD	coronary artery disease
CYP	cytochrome P450
DDAH-1	type 1 dimethylarginine dimethylaminohydrolase
ELISA	enzyme-linked immunosorbent assay

GFR	glomerular filtration rate
HDL	high-density lipoproteins
HO-1	type 1 heme oxygenase
LDL	low-density lipoproteins
NADPH	nicotinamide adenine dinucleotide phosphate
NO	nitric oxide
PPI	proton pump inhibitors
PRMTs-I	type I protein-arginine N-methyltransferases
SD	standard deviation

References

1. Ghebremariam, Y.T.; LePendu, P.; Lee, J.C.; Erlanson, D.A.; Slaviero, A.; Shah, N.H.; Leiper, J.; Cooke, J.P. Unexpected effect of proton pump inhibitors: Elevation of the cardiovascular risk factor asymmetric dimethylarginine. *Circulation* **2013**, *128*, 845–853. [CrossRef] [PubMed]

2. Schnabel, R.; Blankenberg, S.; Lubos, E.; Lackner, K.J.; Rupprecht, H.J.; Espinola-Klein, C.; Jachmann, N.; Post, F.; Peetz, D.; Bickel, C.; *et al.* Asymmetric dimethylarginine and the risk of cardiovascular events and death in patients with coronary artery disease: Results from the Athero*Gene* study. *Circ. Res.* **2005**, *97*, e53–e59. [CrossRef] [PubMed]

3. Meinitzer, A.; Seelhorst, U.; Wellnitz, B.; Halwachs-Baumann, G.; Boehm, B.O.; Winkelmann, B.R.; März, W. Asymmetrical dimethylarginine independently predicts total and cardiovascular mortality in individuals with angiographic coronary artery disease (the Ludwigshafen Risk and Cardiovascular Health study). *Clin. Chem.* **2007**, *53*, 273–283. [CrossRef] [PubMed]

4. Wang, Z.; Tang, W.H.; Cho, L.; Brennan, D.M.; Hazen, S.L. Targeted metabolomic evaluation of arginine methylation and cardiovascular risks: Potential mechanisms beyond nitric oxide synthase inhibition. *Arterioscler. Thromb. Vasc. Biol.* **2009**, *29*, 1383–1391. [CrossRef] [PubMed]

5. Ho, P.M.; Maddox, T.M.; Wang, L.; Fihn, S.D.; Jesse, R.L.; Peterson, E.D.; Rumsfeld, J.S. Risk of adverse outcomes associated with concomitant use of clopidogrel and proton pump inhibitors following acute coronary syndrome. *JAMA* **2009**, *301*, 937–944. [CrossRef] [PubMed]

6. Juurlink, D.N.; Gomes, T.; Ko, D.T.; Szmitko, P.E.; Austin, P.C.; Tu, J.V.; Henry, D.A.; Kopp, A.; Mamdani, M.M. A population-based study of the drug interaction between proton pump inhibitors and clopidogrel. *CMAJ* **2009**, *180*, 713–718. [CrossRef] [PubMed]

7. Charlot, M.; Ahlehoff, O.; Norgaard, M.L.; Jørgensen, C.H.; Sørensen, R.; Abildstrøm, S.Z.; Hansen, P.R.; Madsen, J.K.; Køber, L.; Torp-Pedersen, C.; *et al.* Proton-pump inhibitors are associated with increased cardiovascular risk independent of clopidogrel use: A nationwide cohort study. *Ann. Intern. Med.* **2010**, *153*, 378–386. [CrossRef] [PubMed]

8. Charlot, M.; Grove, E.L.; Hansen, P.R.; Olesen, J.B.; Ahlehoff, O.; Selmer, C.; Lindhardsen, J.; Madsen, J.K.; Køber, L.; Torp-Pedersen, C.; *et al.* Proton pump inhibitor use and risk of adverse cardiovascular events in aspirin treated patients with first time myocardial infarction: Nationwide propensity score matched study. *BMJ* **2011**, *342*, d2690. [CrossRef] [PubMed]

9. Goodman, S.G.; Clare, R.; Pieper, K.S.; Nicolau, J.C.; Storey, R.F.; Cantor, W.J.; Mahaffey, K.W.; Angiolillo, D.J.; Husted, S.; Cannon, C.P.; *et al.* Association of proton pump inhibitor use on cardiovascular outcomes with clopidogrel and ticagrelor: Insights from the platelet inhibition and patient outcomes trial. *Circulation* **2012**, *125*, 978–986. [CrossRef] [PubMed]

10. Kwok, C.S.; Jeevanantham, V.; Dawn, B.; Loke, Y.K. No consistent evidence of differential cardiovascular risk amongst proton-pump inhibitors when used with clopidogrel: Meta-analysis. *Int. J. Cardiol.* **2013**, *167*, 965–974. [CrossRef] [PubMed]

11. Shih, C.J.; Chen, Y.T.; Ou, S.M.; Li, S.Y.; Chen, T.J.; Wang, S.J. Proton pump inhibitor use represents an independent risk factor for myocardial infarction. *Int. J. Cardiol.* **2014**, *177*, 292–297. [CrossRef] [PubMed]

12. Shah, N.H.; LePendu, P.; Bauer-Mehren, A.; Ghebremariam, Y.T.; Iyer, S.V.; Marcus, J.; Nead, K.T.; Cooke, J.P.; Leeper, N.J. Proton pump inhibitor usage and the risk of myocardial infarction in the general population. *PLoS ONE* **2015**, *10*, e0124653. [CrossRef] [PubMed]

13. Agewall, S.; Cattaneo, M.; Collet, J.P.; Andreotti, F.; Lip, G.Y.; Verheugt, F.W.; Huber, K.; Grove, E.L.; Morais, J.; Husted, S.; *et al.* Expert position paper on the use of proton pump inhibitors in patients with cardiovascular disease and antithrombotic therapy. *Eur. Heart J.* **2013**, *34*, 1708–1713. [CrossRef] [PubMed]

14. Melloni, C.; Washam, J.B.; Jones, W.S.; Halim, S.A.; Hasselblad, V.; Mayer, S.B.; Heidenfelder, B.L.; Dolor, R.J. Conflicting results between randomized trials and observational studies on the impact of proton pump inhibitors on cardiovascular events when coadministered with dual antiplatelet therapy: Systematic review. *Circ. Cardiovasc. Qual. Outcomes* **2015**, *8*, 47–55. [CrossRef] [PubMed]

15. Ghebremariam, Y.T.; Cooke, J.P.; Khan, F.; Thakker, R.N.; Chang, P.; Shah, N.H.; Nead, K.T.; Leeper, N.J. Proton pump inhibitors and vascular function: A prospective cross-over pilot study. *Vasc. Med.* **2015**, *20*, 309–316. [CrossRef] [PubMed]

16. Wang, D.; Gill, P.S.; Chabrashvili, T.; Onozato, M.L.; Raggio, J.; Mendonca, M.; Dennehy, K.; Li, M.; Modlinger, P.; Leiper, J.; *et al.* Isoform-specific regulation by N^G,N^G-dimethylarginine dimethylaminohydrolase of rat serum asymmetric dimethylarginine and vascular endothelium-derived relaxing factor/NO. *Circ. Res.* **2007**, *101*, 627–635. [CrossRef] [PubMed]

17. Lind, L.; Ingelsson, E.; Kumar, J.; Syvänen, A.C.; Axelsson, T.; Teerlink, T. Genetic variation in the dimethylarginine dimethylaminohydrolase 1 gene (DDAH1) is related to asymmetric dimethylarginine (ADMA) levels, but not to endothelium-dependent vasodilation. *Vasc. Med.* **2013**, *18*, 192–199. [CrossRef] [PubMed]

18. Seppälä, I.; Kleber, M.E.; Lyytikäinen, L.P.; Hernesniemi, J.A.; Mäkelä, K.M.; Oksala, N.; Laaksonen, R.; Pilz, S.; Tomaschitz, A.; Silbernagel, G.; *et al.* Genome-wide association study on dimethylarginines reveals novel *AGXT2* variants associated with heart rate variability but not with overall mortality. *Eur. Heart J.* **2014**, *35*, 524–531. [CrossRef] [PubMed]

19. Lüneburg, N.; Lieb, W.; Zeller, T.; Chen, M.H.; Maas, R.; Carter, A.M.; Xanthakis, V.; Glazer, N.L.; Schwedhelm, E.; Seshadri, S.; *et al.* Genome-wide association study of L-arginine and dimethylarginines reveals novel metabolic pathway for symmetric dimethylarginine. *Circ. Cardiovasc. Genet.* **2014**, *7*, 864–872. [CrossRef] [PubMed]

20. Delles, C.; Schneider, M.P.; John, S.; Gekle, M.; Schmieder, R.E. Angiotensin converting enzyme inhibition and angiotensin ii AT_1-receptor blockade reduce the levels of asymmetrical N^G,N^G-dimethylarginine in human essential hypertension. *Am. J. Hypertens.* **2002**, *15*, 590–593. [CrossRef]

21. Hetzel, S.; DeMets, D.; Schneider, R.; Borzak, S.; Schneider, W.; Serebruany, V.; Schröder, H.; Hennekens, C.H. Aspirin increases nitric oxide formation in chronic stable coronary disease. *J. Cardiovasc. Pharmacol. Ther.* **2013**, *18*, 217–221. [CrossRef] [PubMed]

22. Serban, C.; Sahebkar, A.; Ursoniu, S.; Mikhailidis, D.P.; Rizzo, M.; Lip, G.Y.; Kees Hovingh, G.; Kastelein, J.J.; Kalinowski, L.; Rysz, J.; *et al.* A systematic review and meta-analysis of the effect of statins on plasma asymmetric dimethylarginine concentrations. *Sci. Rep.* **2015**, *5*, 9902. [CrossRef] [PubMed]

23. Krempl, T.K.; Maas, R.; Sydow, K.; Meinertz, T.; Böger, R.H.; Kähler, J. Elevation of asymmetric dimethylarginine in patients with unstable angina and recurrent cardiovascular events. *Eur. Heart J.* **2005**, *26*, 1846–1851. [CrossRef] [PubMed]

24. Schulze, F.; Lenzen, H.; Hanefeld, C.; Bartling, A.; Osterziel, K.J.; Goudeva, L.; Schmidt-Lucke, C.; Kusus, M.; Maas, R.; Schwedhelm, E.; *et al.* Asymmetric dimethylarginine is an independent risk factor for coronary heart disease: Results from the multicenter Coronary Artery Risk Determination investigating the Influence of ADMA Concentration (CARDIAC) study. *Am. Heart J.* **2006**, *152*. [CrossRef] [PubMed]

25. Napora, M.; Graczykowska, A.; Próchniewska, K.; Zdrojewski, Z.; Całka, A.; Górny, J.; Stompór, T. Relationship between serum asymmetric dimethylarginine and left ventricular structure and function in patients with end-stage renal disease treated with hemodialysis. *Pol. Arch. Med. Wewn.* **2012**, *122*, 226–234. [PubMed]

26. Teerlink, T.; Luo, Z.; Palm, F.; Wilcox, C.S. Cellular ADMA: Regulation and action. *Pharmacol. Res.* **2009**, *60*, 448–460. [CrossRef] [PubMed]

27. Becker, J.C.; Grosser, N.; Waltke, C.; Schulz, S.; Erdmann, K.; Domschke, W.; Schröder, H.; Pohle, T. Beyond gastric acid reduction: Proton pump inhibitors induce heme oxygenase-1 in gastric and endothelial cells. *Biochem. Biophys. Res. Commun.* **2006**, *345*, 1014–1021. [CrossRef] [PubMed]

28. Böger, R.H.; Sydow, K.; Borlak, J.; Thum, T.; Lenzen, H.; Schubert, B.; Tsikas, D.; Bode-Böger, S.M. LDL cholesterol upregulates synthesis of asymmetrical dimethylarginine in human endothelial cells: Involvement of S-adenosylmethionine-dependent methyltransferases. *Circ. Res.* **2000**, *87*, 99–105. [CrossRef] [PubMed]

29. Ito, A.; Tsao, P.S.; Adimoolam, S.; Kimoto, M.; Ogawa, T.; Cooke, J.P. Novel mechanism for endothelial dysfunction: Dysregulation of dimethylarginine dimethylaminohydrolase. *Circulation* **1999**, *99*, 3092–3095. [CrossRef] [PubMed]

30. Palm, F.; Onozato, M.L.; Luo, Z.; Wilcox, C.S. Dimethylarginine dimethylaminohydrolase (DDAH): Expression, regulation, and function in the cardiovascular and renal systems. *Am. J. Physiol. Heart Circ. Physiol.* **2007**, *293*, H3227–H3245. [CrossRef] [PubMed]

31. Kieboom, B.C.; Kiefte-de Jong, J.C.; Eijgelsheim, M.; Franco, O.H.; Kuipers, E.J.; Hofman, A.; Zietse, R.; Stricker, B.H.; Hoorn, E.J. Proton pump inhibitors and hypomagnesemia in the general population: A population-based cohort study. *Am. J. Kidney Dis.* **2015**, *66*, 775–782. [CrossRef] [PubMed]

32. Attwood, S.E.; Ell, C.; Galmiche, J.P.; Fiocca, R.; Hatlebakk, J.G.; Hasselgren, B.; Långström, G.; Jahreskog, M.; Eklund, S.; Lind, T.; *et al.* Long-term safety of proton pump inhibitor therapy assessed under controlled, randomised clinical trial conditions: Data from the SOPRAN and LOTUS studies. *Aliment. Pharmacol. Ther.* **2015**, *41*, 1162–1174. [CrossRef] [PubMed]

33. Würtz, M.; Grove, E.L.; Kristensen, S.D.; Hvas, A.M. The antiplatelet effect of aspirin is reduced by proton pump inhibitors in patients with coronary artery disease. *Heart* **2010**, *96*, 368–371. [CrossRef] [PubMed]

34. Adamopoulos, A.B.; Sakizlis, G.N.; Nasothimiou, E.G.; Anastasopoulou, I.; Anastasakou, E.; Kotsi, P.; Karafoulidou, A.; Stergiou, G.S. Do proton pump inhibitors attenuate the effect of aspirin on platelet aggregation? A randomized crossover study. *J. Cardiovasc. Pharmacol.* **2009**, *54*, 163–168. [CrossRef] [PubMed]

35. Uno, T.; Niioka, T.; Hayakari, M.; Yasui-Furukori, N.; Sugawara, K.; Tateishi, T. Absolute bioavailability and metabolism of omeprazole in relation to CYP2C19 genotypes following single intravenous and oral administrations. *Eur. J. Clin. Pharmacol.* **2007**, *63*, 143–149. [CrossRef] [PubMed]

36. Barter, Z.E.; Tucker, G.T.; Rowland-Yeo, K. Differences in cytochrome p450-mediated pharmacokinetics between Chinese and Caucasian populations predicted by mechanistic physiologically based pharmacokinetic modelling. *Clin. Pharmacokinet.* **2013**, *52*, 1085–1100. [CrossRef] [PubMed]

37. Krajčíová, L.; Petrovič, R.; Déžiová, L.; Chandoga, J.; Turčáni, P. Frequency of selected single nucleotide polymorphisms influencing the warfarin pharmacogenetics in Slovak population. *Eur. J. Haematol.* **2014**, *93*, 320–328. [CrossRef] [PubMed]

38. Kruszelnicka, O.; Surdacki, A.; Golay, A. Differential associations of angiographic extent and severity of coronary artery disease with asymmetric dimethylarginine but not insulin resistance in non-diabetic men with stable angina: A cross-sectional study. *Cardiovasc. Diabetol.* **2013**, *12*, 145. [CrossRef] [PubMed]

39. Kruszelnicka-Kwiatkowska, O.; Surdacki, A.; Goldsztajn, P.; Matysek, J.; Piwowarska, W.; Golay, A. Relationship between hyperinsulinemia and angiographically defined coronary atherosclerosis in non-diabetic men. *Diabetes Metab.* **2002**, *28*, 305–309. [PubMed]

40. Sullivan, D.R.; Marwick, T.H.; Freedman, S.B. A new method of scoring coronary angiograms to reflect extent of coronary atherosclerosis and improve correlation with major risk factors. *Am. Heart J.* **1990**, *119*, 1262–1267. [CrossRef]

9

Coronary Artery Calcium Screening: Does it Perform Better than Other Cardiovascular Risk Stratification Tools?

Irfan Zeb [1,*] and Matthew Budoff [2]

[1] Department of Medicine, Bronx-Lebanon Hospital Center, 1650 Grand Concourse, Bronx, NY 10457, USA
[2] Department of Cardiology, Los Angeles Biomedical Research Institute at Harbor-UCLA Medical Center, Torrance, CA 90502, USA; mbudoff@labiomed.org
*   Correspondence: izeb82@gmail.com;

Academic Editor: Michael Henein

Abstract: Coronary artery calcium (CAC) has been advocated as one of the strongest cardiovascular risk prediction markers. It performs better across a wide range of Framingham risk categories (6%–10% and 10%–20% 10-year risk categories) and also helps in reclassifying the risk of these subjects into either higher or lower risk categories based on CAC scores. It also performs better among population subgroups where Framingham risk score does not perform well, especially young subjects, women, family history of premature coronary artery disease and ethnic differences in coronary risk. The absence of CAC is also associated with excellent prognosis, with 10-year event rate of 1%. Studies have also compared with other commonly used markers of cardiovascular disease risk such as Carotid intima-media thickness and highly sensitive C-reactive protein. CAC also performs better compared with carotid intima-media thickness and highly sensitive C-reactive protein in prediction of coronary heart disease and cardiovascular disease events. CAC scans are associated with relatively low radiation exposure (0.9–1.1 mSv) and provide information that can be used not only for risk stratification but also can be used to track the progression of atherosclerosis and the effects of statins.

Keywords: coronary artery calcium; risk stratification; cardiovascular risk

1. Introduction

Atherosclerosis coronary artery disease is among the leading cause of morbidity and mortality in the Western world. The shear burden of cardiovascular disease on healthcare costs is enormous, with an estimate of 475 billion US dollars spent in the year 2009 alone [1]. By 2030, real total direct medical costs of cardiovascular disease (CVD) are projected to increase to $\approx$ $ 918 billion [2]. In order to drive the cost down, emphasis is on preventive measures and earlier detection of cardiovascular disease. There is a number of risk factors algorithms, biomarkers and imaging studies to screen for cardiovascular diseases. Framingham risk scores (FRS), Reynolds risk score, highly sensitive C-reactive protein (hs-CRP), carotid intima media thickness (CIMT) and coronary artery calcium (CAC) are among the various measures that can be used for screening of cardiovascular disease among asymptomatic population. CAC score has emerged as one of the strongest risk prediction tools. It represents calcific atherosclerosis in the coronary arteries and correlates well with the overall burden of atherosclerosis in the coronary arteries. The current review article will compare CAC score with the remaining risk stratification tools.

2. Framingham Risk Score and Coronary Artery Calcium

Framingham risk score is the most commonly used cardiovascular risk stratification tool in the general population due to its ease of use. It takes into account major cardiovascular risk factors including age, sex, dyslipidemia, smoking and hypertension [3]. This risk scoring system predicts an estimate of population risk for CVD events over 10-years and categorizes individual risk for developing CVD to low (10-year risk of <10%), intermediate (10-year risk of 10%–20%), and high (10-year risk of >20%) risk. FRS is easy to calculate and provides a good overall estimate of patient risk for future cardiovascular problems. However, there are several limitations to the use of this classification for risk assessment in the general population.

Shaw et al. [4] followed up a cohort of 10,377 asymptomatic individuals for mean duration of five years and compared cardiac risk factors such as family history of coronary artery disease, hypercholesterolemia, hypertension, smoking and diabetes mellitus with CAC score (Figure 1). CAC was found to be an independent predictor of mortality ($p < 0.001$) and it provided improved discrimination value compared to the cardiac risk factors alone (concordance index 0.78 vs. 0.72, $p < 0.001$) in a multivariable model for prediction of death. CAC was also superior to estimated Framingham risk score in outcome classification ability (Area under the ROC curve = 0.73 vs. 0.67, $p < 0.001$).

Greenland et al. [5] evaluated predictive value of CAC across increasing levels of FRS categories (0%–9%, 10%–15%, 16%–20% and ≥21%). For low risk FRS categories (0%–9%), CAC >300 did not provide an increased risk. CAC >100 was associated with increased risk among FRS categories 10%–15% and higher. The risk associated with FRS category 10%–15% and CAC score >300 (hazard ratio 17.6, $p < 0.001$) was comparable with the risk associated with FRS category >21% and CAC >300 (hazard ratio 19.1, $p < 0.001$). 2010 American College of Cardiology (ACC) and American Heart Association (AHA) guidelines [6] have incorporated CAC for cardiovascular risk assessment in asymptomatic adults at intermediate risk (10%–20% 10-year risk) (Class II a indication). The current clinical practice guidelines [6] do not recommend the use of CAC for low risk population risk assessment. Okwuosa et al. [7] evaluated the prevalence of CAC in low risk FRS categories and the number needed to screen to detect one individual with CAC score >300. There were 1.7% and 4.4% of the population found to have CAC score ≥300 within FRS categories of 0%–2.5% and 2.6%–5.0%, respectively. The respective number needed to screen were 59.7 and 22.7. The number needed to screen to detect persons with CAC score ≥300 decreased with increasing FRS categories; with only 4.2 and 3.3 individuals needed to be screened with FRS of 15.1%–20% and >20%. Okwuosa et al. [8] evaluated role of novel markers for CAC score progression among patients within low risk FRS category (<10%). They looked at the following variables: LDL particle number (LDLpn), urine albumin, CRP using a high-sensitivity assay, D-dimer, factor VIIIc, total homocysteine (tHcy), fibrinogen, cystatin C, soluble intercellular adhesion molecule-1 (sICAM-1) and carotid intima media thickness (CIMT). The study showed significant association of most of these risk factors with CAC progression in univariate and age adjusted models. This statistical significance was lost after adjustment for traditional cardiovascular risk factors. The study also evaluated predictive value of various combinations of novel markers with CAC progression compared with a base model composed of traditional risk factors. These combination models showed little or no improvement over the base model in discrimination and informativeness. Taylor et al. [9] performed a study evaluating the predictive value of CAC in 2000 healthy young men and women aged 40–50 years of age. A total of nine coronary events occurred, with four in men with 10-year FRS risk <6% and five men with 10-year FRS risk of 6%–10%. None of the events occurred in men with 10-year FRS risk above 10%. Seven out of nine men had CAC among those who suffered coronary heart disease (CHD) events. This study showed that the presence of any CAC was associated with an 11.8-fold increased risk of acute CHD ($p = 0.002$) after controlling for the FRS. 2010 ACC/AHA guidelines [6] suggest use of CAC for cardiovascular risk assessment of individuals with 10-year FRS risk of 6%–10% (Class II b indication). The current clinical practice guidelines do not recommend the use of CAC for low risk individuals (10-year FRS risk <6%) for cardiovascular risk assessment (Class III indication). The study performed by Greenland *et al.* [5] did not show any benefit of cardiovascular risk assessment with CAC score in the 10-year FRS category of less than 10%. The mean age of population at the time of computed tomography (CT) scan in this study was 65.7 years. The population groups in both Taylor *et al.* [9] (mean age 43 years) and Okwuosa *et al.* [7] were younger (mean age: 60.9 years, 53% women). It is already known that the FRS performs poorly in younger patients and women [10–12]. In a multi-ethnic study of atherosclerosis, 90% of the women were classified as low risk based on FRS risk classification [13]. There were 32% of low risk women who were found to have CAC score of more than 0 (four percent had CAC score ≥300). In these women, CAC score of >300 were highly predictive of future CHD and CVD events (6.7% and 8.6% absolute CHD and CVD risk, respectively) over a 3.75 year period. Ninety-five percent of the US women younger than 70 are found to be at low risk for coronary heart disease according to the data from Third National Health and Nutrition Examination Survey (NHANES III) [10] and, thereby, do not qualify for more aggressive medical management for standard risk factors according to the National Cholesterol Education Program Expert Panel on Detection, Evaluation, and Treatment of High Blood Cholesterol in Adults (Adult Treatment Panel III) (NCEP/ATP III) [14]. These persons otherwise may be classified as low-risk, and may not benefit from preventive treatments that can otherwise be offered to them based on CAC scores.

Elias-Smale *et al.* [15] evaluated the effect of CAC in risk assessment of elderly population (2028 subjects, age 69.6 ± 6.2 years and showed that CAC was able to reclassify 52% of men and women in intermediate risk category.

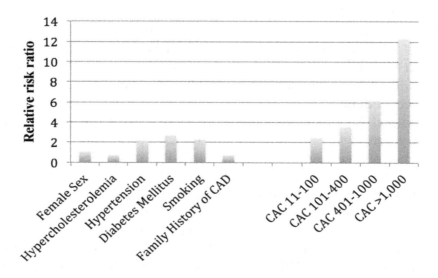

Figure 1. Predictive value of coronary artery calcium [4].

Family history of premature coronary artery disease represents a unique situation. The persons may suffer from cardiovascular events at an earlier age. The usual risk stratification tools such as FRS may perform poorly in these persons. Reynolds risk score includes parental family history of premature CAD and high-sensitivity C-reactive protein (hs-CRP) to traditional risk factors. CAC use has been assessed in this situation as well [16–18]. Nasir *et al.* [16] showed that the age-, gender- and race-adjusted prevalence of CAC >0 was significantly higher with presence of any family history of premature CHD than those with no family history of premature CHD among individuals classified as low risk (35% *vs.* 23%, *p* < 0.0001) and among those at intermediate risk (70% *vs.* 60%, *p* = 0.01). Similar results were seen with CAC ≥75th percentile among individuals at low risk (24% *vs.* 14%, *p* = 0.0003) and intermediate-risk (34% *vs.* 20%, *p* < 0.001) respectively. A *post hoc* analysis from St. Francis Heart study [17] revealed benefit of statin treatment in individuals with a family history of premature CAD and CAC above 80th percentile.

CAC has been shown to perform better across a wide range of FRS categories (6%–10% 10-year risk and 10%–20% 10-year risk). FRS is a population-based risk of 10-year event rates; however, individual persons may not be at the same level of risk in each category as determined by FRS. The individual risk can be further stratified with the use of various markers like hs-CRP and CAC. Polonski et al. [19] showed that addition of CAC to traditional risk factors improves risk prediction significantly compared to traditional risk factors alone. Traditional risk factors were able to classify 69% of the cohort into the highest or lowest risk categories, whereas addition of CAC to this model increased it to 77%. CAC along with traditional risk factors was able to reclassify 23% of those who had cardiac events into high risk and 13% without cardiac events into low risk.

Coronary atherosclerosis burden differs between different ethnic groups [20]. Framingham risk score does not account for the ethnicities. Detrano et al. [20] performed coronary calcium scans on population-based sample of 6722 men and women, of whom 38.6% were white, 27.6% were black, 21.9% were Hispanic, and 11.9% were Chinese. They found that adjusted risk for any coronary events for CAC score categories 1–100, 101–300 and >300 increased by a factor of 3.61-fold, 7.73-fold and 9.67-fold when compared with CAC score of zero ($p < 0.001$, respectively). The adjusted risk for any coronary events for ethnic groups Whites, Chinese, Black and Hispanics was 1.22-fold ($p < 0.001$), 1.36-fold ($p < 0.005$), 1.39-fold ($p < 0.001$) and 1.18-fold ($p < 0.001$), respectively. Across four ethnic groups, a doubling of CAC increased the risk of major coronary event by 15%–35% and the risk of any coronary event by 18%–39%. The areas under the receiver-operating-characteristic curve showed superior predictive value of CAC compared to the standard risk factors for both major and any coronary events.

The predictive value of increasing CAC score is well established. The protective value of CAC score zero is also very promising. A number of studies have consistently reported better outcomes associated with the absence of CAC (Table 1). These persons may require less intensive treatments and further diagnostic testing due to very low event rates in this population group. Blaha et al. [21] evaluated annualized all-cause mortality rates in 44,052 consecutive asymptomatic patients referred for CAC testing. They found that 45% had no CAC on screening and there were 104 deaths in those with CAC score zero. Patients with CAC score of 0 have an excellent prognosis, with a 10-year event rate of about 1%.

Table 1. Predictive value of zero coronary artery calcium score.

Author	Year	Total No. of Participants	Participants with CAC Score 0	Event Rate	Follow up Period
Blaha et al. [21]	2009	44,052	19,898	0.87/1000 person-years	Mean follow-up of 5.6 ± 2.6 years
Arad et al. [22]	2005	4613	1504	1/1000 person-years	4.3 years
Taylor et al. [9]	2005	2000	1263	0.6/1000 person-years	Mean follow-up of 3.0 ±1.4 years
Budoff et al. [23]	2007	25,253	11,046	0.6/1000 person-years	Mean follow-up of 6.8 ± 3 years
Detrano et al. [20]	2009	6722	3409	0.6/1000 person-years	3.7 years
Shaw et al. [4]	2003	10,377	5067	1.5 events/1000 person-years	Mean follow-up of 5.0 years
LaMonte et al. [24]	2005	10,746	2692	1.6 events/1000 person-years	3.5 years

The value of CAC in cardiac disease prediction has been well established. Herman *et al.* [25] evaluated association of CAC with stroke and showed that log10 (CAC + 1) is an independent predictor of stroke (hazards ratio, 1.52 (95% confidence interval, 1.19–1.92); $p = 0.001$) in addition to age, systolic blood pressure and smoking in subjects at low or intermediate vascular risk. This association was independent of atrial fibrillation detected at baseline and follow up exams in prediction of stroke (fully adjusted hazard ratio, 1.31 (1.00–1.71); $p = 0.049$) that may be the underlying cause for cryptogenic strokes. O'Neal *et al.* [26] showed that higher CAC scores were associated with increased risk for atrial fibrillation (CAC = 1–100: Hazard Ratio 1.4, 95% CI 1.01–2.0; CAC = 101–300: HR 1.6, 95% CI 1.1–2.4; CAC > 300: HR 2.1, 95% CI 1.4–2.9) in a model adjusted for sociodemographics, cardiovascular risk factors, and potential confounders.

The recently published ACC/AHA guidelines on the assessment of cardiovascular risk [27] used a different risk tool to estimate 10-year and long term risk of atherosclerotic cardiovascular disease (ASCVD) that incorporates age, sex, race, HDL-cholesterol, total cholesterol, diabetes, systolic blood pressure or treatment for hypertension and smoking status. This new risk stratification tool may replace FRS for risk prediction. However there are currently no studies available that compare CAC with 10-year ASCVD risk tool.

3. Reynolds Risk Score and Coronary Artery Calcium

Reynolds risk score (RRS) includes traditional risk factors used in FRS and adds parental family history of premature CAD and high-sensitivity C-reactive protein (hs-CRP) [28]. It provides improved prediction of CVD events in both men and women and has been proposed as an alternative to FRS in risk stratification [28,29]. DeFillepis *et al.* [30] compared the performance of FRS and RRS in predicting CAC incidence and progression among 5140 individuals in MESA population. Both FRS and RRS were predictive of incident CAC (relative risk: 1.40 and 1.41 per 5% increase in risk, respectively) and CAC progression (relative risk 6.92 and 6.82 per 5% increase in risk, respectively). There was discordance in risk category classification (<10% and >10% per 10-year HD risk) in 13.7% of patients. RRS was found superior to FRS in providing additional predictive information for incidence and progression of CAC when discordance between the scoring systems existed. Desai *et al.* [31] evaluated whether CAC leads to reclassification of RRS risk assessment in patients without prior CHD. There were 72% of patients with CAC score >400 and 88% of patients with high CAC percentile had low or intermediate risk by RRS risk classification. CAC can potentially improve risk reclassification for RRS risk assessment.

4. Carotid Intima Media Thickness and Coronary Artery Calcium

Carotid intima-media thickness (CIMT) represents carotid atherosclerosis and is being used as a surrogate marker for atherosclerosis. Its utility relies on its ability to predict future adverse cardiovascular events [32]. Lorenz *et al.* [33] performed a meta-analysis of eight studies where they showed that the age- and sex-adjusted overall estimates of the relative risk of 1.26 (95% CI 1.21–1.30) for myocardial infarction and 1.32 (95% CI 1.27–1.38) for stroke for each one-standard deviation difference of common carotid IMT. CIMT does predict future CHD events but is a slightly better predictor for cerebrovascular events. Folsom *et al.* [34] compared CAC with CIMT in a cohort of 6698 subjects aged 45–84 years of age in four ethnic groups enrolled in MESA study and showed that the hazard of CVD increased 2.1 (95% CI 1.8–2.5) fold for log-transformed CAC *vs.* 1.3-fold (95% CI 1.1–1.4) for maximum CIMT for each standard deviation increment of log-transformed CAC and maximum CIMT. For coronary heart disease, the hazard ratios per 1-SD increment increased 2.5-fold (95% CI 2.1–3.1) for CAC score and 1.2-fold (95% CI 1.0–1.4) for IMT. The study also showed CAC to be a superior predictor of incident CVD compared with CIMT (area under the curve 0.81 *vs.* 0.78), respectively. Terry *et al.* [35] compared the performance of CAC and CIMT for non-invasive detection of prevalent CAD (≥50% stenosis in one or more coronary arteries identified on coronary angiography). CAC performed better than CIMT in terms of prevalent CAD for each quartile increase in both measures (odds ratio: 8-fold *vs.* 1.7-fold, respectively).

CAC seems to be better than CIMT in patients with atherosclerosis CAD. However, among patients with coronary micro-vascular dysfunction, CIMT seem to perform better than CAC score. Danad *et al.* [36] evaluated 120 patients without documented evidence of CAD to compare CAC with CIMT for prediction of minimal coronary vascular resistance, a measure used to detect coronary micro-vascular disease [37]. Using bivariate and multivariable regression analysis using backward elimination revealed that only CIMT was a predictor of minimal coronary vascular resistance. Naqvi *et al.* [38] showed that CIMT based mean vascular age (61.6 ± 11.4 years) was significantly higher than coronary calcium age (58.3 ± 11.1 years) ($p = 0.001$); both of these were significantly higher than mean chronological age ($p < 0.0001$ and $p < 0.04$, respectively). CIMT was able to upgrade or downgrade FRS by >5% compared with CAC (42% of CIMT cases *vs.* 17% of CAC cases).

Studies comparing CAC with CIMT in younger population groups, where the prevalence of CAC is very low, CIMT may perform better in those population groups. Davis *et al.* [39] performed a study in young population (33–42 years of age) evaluating the relationship of CAC with CIMT. The multivariate model showed low density cholesterol-C ($p < 0.001$), pack-year smoking ($p < 0.005$) and CAC ($p < 0.05$) were significant in men; and low density cholesterol-C ($p < 0.001$), systolic blood pressure ($p < 0.01$) and CAC ($p < 0.05$) were significant in women and were predictive of CIMT in this population.

Lester *et al.* [40] performed a study on relatively younger population, aged 36–59 years of age, comparing CAC and CIMT to detect subclinical atherosclerosis. A large proportion of population had a CAC score of zero (75%). There was evidence of carotid atherosclerosis in 47% of the population with CAC score of zero, showing the role of CIMT in low risk, relatively younger population group with CAC score of zero.

5. C-Reactive Protein and Coronary Artery Calcium

AHA/ACC recommends measurement of C-reactive protein (CRP) in men 50 years of age or older or women 60 years of age or older with low-density lipoprotein cholesterol less than 130 mg/dL can be useful in selection of patients for statin therapy [41]. These recommendations are based on JUPITER trial [42] assessing the benefit of statin treatment in apparently healthy persons with hyperlipidemia (LDL-C < 130 mg/dL) but with elevated high-sensitivity CRP levels (hs-CRP ≥ 2 mg/dL). Measurement of hs-CRP has been shown as an independent prediction of future vascular events and improves global classification of risk, regardless of the LDL cholesterol level [43–49]. Arad *et al.* [22] performed a study evaluating 4903 apparently healthy middle-aged persons comparing CAC to standard coronary disease risk factors and CRP that were followed for a period of 4.3 years. CAC was shown to perform better than CRP and to highly correlate with future CAD events in this study. Park *et al.* [50] performed a study evaluating 1461 subjects without coronary heart disease comparing CAC and CRP in predicting cardiovascular events in non-diabetic individuals. The study showed that both CAC was predictive of non-fatal myocardial infarction or coronary death and any cardiovascular events ($p < 0.005$) whereas CRP was only predictive of cardiovascular events ($p = 0.03$). Risk group analysis that are defined by increasing tertiles for CAC (<3.7, 3.7–142.1, >142.1) and the 75th percentile for CRP (>4.05 mg/L) were associated with increasing risk with increasing CAC and CRP. Relative risks for the medium-calcium/low-CRP risk group to high-calcium/high-CRP risk group ranged from 1.8 to 6.1 for MI/coronary death ($p = 0.003$) and 2.8–7.5 for any cardiovascular event ($p < 0.001$). Lakoski *et al.* [51] examined the MESA participants to determine how many individuals risk can be reclassified with the use of CAC and CRP. The study showed that 30% of the intermediate-risk subjects by FRS had CRP concentration greater than 3 mg/L and 33% had CAC scores more than 100 AU. In gender specific analysis, 49% of intermediate-risk women and 27% of intermediate-risk men had CRP >3 mg/L, compared with 33% of intermediate-risk men and women had CAC >100 AU. When gender specific cut points for CRP and CAC were use, the same percentage of intermediate risk women and men had CRP above 75th percentile (28% and 27%, respectively) whereas more intermediate-risk women 40%, CAC > 50) than men (25%, CAC > 180) had a high CAC score.

Blaha *et al.* [52] performed a study evaluating whether CAC score may further risk stratify a JUPITER-eligible population (LDL-C < 130 mg/dL and hs-CRP $\geq$ 2.0 mg/dL) in participants enrolled in MESA study. For CHD events, the five-year number needed to treat for CAC scores of 0, 1–100 and >100 was 549, 94 and 24, respectively. In JUPITOR trial, the five-year number needed to prevent the occurrence of one primary end point was 25 [42]. The presence of CAC was associated with 4.3-fold increased CHD (95% CI 2.0–9.3) and 2.6-fold increased CVD (95% CI 1.5–4.5), while hs-CRP was not associated with either CHD or CVD after multivariable adjustment [52].

Möhlenkamp *et al.* [53] performed a study involving 3966 subjects without known CAD or acute inflammation, followed for 5.1 ± 0.3 years, to determine whether combined presence of CAC and hs-CRP improves discrimination and stratification of coronary events and all-cause mortality. For coronary events, net reclassification improvement (NRI) was 23.8% ($p = 0.0007$) for CAC and 10.5% ($p = 0.026$) for hs-CRP. Addition of CAC to Framingham risk variables and hs-CRP improved discrimination of coronary risk but not *vice versa*. Among persons with CAC score of zero, hs-CRP >3 mg/L was associated with a significantly higher coronary event risk compared with hs-CRP <3.0 mg/L ($p = 0.006$). Reilly *et al.* [54] performed a study involving 914 participants from the Study of Inherited Risk of Coronary Atherosclerosis (SIRCA) who were free of clinical CAD and had a family history of premature CAD. The study showed that median CAC scores increased across ordinal CRP categories in women but not in men (Krushal-Wallis $\chi^2 = 22.5$, $p < 0.001$ in women, $\chi^2 = 2.5$, $p < 0.29$ in men, respectively). CRP levels were found to be significant predictors of CAC scores in women after adjusting for traditional risk factors, which was lost after adjustment for body mass index. There was no such association found between CRP and CAC in men.

6. Coronary Artery Calcium and Other Imaging Parameters for Risk Prediction

Various imaging markers that can be easily obtained from coronary artery calcium scan have been proposed for prediction of CHD and CVD events. Pericardial fat is present around the heart—encompassing the coronary arteries—has been shown to be a predictor of coronary events [55]. Budoff *et al.* [56] showed that thoracic aortic wall calcification to be a significant predictor of incident coronary events in women, independent of CAC. Zeb *et al.* [57] showed liver fat measured by CT scans to be an independent predictor of incident coronary heart disease events. Yeboah *et al.* [58] performed a study to assess whether addition of computed tomography risk markers thoracic aorta calcium (TAC), aortic valve calcification (AVC), mitral annular calcification (MAC), pericardial adipose tissue volume (PAT), and liver attenuation (LA) to FRS + CAC provide improved discrimination for incident CHD and incident CVD events. CAC, TAC, AVC and MAC were all significantly associated with incident CVD/CHD/mortality among intermediate risk subjects; CAC had the strongest association. The addition of CAC to the FRS provides superior discrimination especially in intermediate-risk individuals. Among participants with intermediate FRS risk, the addition of TAC, AVC, MAC, PAT, or LA to FRS + CAC resulted in a significant reduction in area of the curve for incident CHD (0.712 *vs.* 0.646, 0.655, 0.652, 0.648 and 0.569; all $p < 0.01$, respectively). The addition of CAC to FRS resulted in a superior discrimination for incident CHD in the intermediate-risk groups compared to when TAC, AVC, MAC, PAT and LA were added to FRS + CAC (0.024, 0.026, 0.019, 0.012 and 0.012, respectively). These risk markers are unlikely to be useful for improving cardiovascular risk prediction.

7. Conclusions

CAC score has been shown as the strongest predictor of incident coronary events and is able to reclassify low-to-intermediate risk groups and certain subgroups, especially women and young adults most of which may be classified as low risk by FRS risk stratification. Most of the adult population will have CAC scores of zero (Table 1). The prevalence of CAC scores increases with increasing age. There is a number of different cutoffs that are used to denote increased CHD risk [20,59], however, the most commonly used cutoffs of increased CHD risk are CAC score 1–100, CAC 101–300 and CAC > 300 [20]. Studies have shown that subjects who undergo CAC scans tend to have better compliance rates with medications compared with other groups, and promote a healthy behavior in these patients (a picture equals a thousand words) [60,61]. CAC scans can be used to evaluate the efficacy of treatment regimens over time. The accelerated progression of CAC is associated with adverse cardiovascular events [62–65]. There are certain concerns associated with the use of CAC scores. Among them, the foremost concern associated with CAC use is radiation exposure. The recent advances in imaging techniques has lowered the radiation exposure associated with CAC scans and is comparable to mammograms in terms in radiation exposure (0.9 to 1.1 mSv) [66,67]. The scan can be easily performed in an outpatient setting without any prior preparation. Medicare is currently reimbursing the cost of CAC scans for selected population groups. Another issue that can arise with the use of CAC scans are incidental findings which can drive the cost upward due to further downstream testing as a result of these incidental findings. The prevalence of incidental findings can range from 4% to 8% [68–70]. There is a number of cost effectiveness analysis studies that are looking at the cost associated with the use of CAC scans. However, the information obtained with CAC can be very useful for earlier detection, institution of statins and prevention of adverse cardiovascular events.

Author Contributions: Irfan Zeb and Matthew Budoff contributed to the preparation of this review article.

References

1. Lloyd-Jones, D.; Adams, R.; Carnethon, M.; de Simone, G.; Ferguson, T.B.; Flegal, K.; Ford, E.; Furie, K.; Go, A.; Greenlund, K.; *et al.* Heart disease and stroke statistics—2009 Update: A report from the American Heart Association Statistics Committee and Stroke Statistics Subcommittee. *Circulation* **2009**, *119*, 480–486. [CrossRef] [PubMed]

2. Go, A.S.; Mozaffarian, D.; Roger, V.L.; Benjamin, E.J.; Berry, J.D.; Blaha, M.J.; Dai, S.; Ford, E.S.; Fox, C.S.; Franco, S.; *et al.* Heart disease and stroke statistics—2014 Update: A report from the American Heart Association. *Circulation* **2014**, *129*, e28–e292. [CrossRef] [PubMed]

3. Grundy, S.M.; Pasternak, R.; Greenland, P.; Smith, S., Jr.; Fuster, V. Assessment of cardiovascular risk by use of multiple-risk-factor assessment equations: A statement for healthcare professionals from the American Heart Association and the American College of Cardiology. *Circulation* **1999**, *100*, 1481–1492. [CrossRef] [PubMed]

4. Shaw, L.J.; Raggi, P.; Schisterman, E.; Berman, D.S.; Callister, T.Q. Prognostic value of cardiac risk factors and coronary artery calcium screening for all-cause mortality. *Radiology* **2003**, *228*, 826–833. [CrossRef] [PubMed]

5. Greenland, P.; LaBree, L.; Azen, S.P.; Doherty, T.M.; Detrano, R.C. Coronary artery calcium score combined with Framingham score for risk prediction in asymptomatic individuals. *JAMA* **2004**, *291*, 210–215. [CrossRef] [PubMed]

6. Greenland, P.; Alpert, J.S.; Beller, G.A.; Benjamin, E.J.; Budoff, M.J.; Fayad, Z.A.; Foster, E.; Hlatky, M.A.; Hodgson, J.M.; Kushner, F.G.; *et al.* 2010 ACCF/AHA guideline for assessment of cardiovascular risk in asymptomatic adults: A report of the American College of Cardiology Foundation/American Heart Association task force on practice guidelines. *J. Am. Coll. Cardiol.* **2010**, *56*, e50–e103. [CrossRef] [PubMed]

7. Okwuosa, T.M.; Greenland, P.; Ning, H.; Liu, K.; Bild, D.E.; Burke, G.L.; Eng, J.; Lloyd-Jones, D.M. Distribution of coronary artery calcium scores by Framingham 10-year risk strata in the MESA (Multi-Ethnic Study of Atherosclerosis) potential implications for coronary risk assessment. *J. Am. Coll. Cardiol.* **2011**, *57*, 1838–1845. [CrossRef] [PubMed]

8. Okwuosa, T.M.; Greenland, P.; Burke, G.L.; Eng, J.; Cushman, M.; Michos, E.D.; Ning, H.; Lloyd-Jones, D.M. Prediction of coronary artery calcium progression in individuals with low Framingham Risk Score: The Multi-Ethnic Study of Atherosclerosis. *JACC Cardiovasc. Imaging* **2012**, *5*, 144–153. [CrossRef] [PubMed]

9. Taylor, A.J.; Bindeman, J.; Feuerstein, I.; Cao, F.; Brazaitis, M.; O'Malley, P.G. Coronary calcium independently predicts incident premature coronary heart disease over measured cardiovascular risk factors: Mean three-year outcomes in the Prospective Army Coronary Calcium (PACC) project. *J. Am. Coll. Cardiol.* **2005**, *46*, 807–814. [CrossRef] [PubMed]

10. Ford, E.S.; Giles, W.H.; Mokdad, A.H. The distribution of 10-year risk for coronary heart disease among US adults: Findings from the National Health and Nutrition Examination Survey III. *J. Am. Coll. Cardiol.* **2004**, *43*, 1791–1796. [CrossRef] [PubMed]

11. Berry, J.D.; Lloyd-Jones, D.M.; Garside, D.B.; Greenland, P. Framingham risk score and prediction of coronary heart disease death in young men. *Am. Heart J.* **2007**, *154*, 80–86. [CrossRef] [PubMed]

12. Akosah, K.O.; Schaper, A.; Cogbill, C.; Schoenfeld, P. Preventing myocardial infarction in the young adult in the first place: How do the National Cholesterol Education Panel III guidelines perform? *J. Am. Coll. Cardiol.* **2003**, *41*, 1475–1479. [CrossRef] [PubMed]

13. Lakoski, S.G.; Greenland, P.; Wong, N.D.; Schreiner, P.J.; Herrington, D.M.; Kronmal, R.A.; Liu, K.; Blumenthal, R.S. Coronary artery calcium scores and risk for cardiovascular events in women classified as "low risk" based on Framingham risk score: The Multi-Ethnic Study of Atherosclerosis (MESA). *Arch. Intern. Med.* **2007**, *167*, 2437–2442. [CrossRef] [PubMed]

14. Expert Panel on Detection, Evaluation, and Treatment of High Blood Cholesterol in Adult. Executive summary of the third report of the National Cholesterol Education Program (NCEP) expert panel on detection, evaluation, and treatment of high blood cholesterol in adults (Adult Treatment Panel III). *JAMA* **2001**, *285*, 2486–2497.

15. Elias-Smale, S.E.; Proenca, R.V.; Koller, M.T.; Kavousi, M.; van Rooij, F.J.; Hunink, M.G.; Steyerberg, E.W.; Hofman, A.; Oudkerk, M.; Witteman, J.C. Coronary calcium score improves classification of coronary heart disease risk in the elderly: The Rotterdam study. *J. Am. Coll. Cardiol.* **2010**, *56*, 1407–1414. [CrossRef] [PubMed]

16. Nasir, K.; Budoff, M.J.; Wong, N.D.; Scheuner, M.; Herrington, D.; Arnett, D.K.; Szklo, M.; Greenland, P.; Blumenthal, R.S. Family history of premature coronary heart disease and coronary artery calcification: Multi-Ethnic Study of Atherosclerosis (MESA). *Circulation* **2007**, *116*, 619–626. [CrossRef] [PubMed]

17. Mulders, T.A.; Sivapalaratnam, S.; Stroes, E.S.; Kastelein, J.J.; Guerci, A.D.; Pinto-Sietsma, S.J. Asymptomatic individuals with a positive family history for premature coronary artery disease and elevated coronary calcium scores benefit from statin treatment: A *post hoc* analysis from the St. Francis Heart Study. *JACC Cardiovasc. Imaging* **2012**, *5*, 252–260. [CrossRef] [PubMed]

18. Pandey, A.K.; Blaha, M.J.; Sharma, K.; Rivera, J.; Budoff, M.J.; Blankstein, R.; Al-Mallah, M.; Wong, N.D.; Shaw, L.; Carr, J.; *et al.* Family history of coronary heart disease and the incidence and progression of coronary artery calcification: Multi-Ethnic Study of Atherosclerosis (MESA). *Atherosclerosis* **2014**, *232*, 369–376. [CrossRef] [PubMed]

19. Polonsky, T.S.; McClelland, R.L.; Jorgensen, N.W.; Bild, D.E.; Burke, G.L.; Guerci, A.D.; Greenland, P. Coronary artery calcium score and risk classification for coronary heart disease prediction. *JAMA* **2010**, *303*, 1610–1016. [CrossRef] [PubMed]

20. Detrano, R.; Guerci, A.D.; Carr, J.J.; Bild, D.E.; Burke, G.; Folsom, A.R.; Liu, K.; Shea, S.; Szklo, M.; Bluemke, D.A.; *et al.* Coronary calcium as a predictor of coronary events in four racial or ethnic groups. *New Engl. J. Med.* **2008**, *358*, 1336–1345. [CrossRef] [PubMed]

21. Blaha, M.; Budoff, M.J.; Shaw, L.J.; Khosa, F.; Rumberger, J.A.; Berman, D.; Callister, T.; Raggi, P.; Blumenthal, R.S.; Nasir, K. Absence of coronary artery calcification and all-cause mortality. *JACC Cardiovasc. Imaging* **2009**, *2*, 692–700. [CrossRef] [PubMed]

22. Arad, Y.; Goodman, K.J.; Roth, M.; Newstein, D.; Guerci, A.D. Coronary calcification, coronary disease risk factors, C-reactive protein, and atherosclerotic cardiovascular disease events: The St. Francis Heart Study. *J. Am. Coll. Cardiol.* **2005**, *46*, 158–165. [CrossRef] [PubMed]

23. Budoff, M.J.; Shaw, L.J.; Liu, S.T.; Weinstein, S.R.; Mosler, T.P.; Tseng, P.H.; Flores, F.R.; Callister, T.Q.; Raggi, P.; Berman, D.S. Long-term prognosis associated with coronary calcification: Observations from a registry of 25,253 patients. *J. Am. Coll. Cardiol.* **2007**, *49*, 1860–1870. [CrossRef] [PubMed]

24. LaMonte, M.J.; FitzGerald, S.J.; Church, T.S.; Barlow, C.E.; Radford, N.B.; Levine, B.D.; Pippin, J.J.; Gibbons, L.W.; Blair, S.N.; Nichaman, M.Z. Coronary artery calcium score and coronary heart disease events in a large cohort of asymptomatic men and women. *Am. J. Epidemiol.* **2005**, *162*, 421–429. [CrossRef] [PubMed]

25. Hermann, D.M.; Gronewold, J.; Lehmann, N.; Moebus, S.; Jockel, K.H.; Bauer, M.; Erbel, R. Coronary artery calcification is an independent stroke predictor in the general population. *Stroke* **2013**, *44*, 1008–1013. [CrossRef] [PubMed]

26. O'Neal, W.T.; Efird, J.T.; Dawood, F.Z.; Yeboah, J.; Alonso, A.; Heckbert, S.R.; Soliman, E.Z. Coronary artery calcium and risk of atrial fibrillation (from the multi-ethnic study of atherosclerosis). *Am. J. Cardiol.* **2014**, *114*, 1707–1712. [CrossRef] [PubMed]

27. Goff, D.C., Jr.; Lloyd-Jones, D.M.; Bennett, G.; Coady, S.; D'Agostino, R.B.; Gibbons, R.; Greenland, P.; Lackland, D.T.; Levy, D.; O'Donnell, C.J.; *et al.* 2013 ACC/AHA guideline on the assessment of cardiovascular risk: A report of the American College of Cardiology/American Heart Association Task Force on Practice Guidelines. *Circulation* **2014**, *129*, S49–S73. [CrossRef] [PubMed]

28. Ridker, P.M.; Buring, J.E.; Rifai, N.; Cook, N.R. Development and validation of improved algorithms for the assessment of global cardiovascular risk in women: The Reynolds Risk Score. *JAMA* **2007**, *297*, 611–619. [CrossRef] [PubMed]

29. Ridker, P.M.; Paynter, N.P.; Rifai, N.; Gaziano, J.M.; Cook, N.R. C-reactive protein and parental history improve global cardiovascular risk prediction: The Reynolds Risk Score for men. *Circulation* **2008**, *118*, 2243–2251. [CrossRef] [PubMed]

30. DeFilippis, A.P.; Blaha, M.J.; Ndumele, C.E.; Budoff, M.J.; Lloyd-Jones, D.M.; McClelland, R.L.; Lakoski, S.G.; Cushman, M.; Wong, N.D.; Blumenthal, R.S.; *et al.* The association of Framingham and Reynolds Risk Scores with incidence and progression of coronary artery calcification in MESA (Multi-Ethnic Study of Atherosclerosis). *J. Am. Coll. Cardiol.* **2011**, *58*, 2076–2083. [CrossRef] [PubMed]

31. Desai, MY; Halliburton, S.; Masri, A.; Kottha, A.; Kuzmiak, S.; Flamm, S.; Schoenhagen, P. Reclassification of cardiovascular risk with coronary calcium scoring in subjects without documented coronary heart disease: Comparison with risk assessment based on Reynolds Risk Score. *J. Am. Coll. Cardiol.* **2012**, *59*, E1186. [CrossRef]

32. Naqvi, T.Z.; Lee, M.S. Carotid Intima-media thickness and plaque in cardiovascular risk assessment. *JACC Cardiovasc. Imaging* **2014**, *7*, 1025–1038. [CrossRef] [PubMed]

33. Lorenz, M.W.; Markus, H.S.; Bots, M.L.; Rosvall, M.; Sitzer, M. Prediction of clinical cardiovascular events with carotid intima-media thickness: A systematic review and meta-analysis. *Circulation* **2007**, *115*, 459–467. [CrossRef] [PubMed]

34. Folsom, A.R.; Kronmal, R.A.; Detrano, R.C.; O'Leary, D.H.; Bild, D.E.; Bluemke, D.A.; Budoff, M.J.; Liu, K.; Shea, S.; Szklo, M.; *et al.* Coronary artery calcification compared with carotid intima-media thickness in the prediction of cardiovascular disease incidence: The Multi-Ethnic Study of Atherosclerosis (MESA). *Arch. Int. Med.* **2008**, *168*, 1333–1339. [CrossRef]

35. Terry, J.G.; Carr, J.J.; Tang, R.; Evans, G.W.; Kouba, E.O.; Shi, R.; Cook, D.R.; Vieira, J.L.; Espeland, M.A.; Mercuri, M.F.; *et al.* Coronary artery calcium outperforms carotid artery intima-media thickness as a noninvasive index of prevalent coronary artery stenosis. *Arterioscler. Thromb. Vasc. Biol.* **2005**, *25*, 1723–1728. [CrossRef] [PubMed]

36. Danad, I.; Raijmakers, P.G.; Kamali, P.; Harms, H.J.; de Haan, S.; Lubberink, M.; van Kuijk, C.; Hoekstra, O.S.; Lammertsma, A.A.; Smulders, Y.M.; *et al.* Carotid artery intima-media thickness, but not coronary artery calcium, predicts coronary vascular resistance in patients evaluated for coronary artery disease. *Eur. Heart J. Cardiovasc. Imaging* **2012**, *13*, 317–323. [CrossRef] [PubMed]

37. Knaapen, P.; Camici, P.G.; Marques, K.M.; Nijveldt, R.; Bax, J.J.; Westerhof, N.; Gotte, M.J.; Jerosch-Herold, M.; Schelbert, H.R.; Lammertsma, A.A.; *et al.* Coronary microvascular resistance: Methods for its quantification in humans. *Basic Res. Cardiol.* **2009**, *104*, 485–498. [CrossRef] [PubMed]

38. Naqvi, T.Z.; Mendoza, F.; Rafii, F.; Gransar, H.; Guerra, M.; Lepor, N.; Berman, D.S.; Shah, P.K. High prevalence of ultrasound detected carotid atherosclerosis in subjects with low Framingham Risk Score: Potential implications for screening for subclinical atherosclerosis. *J. Am. Soc. Echocardiogr.* **2010**, *23*, 809–815. [CrossRef] [PubMed]

39. Davis, P.H.; Dawson, J.D.; Mahoney, L.T.; Lauer, R.M. Increased carotid intimal-medial thickness and coronary calcification are related in young and middle-aged adults: The Muscatine study. *Circulation* **1999**, *100*, 838–842. [CrossRef] [PubMed]

40. Lester, S.J.; Eleid, M.F.; Khandheria, B.K.; Hurst, R.T. Carotid intima-media thickness and coronary artery calcium score as indications of subclinical atherosclerosis. *Mayo Clin. Proc.* **2009**, *84*, 229–233. [CrossRef] [PubMed]

41. Greenland, P.; Alpert, J.S.; Beller, G.A.; Benjamin, E.J.; Budoff, M.J.; Fayad, Z.A.; Foster, E.; Hlatky, M.A.; Hodgson, J.M.; Kushner, F.G.; *et al.* 2010 ACCF/AHA guideline for assessment of cardiovascular risk in asymptomatic adults: Executive summary: A report of the American College of Cardiology Foundation/American Heart Association task force on practice guidelines. *Circulation* **2010**, *122*, 2748–2764. [CrossRef] [PubMed]

42. Ridker, P.M.; Danielson, E.; Fonseca, F.A.; Genest, J.; Gotto, A.M., Jr.; Kastelein, J.J.; Koenig, W.; Libby, P.; Lorenzatti, A.J.; MacFadyen, J.G.; *et al.* Rosuvastatin to prevent vascular events in men and women with elevated C-reactive protein. *N. Engl. J. Med.* **2008**, *359*, 2195–2207. [CrossRef] [PubMed]

43. Ridker, P.M.; Cushman, M.; Stampfer, M.J.; Tracy, R.P.; Hennekens, C.H. Inflammation, aspirin, and the risk of cardiovascular disease in apparently healthy men. *N. Engl. J. Med.* **1997**, *336*, 973–979. [CrossRef] [PubMed]

44. Ridker, P.M.; Hennekens, C.H.; Buring, J.E.; Rifai, N. C-reactive protein and other markers of inflammation in the prediction of cardiovascular disease in women. *N. Engl. J. Med.* **2000**, *342*, 836–843. [CrossRef] [PubMed]

45. Ridker, P.M.; Rifai, N.; Rose, L.; Buring, J.E.; Cook, N.R. Comparison of C-reactive protein and low-density lipoprotein cholesterol levels in the prediction of first cardiovascular events. *N. Engl. J. Med.* **2002**, *347*, 1557–1565. [CrossRef] [PubMed]

46. Koenig, W.; Lowel, H.; Baumert, J.; Meisinger, C. C-reactive protein modulates risk prediction based on the Framingham Score: Implications for future risk assessment: Results from a large cohort study in southern Germany. *Circulation* **2004**, *109*, 1349–1353. [CrossRef] [PubMed]

47. Pai, J.K.; Pischon, T.; Ma, J.; Manson, J.E.; Hankinson, S.E.; Joshipura, K.; Curhan, G.C.; Rifai, N.; Cannuscio, C.C.; Stampfer, M.J.; *et al.* Inflammatory markers and the risk of coronary heart disease in men and women. *New Engl. J. Med.* **2004**, *351*, 2599–2610. [CrossRef] [PubMed]

48. Boekholdt, S.M.; Hack, C.E.; Sandhu, M.S.; Luben, R.; Bingham, S.A.; Wareham, N.J.; Peters, R.J.; Jukema, J.W.; Day, N.E.; Kastelein, J.J.; *et al.* C-reactive protein levels and coronary artery disease incidence and mortality in apparently healthy men and women: The EPIC-Norfolk prospective population study 1993–2003. *Atherosclerosis* **2006**, *187*, 415–422. [CrossRef] [PubMed]

49. Ballantyne, C.M.; Hoogeveen, R.C.; Bang, H.; Coresh, J.; Folsom, A.R.; Heiss, G.; Sharrett, A.R. Lipoprotein-associated phospholipase A2, high-sensitivity C-reactive protein, and risk for incident coronary heart disease in middle-aged men and women in the Atherosclerosis Risk in Communities (ARIC) study. *Circulation* **2004**, *109*, 837–842. [CrossRef] [PubMed]

50. Park, R.; Detrano, R.; Xiang, M.; Fu, P.; Ibrahim, Y.; LaBree, L.; Azen, S. Combined use of computed tomography coronary calcium scores and C-reactive protein levels in predicting cardiovascular events in nondiabetic individuals. *Circulation* **2002**, *106*, 2073–2077. [CrossRef] [PubMed]

51. Lakoski, S.G.; Cushman, M.; Blumenthal, R.S.; Kronmal, R.; Arnett, D.; D'Agostino, R.B., Jr.; Detrano, R.C.; Herrington, D.M. Implications of C-reactive protein or coronary artery calcium score as an adjunct to global risk assessment for primary prevention of CHD. *Atherosclerosis* **2007**, *193*, 401–407. [CrossRef] [PubMed]

52. Blaha, M.J.; Budoff, M.J.; DeFilippis, A.P.; Blankstein, R.; Rivera, J.J.; Agatston, A.; O'Leary, D.H.; Lima, J.; Blumenthal, R.S.; Nasir, K. Associations between C-reactive protein, coronary artery calcium, and cardiovascular events: Implications for the JUPITER population from MESA, a population-based cohort study. *Lancet* **2011**, *378*, 684–692. [CrossRef] [PubMed]

53. Mohlenkamp, S.; Lehmann, N.; Moebus, S.; Schmermund, A.; Dragano, N.; Stang, A.; Siegrist, J.; Mann, K.; Jockel, K.H.; Erbel, R.; *et al.* Quantification of coronary atherosclerosis and inflammation to predict coronary events and all-cause mortality. *J. Am. Coll. Cardiol.* **2011**, *57*, 1455–1464. [CrossRef] [PubMed]

54. Reilly, M.P.; Wolfe, M.L.; Localio, A.R.; Rader, D.J. Study of inherited risk of coronary A. C-reactive protein and coronary artery calcification: The study of Inherited Risk of Coronary Atherosclerosis (SIRCA). *Arterioscler. Thromb. Vasc. Biol.* **2003**, *23*, 1851–1856. [CrossRef] [PubMed]

55. Ding, J.; Hsu, F.C.; Harris, T.B.; Liu, Y.; Kritchevsky, S.B.; Szklo, M.; Ouyang, P.; Espeland, M.A.; Lohman, K.K.; Criqui, M.H.; *et al.* The association of pericardial fat with incident coronary heart disease: The Multi-Ethnic Study of Atherosclerosis (MESA). *Am. J. Clin. Nutr.* **2009**, *90*, 499–504. [CrossRef] [PubMed]

56. Budoff, M.J.; Nasir, K.; Katz, R.; Takasu, J.; Carr, J.J.; Wong, N.D.; Allison, M.; Lima, J.A.; Detrano, R.; Blumenthal, R.S.; *et al.* Thoracic aortic calcification and coronary heart disease events: The Multi-Ethnic Study of Atherosclerosis (MESA). *Atherosclerosis* **2011**, *215*, 196–202. [CrossRef] [PubMed]

57. Zeb, I.; Budoff, M.J.; Katz, R.; Lloyd-Jones, D.; Agatston, A.; Blumenthal, R.S.; Blaha, M.; Blankstein, R.; Carr, J.J.; Nasir, K. Non-alcoholic fatty liver disease is an independent predictor of long-term incident coronary heart disease events—The Multi-Ethnic Study of Atherosclerosis. *Circulation* **2012**, *126*, A13688.

58. Yeboah, J.; Carr, J.J.; Terry, J.G.; Ding, J.; Zeb, I.; Liu, S.; Nasir, K.; Post, W.; Blumenthal, R.S.; Budoff, M.J. Computed tomography-derived cardiovascular risk markers, incident cardiovascular events, and all-cause mortality in nondiabetics: The Multi-Ethnic Study of Atherosclerosis. *Eur. J. Prev. Cardiol.* **2014**, *21*, 1233–1241. [CrossRef] [PubMed]

59. Budoff, M.J.; Nasir, K.; McClelland, R.L.; Detrano, R.; Wong, N.; Blumenthal, R.S.; Kondos, G.; Kronmal, R.A. Coronary calcium predicts events better with absolute calcium scores than age-sex-race/ethnicity percentiles: MESA (Multi-Ethnic Study of Atherosclerosis). *J. Am. Coll. Cardiol.* **2009**, *53*, 345–352. [CrossRef] [PubMed]

60. Kalia, N.K.; Miller, L.G.; Nasir, K.; Blumenthal, R.S.; Agrawal, N.; Budoff, M.J. Visualizing coronary calcium is associated with improvements in adherence to statin therapy. *Atherosclerosis* **2006**, *185*, 394–399. [CrossRef] [PubMed]

61. Taylor, A.J.; Bindeman, J.; Feuerstein, I.; Le, T.; Bauer, K.; Byrd, C.; Wu, H.; O'Malley, P.G. Community-based provision of statin and aspirin after the detection of coronary artery calcium within a community-based screening cohort. *J. Am. Coll. Cardiol.* **2008**, *51*, 1337–1341. [CrossRef] [PubMed]

62. Budoff, M.J.; Hokanson, J.E.; Nasir, K.; Shaw, L.J.; Kinney, G.L.; Chow, D.; Demoss, D.; Nuguri, V.; Nabavi, V.; Ratakonda, R.; *et al.* Progression of coronary artery calcium predicts all-cause mortality. *JACC Cardiovasc. Imaging* **2010**, *3*, 1229–1236. [CrossRef] [PubMed]

63. Berry, J.D.; Liu, K.; Folsom, A.R.; Lewis, C.E.; Carr, J.J.; Polak, J.F.; Shea, S.; Sidney, S.; O'Leary, D.H.; Chan, C.; *et al.* Prevalence and progression of subclinical atherosclerosis in younger adults with low short-term but high lifetime estimated risk for cardiovascular disease: The coronary artery risk development in young adults study and multi-ethnic study of atherosclerosis. *Circulation* **2009**, *119*, 382–389. [CrossRef] [PubMed]

64. Raggi, P.; Cooil, B.; Shaw, L.J.; Aboulhson, J.; Takasu, J.; Budoff, M.; Callister, T.Q. Progression of coronary calcium on serial electron beam tomographic scanning is greater in patients with future myocardial infarction. *Am. J. Cardiol.* **2003**, *92*, 827–829. [CrossRef] [PubMed]

65. Budoff, M.J.; Young, R.; Lopez, V.A.; Kronmal, R.A.; Nasir, K.; Blumenthal, R.S.; Detrano, R.C.; Bild, D.E.; Guerci, A.D.; Liu, K.; *et al.* Progression of coronary calcium and incident coronary heart disease events: MESA (Multi-Ethnic Study of Atherosclerosis). *J. Am. Coll. Cardiol.* **2013**, *61*, 1231–1239. [CrossRef] [PubMed]

66. Budoff, M.J.; Achenbach, S.; Blumenthal, R.S.; Carr, J.J.; Goldin, J.G.; Greenland, P.; Guerci, A.D.; Lima, J.A.; Rader, D.J.; Rubin, G.D.; *et al.* Assessment of coronary artery disease by cardiac computed tomography: A scientific statement from the American Heart Association Committee on Cardiovascular Imaging and Intervention, Council on Cardiovascular Radiology and Intervention, and Committee on Cardiac Imaging, Council on Clinical Cardiology. *Circulation* **2006**, *114*, 1761–1791. [CrossRef] [PubMed]

67. Parker, M.S.; Hui, F.K.; Camacho, M.A.; Chung, J.K.; Broga, D.W.; Sethi, N.N. Female breast radiation exposure during CT pulmonary angiography. *AJR Am. J. Roentgenol.* **2005**, *185*, 1228–1233. [CrossRef] [PubMed]

68. Horton, K.M.; Post, W.S.; Blumenthal, R.S.; Fishman, E.K. Prevalence of significant noncardiac findings on electron-beam computed tomography coronary artery calcium screening examinations. *Circulation* **2002**, *106*, 532–534. [CrossRef] [PubMed]

69. Schragin, J.G.; Weissfeld, J.L.; Edmundowicz, D.; Strollo, D.C.; Fuhrman, C.R. Non-cardiac findings on coronary electron beam computed tomography scanning. *J. Thora. Imaging* **2004**, *19*, 82–86. [CrossRef]

70. Machaalany, J.; Yam, Y.; Ruddy, T.D.; Abraham, A.; Chen, L.; Beanlands, R.S.; Chow, B.J. Potential clinical and economic consequences of noncardiac incidental findings on cardiac computed tomography. *J. Am. Coll. Cardiol.* **2009**, *54*, 1533–1541. [CrossRef] [PubMed]

10

Validating Intravascular Imaging with Serial Optical Coherence Tomography and Confocal Fluorescence Microscopy

Pier-Luc Tardif [1,2,*], Marie-Jeanne Bertrand [2,3], Maxime Abran [1,2], Alexandre Castonguay [1], Joël Lefebvre [1], Barbara E. Stähli [2], Nolwenn Merlet [2], Teodora Mihalache-Avram [2], Pascale Geoffroy [2], Mélanie Mecteau [2], David Busseuil [2], Feng Ni [4], Abedelnasser Abulrob [4], Éric Rhéaume [2,3], Philippe L'Allier [2,3], Jean-Claude Tardif [2,3] and Frédéric Lesage [1,2,*]

[1]   Département de Génie Électrique et Institut de Génie Biomédical, École Polytechnique de Montréal, Montreal, QC H3T 1J4, Canada; maxime.abran@gmail.com (M.A.); alexandre.castonguay87@gmail.com (A.C.); joel.lefebvre@gmail.com (J.L.);
[2]   Montreal Heart Institute, Montreal, QC H1T 1C8, Canada; mariejeanne.bertrand@gmail.com (M.-J.B.); barbarastaehli@hotmail.com (B.E.S.); nolwenn.merlet@gmail.com (N.M.); Teodora.Mihalache-Avram@icm-mhi.org (T.M.-A.); Pascale.Geoffroy@icm-mhi.org (P.G.); melanie.mecteau@icm-mhi.org (M.M.); david.busseuil@icm-biobanque.org (D.B.); Eric.Rheaume@icm-mhi.org (É.R.); philippe.l_lallier@icloud.com (P.L.); jean-claude.tardif@icm-mhi.org (J.-C.T.)
[3]   Département de Médecine, Université de Montréal, Montreal, QC H3C 3J7, Canada
[4]   National Research Council Canada (NRCC), Montreal, QC H3A 1A3, Canada; Feng.Ni@cnrc-nrc.gc.ca (F.N.); abedelnasser.abulrob@nrc-cnrc.gc.ca (A.A.)
*   Correspondence: pierluctardif@gmail.com (P.-L.T.); frederic.lesage@polymtl.ca (F.L.);

Academic Editors: Michael Henein and Joseph V. Moxon

Abstract: Atherosclerotic cardiovascular diseases are characterized by the formation of a plaque in the arterial wall. Intravascular ultrasound (IVUS) provides high-resolution images allowing delineation of atherosclerotic plaques. When combined with near infrared fluorescence (NIRF), the plaque can also be studied at a molecular level with a large variety of biomarkers. In this work, we present a system enabling automated volumetric histology imaging of excised aortas that can spatially correlate results with combined IVUS/NIRF imaging of lipid-rich atheroma in cholesterol-fed rabbits. Pullbacks in the rabbit aortas were performed with a dual modality IVUS/NIRF catheter developed by our group. Ex vivo three-dimensional (3D) histology was performed combining optical coherence tomography (OCT) and confocal fluorescence microscopy, providing high-resolution anatomical and molecular information, respectively, to validate in vivo findings. The microscope was combined with a serial slicer allowing for the imaging of the whole vessel automatically. Colocalization of in vivo and ex vivo results is demonstrated. Slices can then be recovered to be tested in conventional histology.

Keywords: intravascular ultrasound (IVUS); near-infrared fluorescence (NIRF); atherosclerosis; ex vivo three-dimensional (3D) histology; optical coherence tomography (OCT); confocal fluorescence microscopy

---

1. Introduction

Atherosclerosis is a chronic immune-mediated inflammatory disease that arises from a series of complex events triggered by endothelial dysfunction, lipid accumulation in the arterial wall, and infiltration of monocyte-derived macrophages [1,2]. Acute coronary syndromes (ACS) occur mostly from the rupture of modestly stenotic lipid-rich "vulnerable" plaques, which leads to endoluminal thrombus formation, myocardial ischemia, and sudden cardiac death [3,4]. Although coronary angiography remains the gold standard for epicardial coronary stenoses assessment and treatment, it frequently underestimates true plaque burden and provides no information regarding plaque composition [5]. Intravascular ultrasound (IVUS) imaging has been established as an adjunct imaging technology to coronary angiography, widely used in both clinical and research applications [6]. By generating in vivo cross-sectional images of the vessel wall and lumen, IVUS enables the characterization of atherosclerotic vessel segments by providing accurate lumen and vessel dimensions, as well as non-protruding plaques, positive vascular remodeling, and plaque burden assessment [7,8]. Conventional grayscale IVUS is, however, limited with regards to the analysis of plaque composition [9], whereas emerging molecular imaging technologies, such as fluorescence imaging, have been developed to overcome these limitations. Multimodality imaging systems, such as the dual-modality IVUS/near-infrared fluorescence (NIRF) imaging catheter previously engineered by our group and others [10–13], were designed for integrated microstructural and molecular plaque imaging, thus enabling a more detailed plaque characterization. The use of molecular probes in conjunction with fluorescence imaging has been shown to provide complementary information with regards to plaque activity and inflammation [14–19]. Translation of molecular imaging results to clinical applications, however, requires validation; and despite impressive advances in intravascular imaging over the past decade, histology remains the gold standard for determining plaque composition and geometry. Although providing high-resolution cross-sectional images of the arterial wall, histology remains limited to the number of tissue sections analyzed and by the lack of anatomical context; thus resulting in missed valuable data. When comparing in vivo intravascular imaging applications with histology, colocalization is often challenged by geometric distortions and tissue shrinkage, as well as the lack of anatomical landmarks and the limited resolution of IVUS imaging.

OCT-based block-face three-dimensional (3D) histology combined with serial cutting of tissues has been proven in the past to be an efficient technique to reconstruct and visualize whole intact organs or tissues [20,21]. Previous work has demonstrated the use of serial OCT imaging primarily for brain imaging. However, this method has so far never been used for cardiovascular imaging. From the spatial resolution of optical coherence tomography (OCT), largely superior to IVUS [6], and the capacity of confocal fluorescence microscopy to efficiently identify the same molecular biomarkers as NIRF imaging [22], we developed a novel ex vivo automated 3D histology platform comprising a dual-modality imaging system based on OCT-coupled fluorescence sensitive confocal microscopy [21]. In this work we detail the process of image reconstruction using this system and, for the first time, describe its use for the purpose of atherosclerosis detection and localization in iliac arteries and aortas of an atherosclerotic rabbit model. Fluorescent signal colocalization obtained from in vivo and ex vivo imaging was performed to validate the potential of these methods to be co-registered and for OCT-combined fluorescence sensitive confocal microscopy to serve as a future histology add-on validation tool in the development of novel molecular probes.

2. Results

2.1. In Vitro Affinity of Anti-ICAM-1 Antibody

A fluorescently labelled anti-intercellular adhesion molecule-1 (ICAM-1) antibody was used as a marker of inflammation below. Four ICAM-1 probes were initially tested in vitro, but only one showed positive affinity with inflammation (Figure 1). Fluorescence confocal microscopy images were taken to evaluate the affinity of the anti-ICAM-1 antibody with mammalian cells. Human Umbilical Vein Cells (HUVEC) were imaged before and after being activated by Tumor Necrosis Factor Alpha (TNF-alpha), which induces inflammation. Placing the fluorophore bound to the ICAM-1 antibody in the cell growth medium followed by flushing, it was observed that the signal was far more present for the TNF-alpha activated cells, suggesting that the ICAM-1 antibody does in fact have affinity with inflammation (Figure 1). Deconvolution was also performed to form a transverse image of the cell to show that the signal was localized on the cellular membrane and not in the growth medium or the cytoplasm (Figure 1C).

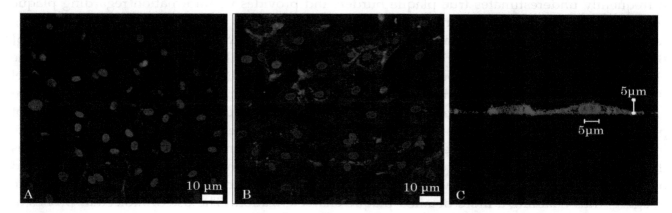

Figure 1. Florescent confocal images of in vitro affinity of the intercellular adhesion molecule-1 (ICAM-1) antibody: (**A**) Inactivated and (**B**) Tumor Necrosis Factor Alpha (TNF-α) activated Human Umbilical Vein Cells (HUVEC). The nuclei (blue) were stained with DAPI (4′,6-Diamidino-2-Phenylindole, Dilactate) (**C**) deconvolved image of a cell. The fluorescence signal (red) is not present in the cytoplasm or the nucleus, but is, rather, located on the cell membrane.

2.2. In Vivo Catheter Imaging

Five atherosclerotic rabbits were imaged following either an in vivo targeted molecular probes injection (model 1) or an intravenous indocyanine green (ICG) (model 2) injection with a dual IVUS/NIRF imaging catheter designed by our group (Figure 2). The IVUS had a frequency of 45 MHz and the excitation wavelength of the NIRF was 780 nm. As shown in Figure 2B,C, a strong in vivo signal was obtained following injection of an ICAM-1 nanobody probe at 30.05 mm of pullback in model 1, with partial correlation with the echolucent region on IVUS imaging. Other ICAM-1 nanobodies that did not show affinity in vitro were also injected with the purpose of evaluating their targeting ability. For these, weak signals were detected by in vivo NIRF/IVUS imaging, despite the presence of plaque on IVUS. In model 2, a strong but localized signal was seen at 8.4 mm of catheter pullback correlated with IVUS imaging, with the plaque pointed by the red arrow (Figure 2E). The pulse generated by the ultrasound (US), created an artifact and a mask was applied to hide the catheter on the images up to the artifact radial position, which extended 50 μm past the wall of the catheter. Thus, part of the mask intersected the vessel wall (Figure 2E) in smaller vessels, but not in bigger ones (Figure 2C). A ring artifact that can be seen of Figure 2C was caused by a reflection on the sheath surrounding the catheter.

2.3. Serial Imaging System, Ex Vivo OCT Reconstructions and Fluorescence Alignment

A serial microscopy imaging system was designed combining OCT and confocal fluorescence imaging (Figure 3A). Micrometer-precise motors and a razor blade attached to a custom vibratome allowed automatic serial mosaic imaging of agarose-embedded artery sections to be performed. OCT and fluorescence data were measured simultaneously which enabled co-registration of OCT imaging with fluorescence. OCT provided 3D volumes for each slice (200 μm thickness) while a single confocal image was taken (2D) with focus centered in the slice. For confocal fluorescence, a trade-off was required in the system to enable the combination of OCT (which requires a long focal depth for accurate 3D images) and confocal microscopy requiring filling the objective for optimal resolution. In this design, the confocal beam under-filled the objective, leading to a fluorescent point-spread-function that extended in depth.

The model 1 rabbits were imaged with a 3× objective whereas the model 2 rabbit was imaged with a 10× water immersion objective. The former being designed to work in air, a chamber was built between the end of the objective and water by gluing a glass window to the aluminum lens tube. Typical results are presented in Figure 3B–D for raw, processed, and 3D reconstruction data, respectively. Fluorescence signal was higher at the surface or near the arterial wall, which suggests that the ICAM-1 nanobodies bind to lipid plaques and that these molecular probes are sources of specific signals. The processed slices can then be recovered after slicing and imaged in standard histology (Figure 3E,F), here, with Masson Trichrome (Figure 2E) and Von Kossa (Figure 3F) to detect calcification.

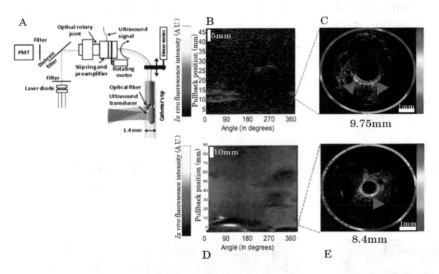

Figure 2. In vivo imaging system and typical images. (**A**) Overview of the bimodal catheter system with a detailed view of the catheter's tip. PMT stands for photomultiplier tube; (**B**) Paired in vivo near-infrared fluorescence signal detected over 360 degrees with 50 mm pullback length; and (**C**) integrated NIRF-IVUS cross-sectional imaging with partial fluorescence signal and echolucent plaque colocalization (shown by red arrows) in model 1. Atherosclerotic plaque, shown by echolucent signal on IVUS (**D,E**), was partly correlated with indocyanine green (ICG)-fluorescence signal at 8.4 mm of pullback (red arrow) in model 2.

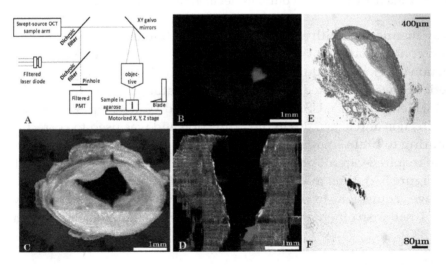

Figure 3. Ex vivo optical coherence tomography (OCT) and confocal reconstruction for a model 1-type rabbit. (**A**) Overview of the serial histology imaging system; (**B**) Example of an averaged slice (raw data) with the fluorescence image superimposed on it (i.e., red signal); (**C**) Example of the same slice after Beer-Lambert corrections, contrast adjustment, and deconvolution (Log-scale), with superimposed fluorescence image (red); (**D**) Localization of the tissue slice (c) on a 3D reconstruction (shown by red arrow); (**E**) Histology slice colored with Masson Trichrome and a 4× objective (**F**) Same slice imaged with VonKossa and a 20× objective.

Data Reconstruction

Due to tissue attenuation of the OCT signal and serial mosaic acquisitions, specific algorithms were developed to reconstruct full 3D volumes. A custom Python stitching and signal correction algorithm was developed, allowing complete artery reconstructions and atherosclerosis localization based on both modalities. The following steps were implemented:

- For each tissue slice, the volume position in the mosaic reference frame was estimated using microscope acquisition data;
- Volumes were then stitched for each tissue slice;
- Post processing was performed that included cropping of the field of view, identification of lumen mask and Beer-Lambert intensity correction;
- After post processing steps, slices were assembled together in order to form a longitudinal 3D volume.

Figure 4A,B show typical images after the post processing steps (masks, Beer-Lambert correction, intensity artifacts correction, and cropping) applied to an averaged OCT slice and fluorescence image, respectively. Figure 4C shows the attenuation map used for Beer-Lambert correction for a particular slice.

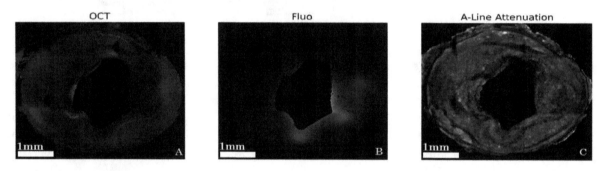

Figure 4. Corrected images for model 1 rabbit for OCT (**A**); and fluorescence (**B**); A-line attenuation map used for OCT intensity correction outlines detailed tissue structures (**C**).

As previously mentioned, with an under-filled objective used in fluorescence imaging, deeper tissue slices could contaminate the signal of the imaged slice in fluorescence due to the extended point-spread function (PSF), thus, requiring a deconvolution algorithm to generate precise fluorescence images. A synthetic PSF was generated using the PSF generator plugin in the ImageJ software (National Institutes of Health, New York, NY, USA) using the Born and Wolf 3D optical model. It had a FWHM of 4.4 μm in the x-y direction and of 146 μm in the z direction and was used to correct fluorescence images.

When comparing to brain imaging obtained from a similar technology, the automatic ex vivo imaging technique required careful preparation of arterial tissues, as conjunctive tissues could cause cutting artifacts (Figure 5A), thus making it challenging to obtain uniform cuts. An algorithm was applied during image acquisitions to ensure fine control of the focal depth and to avoid placing tissues in areas where OCT had instrumental artifacts (spurious reflections) or outside the focal zone of the objective (Figure 5B,C).

2.4. Alignment and Tissue Deformation

Due to ex vivo tissue fixation and a lack of intra-arterial pressure, which led to tissue dehydration and shrinkage, the comparison of in vivo and corresponding ex vivo vessel segments was challenging. Despite the average tissue shrinkage ratio of 61% that was calculated in our experiments, imaging colocalization was possible using landmarks. Longitudinal views of both IVUS and OCT anatomical imaging of an arterial segment are presented in Figure 6. The abdominal aorta and iliac arteries were visualized with both modalities, which served as reference points for colocalization. While longitudinal co-registration was possible, precise pixel-wise deformation models could not be applied since the arterial wall was highly distorted in ex vivo OCT images given the lack of blood flow in fixed tissues. Nevertheless, longitudinal segments could be identified accurately, which enabled comparisons of pullback in vivo results to ex vivo data.

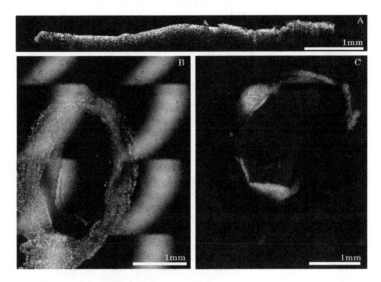

Figure 5. Sources of imaging artifacts and their effects during acquisitions: (**A**) Unevenly cut slice; (**B**) Artifact caused by the glass when the reference arm was not properly placed; (**C**) Slice that was imaged while not placed at the focal point of the lens.

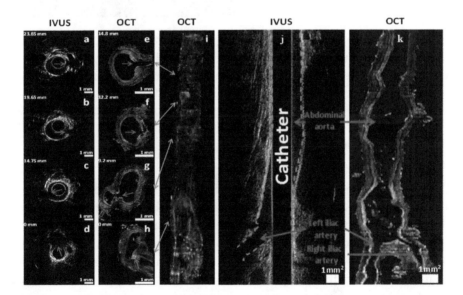

Figure 6. Intravascular ultrasound (IVUS) and OCT colocalization of anatomical landmarks in model 2. (**a–d**) In vivo IVUS cross-sectional images; (**e–h**) Ex vivo OCT cross-sectional images; (**i**) 3D reconstruction in OCT using a maximum intensity projection algorithm. Indicated numbers in mm (upper left of each image) represent the distances between the cross-section and the iliac bifurcation. The catheter was introduced in the right iliac artery, located at the bottom-right in the OCT image in (**h,i**). Green arrows indicate the location of the cross-section slices on 3D reconstruction. Red arrows denote side branches (anatomical landmarks) used for colocalization. Longitudinal view of the abdominal aorta and iliac arteries in IVUS and OCT imaging in model 2; (**j**) In vivo IVUS image of a 50 mm artery segment (green dashed lines delineates the arterial wall); (**k**) Ex vivo OCT image of the same segment, which shrunk to a length of 30 mm after ex vivo tissue fixation. Scale bars represent a region of 1 mm by 1 mm.

2.5. Validation of Intravascular Molecular Imaging

Using the methodological steps outlined above, in vivo ICG accumulation identified with NIRF imaging was confirmed using high-resolution fluorescence confocal imaging, as shown in Figure 7. Intimal thickening was also observed on ex vivo OCT, an indication of the presence of plaque. Figure 7b shows that the intimal thickness varied from 100 μm to 200 μm (red arrows), a difference not perceptible in IVUS, which has a resolution of about 100 μm.

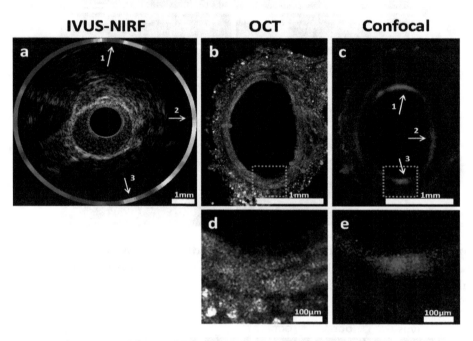

Figure 7. Cross-sectional view of the abdominal aorta in model 2. (**a**) IVUS-NIRF imaging in vivo; (**b**) OCT imaging ex vivo; (**c**) Confocal fluorescence microscopy imaging ex vivo; (**d,e**) Enlarged sections of the green region of (**b,c**). Red arrows identify the intimal thickness at two locations in the OCT image. White arrows indicate colocalization between in vivo and ex vivo fluorescence. Arrow 3 shows a weaker colocalization due to the limitation of our blood attenuation compensation algorithm [19], further supporting the need for co-registered ex vivo validation.

3. Discussion

Combining IVUS and fluorescence imaging (NIRF) within a single catheter may yield a reliable method that could be used to detect and locate atherosclerotic plaques in the arterial wall. This imaging method overcomes the shortcomings of coronary angiography, whereas fluorescence provides information regarding plaque composition and biology. Translation of such imaging technology to clinical applications requires robust preclinical validation, and co-registration of in vivo data to ex vivo assessments is essential for better plaque assessment. In the present work, we demonstrated that multimodal custom serial imaging of tissue sections can be used to corroborate in vivo findings using OCT and confocal imaging to provide high spatial resolution. Our system is also compatible with conventional histology, as the slices from the vibratome can be recovered in the correct order using a small container placed in front of the agarose block and stained using standard procedures.

The main shortcoming of conventional histology is that although it offers information on molecular tissue composition, it does not provide accurate anatomical localization of said tissues. There is, at the moment, no existing method that can reliably corroborate the in vivo plaque localization and composition measurements done with an intravascular catheter during pullbacks. The method described here can, however, combine the molecular composition determination aspect of conventional histology, while the 3D reconstructions allow colocalization to be performed. Furthermore, in conventional histology, images are formed after the tissue is sliced, which leads to additional deformations and difficulties in reconstructing the 3D view. With the block-face OCT technique, images are taken before slicing, facilitating 3D assembly. Our method, while not a substitute for standard histology, is projected to be a complementary method that can help to bridge in vivo and histological data. The ability to co-localize tissues between the in vivo and ex vivo tissues offers a novel approach that could be used to validate future intravascular molecular imaging studies. Having a reliable way to confirm the data gathered in in vivo scans will smooth the transition between the fundamental research and clinical domains, leading to more effective, invasive imagery techniques and eventually better treatments for patients.

3.1. Slicing Optimization

One of the most challenging aspect of the ex vivo imaging process was to obtain uniform flat slices with the vibratome, as the connective tissue surrounding the artery rendered slicing more difficult. Residual connective tissue remaining above the sample after slicing appeared to block the light and/or cause inaccurate surface detection, thus, leading to some slices being imaged while being out of focus. Furthermore, slice stitching in the z-direction was very sensitive to the flatness of the slices. Keeping the slicer blade completely flat and straight at all times was difficult and resulted in different slice thicknesses. Crooked or uneven slices were problematic during reconstructions, since stitching was based on surface detection. To overcome these difficulties, a fixed overlap between slices was imposed. However, this could create gaps, which sometimes led to the presence of dark bands between slices in the longitudinal reconstruction of the aorta. It should be noted that those overlaps may also induce a small bias when approximating tissue shrinkage as the z-stitching was highly dependent on these. Finally, evaluating the shrinking factor was also made more difficult by the fact that our method relied on finding landmarks, which were sometimes sparse. Optimizing tissue embedding and a careful removal of connective tissue is, thus, key to gathering quality data.

3.2. Optical Optimization

In the case of the $3\times$ objective, the glass used to protect it from water where the sample was imaged was a source of artifacts, since a reflection and its harmonics could be seen with the OCT scanner. While adjusting the reference arm's length could minimize the effect of the glass by imaging in the opportune zones, it was never possible to fully remove its effects since the automatic imaging process, which takes a few days to perform, always yielded a few images that were not situated in the ideal zone. Since the glass has very high reflectivity, the artifact often saturated the detector and information was lost when it could be observed within the imaged tissue. It was, thus, very important for the experimenter to place the glass at a position that did not create an artifact near the focal point of the objective.

3.3. Big-Data Processing

The size of the datasets acquired was a factor that rendered data analysis quite cumbersome. A raw dataset of 500 GB for a single artery section required significant computing power to process and disk space for storage. Even lowering the resolution by going from a $10\times$ to a $3\times$ objective, the image sizes only decreased by half. Improvement in processing in terms of efficiency and storage will be required to enable large-scale studies.

4. Materials and Methods

4.1. Animal Model for Atherosclerosis

Six adult, male, New Zealand White rabbits (3–4 kg, 3 months old; Charles River Laboratories, Saint-Constant, QC, Canada) were fed a 0.5% cholesterol diet (Harlan Techlab Diets, Madison, WI, USA) to induce atherosclerosis. Two rabbit models were used: model 1 ($n = 5$), balloon injury performed at week 0, followed by 14-weeks cholesterol-enriched diet; model 2 ($n = 1$), 14-weeks of high-cholesterol diet. One rabbit did not complete the study due to neurologic complications after completion of balloon denudation. The experimental protocols were approved by the animal ethics committee of the Montreal Heart Institute Research Center (Projet ID code: 2015-1827, 2015-32-02, accepted on 24 March 2015) according to the guidelines of the Canadian Council on Animal Care.

4.2. Balloon Dilatation Procedures

Under general anesthesia (ketamine (35 mg/kg) and buprenorphine (10 mg/kg) administered intramuscularly, inhaled isoflurane (3% v/v, Baxter, Deerfield, IL, USA) and supplemental oxygen), balloon injury of the abdominal arterial wall was performed using a 5 French (F) radial introducer catheter (Cordis Corporation, Fremont, CA, USA) introduced through the right carotid artery. Under fluoroscopic guidance (Siemens, Berlin, Germany), a 4.0 mm PTCA balloon catheter (Boston Scientific, Marlborough, MA, USA) was advanced at the iliac bifurcation over a 0.014 inch guidewire (Abbott Vascular, Santa Clara, CA, USA), inflated with 8 atm and retracted three times in the distal 40 mm of the abdominal aorta. The right carotid artery was ligated at the end of the procedure.

4.3. Bimodal Near-Infrared Fluorescence (NIRF)/Intravascular Ultrasound (IVUS) Imaging Catheter System

The in vivo imaging system (Figure 3A) used in this study, designed as an ultrasound-optical imaging catheter linked to an optical assembly and custom-made electronics, was previously described in [10]. The catheter combines an optical fiber for fluorescence imaging and an ultrasound transducer for acoustic imaging. An electronic circuit synchronizes the acquisition with two motors driving the rotating/translating catheter assembly, and raw data is transferred directly to a laptop via a universal serial bus (USB) connection at rates of up to 250 Mbps. A custom Matlab (The MathWorks, Inc., Natick, MA, USA) user interface filters the signals and reconstructs and displays the images in real time during acquisition. Fluorescence excitation was performed using a 780 nm laser diode and emission was detected by a photomultiplier tube (Hamamatsu Photonics, Hamamatsu City, Japan), combined with a bandpass optical filter (832 ± 19 nm). A compensation algorithm was used to adjust the fluorescence signal amplitude for blood attenuation [10].

4.4. In Vivo NIRF Imaging Procedure

In vivo NIRF imaging was performed under anesthesia, as previously described, using a 5 F introducer (Cordis Corporation, Fremont, CA, USA) placed in the left carotid artery (model 1; $n = 4$). Four novel tentative imaging probes (nanobodies) targeting ICAM-1 receptors (National Research Council Canada, Ottawa, CA, USA), labeled with infrared dye 800CW, were injected under fluoroscopic guidance (Siemens, Germany) in the denuded segment of the abdominal aorta of model 1, followed by intravascular IVUS/NIRF imaging. Intravenous indocyanine green (ICG, 10 mg/kg) was injected in model 2 ($n = 1$) and intravascular imaging was performing through a right carotid artery access 40 min after dye injection. Automated imaging pullbacks were performed in the abdominal aorta of both animal models and in the right iliac artery of model 2 at a pullback speed of 0.5 mm/s and a frame rate of 10 images/s over a total length of 50 and 100 mm, respectively. After in vivo imaging procedures, the animals were sacrificed by exsanguination under anesthesia and then underwent abdominal aorta and iliac arteries resection. The samples were fixed in 4% formaldehyde and kept at 4 °C.

4.5. Ex Vivo Imaging System and Methods

Prior to ex vivo imaging, the distal 40 mm of the abdominal aorta and iliac arteries were mounted in a 4% cylindrical agarose block with 0.5% ethylenediaminetetraacetic acid (EDTA). Ex vivo imaging was performed using a custom made automated serialized dual-modality setup for OCT and confocal fluorescence microscopy, incorporating a swept-source laser with a central wavelength of 1310 nm and a tuning bandwidth of 100 nm for OCT. The confocal laser passed through a filter cube before being reflected at a 90° angle by a long pass dichroic mirror at 875 nm which allowed for it to be combined with the OCT laser beam (Figure 3), allowing simultaneous acquisition of OCT and confocal data.

To overcome limited light penetration in the tissue and scattering from microscopic imaging, a vibratome allowed sequential sectioning of the tissue block face in order to reveal new tissue regions to image. Following a previously described design, a dual flexure part isolated vibration of the blade from a direct current (DC) motor on a one-axis yielding precise cutting of the tissue. X and Y stages allowed moving the sample relative to the objective and imaging every sub-region (1 by 1 mm). Tissue samples embedded in agarose blocks were placed underneath a $10\times$ water immersion objective for model 2. After an entire section was imaged, a 200-μm slice of tissue was removed and the process was repeated automatically. For each slice, the Z position of the sample was adjusted in order to have the focus approximately 50 μm under the tissue surface, thus avoiding imaging of deformed tissue due to its slicing. The images from both in vivo and ex vivo systems were analyzed using Matlab. Anatomical landmarks allowed for a precise sub-millimeter colocalization of in vivo and ex vivo images, along with the calculation of the shrinkage ratio of the excised tissue. To obtain three-dimensional (3D) reconstructions, imaging data was downsampled to a voxel size of 4 μm by 4 μm by 200 μm, converted in DICOM and loaded with Osirix (Pixmeo, Geneva, Switzerland). A maximum intensity projection algorithm was applied to generate a three-dimensional view of the vessels. The ex vivo imaging system generated cross-sectional OCT image slices with a pixel size of 2 μm by 2 μm and a depth of 6.5 μm. The resulting dataset had a size of over 500 GB. In fluorescence confocal microscopy, one cross-sectional image was obtained for each 200-μm depth. Colocalization between the IVUS and OCT images was performed. Figure 6 compares the OCT reconstruction with the IVUS scan for rabbit 1. Colocalization between images relied on finding biological landmarks, primarily bifurcations. Pullbacks began at the bifurcation between the left and right iliac artery and could be seen on both types of scans, providing a good starting point.

For model 1, aortas were imaged using the aforementioned OCT/confocal microscope, but with a $3\times$ air objective and a 5 μm $\times$ 5 μm pixel size. Axial resolution was unchanged. A glass was added between the objective and the water to create an air chamber. The field of view (FOV) in the lateral directions was set to 2.5 mm $\times$ 2.5 mm. The ICAM-1 fluorophore was sensitive to a 776 nm wavelength. The $3\times$ objective did not allow for a high enough signal-to-noise ratio (SNR) with a small pinhole (100 μm), and an iris was used instead. This, however, came at the cost of lateral resolution (4.4 μm). The vibratome blade was inclined at an approximately 20-degree angle with the plane of the agarose gel. Connective tissue was removed before embedding the aorta in agarose with a razor blade. Three-dimensional reconstructions of the aortas were done using custom Python algorithms developed for this purpose. Since an iris was used instead of a pinhole, deconvolution was performed on the fluorescence images in order to locate more accurately the sources of signal.

For OCT images, the first reconstruction step was to find the volumes position within the mosaic reference frame. A displacement model of the sample-motorized stage was used to estimate each XY tile position within the mosaic. The model parameters were estimated from the data by computing the phase-correlation based pairwise registration [23] of all neighboring tiles within the mosaic and by inverting the model, solving for each parameter. The next step was to stitch together the volumes for each slice. Adjacent volumes were blended together by finding the medial axis of their 2D overlap region and by applying a small Gaussian feathering to ensure a smooth transition between tiles. Each tissue slice was stitched separately.

A few post processing steps were then applied on each slice to remove intensity artifacts, to limit the field of view to the tissue, to compute the lumen mask, and, finally, to estimate and compensate the light attenuation with depth in the OCT volumes. This last step was done by fitting a Beer-Lambert law on each A-Line and by estimating the attenuation coefficient from this fit [24]. The Beer-Lambert law was then used again with the average tissue attenuation coefficient to normalize the OCT volume and thus reduce its contrast variation with depth.

The last reconstruction step was to stitch the slices together in the z direction to get a complete 3D volume. This was done by computing the shift between adjacent slices using the cross-correlation of their 2D image gradient magnitude. Then, the slices were stitched together by solving the Laplace equation with Dirichlet boundary conditions over their masked overlap region. The tissue mask was used to remove the gaps introduced by the slice cutting artifacts.

Colocalization between the IVUS and OCT images was performed. Colocalization between images relied on finding biological landmarks, primarily vessel bifurcations. Pullbacks began at the bifurcation between the left and right iliac artery and could be seen on both types of scans for model 2, providing a good starting point. The distance between the same landmarks was measured by knowing the pixel size (6.5 μm) for OCT, and by comparing it to the distance found on the IVUS data, which was recorded during acquisition.

5. Conclusions

In conclusion, a method for atherosclerotic plaque detection and molecular characterization has been investigated both in vivo and ex vivo in a rabbit model. The in vivo method relied on an intravascular catheter that combined IVUS and fluorescence imaging, while the ex vivo method combined an OCT and a fluorescence confocal microscope with a custom serial slicer and stitching algorithm to reconstruct whole 3D segments of aortas and locate the presence of plaque with great accuracy. Colocalization between the in vivo and ex vivo data was performed by finding landmarks between the IVUS and OCT volumes. This massive histology method is a promising approach to validating future intravascular catheters; it could potentially become a new gold standard to validate intravascular molecular imaging, and it is a great addition to the currently used histology methods.

Acknowledgments: This study was supported by CIHR operating grant 273578 to Frédéric Lesage.

Author Contributions: Pier-Luc Tardif, Maxime Abran, Alexandre Castonguay, and Joël Lefebvre acquired the 3D histology data and performed image reconstruction; Philippe L'Allier, Marie-Jeanne Bertrand, Maxime Abran, Nolwenn Merlet, Teodora Mihalache-Avram, Pascale Geoffroy, Mélanie Mecteau, and David Busseuil performed the catheter experiments; Feng Ni and Abedelnasser Abulrob synthesized the molecular probes; Éric Rhéaume and Teodora Mihalache-Avram performed histological validations; Philippe L'Allier, Marie-Jeanne Bertrand, Barbara E. Stähli and Frédéric Lesage wrote the article; Philippe L'Allier, Jean-Claude Tardif, and Frédéric Lesage designed and supervised the study.

References

1.   Libby, P.; Okamoto, Y.; Rocha, V.Z.; Folco, E. Inflammation in atherosclerosis transition from theory to practice. *Circ. J.* **2010**, *74*, 213–220. [CrossRef] [PubMed]

2.   Libby, P.; Ridker, P.M.; Hansson, G.K. Progress and challenges in translating the biology of atherosclerosis. *Nature* **2011**, *473*, 317–325. [CrossRef] [PubMed]

3.   Bentzon, J.F.; Otsuka, F.; Virmani, R.; Falk, E. Mechanisms of plaque formation and rupture. *Circ. Res.* **2014**, *114*, 1852–1866. [CrossRef] [PubMed]

4.   Muller, J.E.; Tofler, G.H.; Stone, P.H. Circadian variation and triggers of onset of acute cardiovascular disease. *Circulation* **1989**, *79*, 733–743. [CrossRef] [PubMed]

5.   Mintz, G.S.; Painter, J.A.; Pichard, A.D.; Kent, K.M.; Satler, L.F.; Popma, J.J.; Chuang, Y.C.; Bucher, T.A.; Sokolowicz, L.E.; Leon, M.B. Atherosclerosis in angiographically "normal" coronary artery reference segments: An intravascular ultrasound study with clinical correlations. *J. Am. Coll. Cardiol.* **1995**, *25*, 1479–1485. [CrossRef]

6.   Tardif, J.C.; Lesage, F.; Harel, F.; Romeo, P.; Pressacco, J. Imaging biomarkers in atherosclerosis trials. *Circ. Cardiovasc. Imaging* **2011**, *4*, 319–333. [CrossRef] [PubMed]

7.   Berry, C.L.; L'Allier, P.; Grégoire, J.; Lespérance, J.; Lévesque, S.; Ibrahim, R.; Tardif, J.C. Comparison of intravascular ultrasound and quantitative coronary angiography for the assessment of coronary artery disease progression. *Circulation* **2007**, *115*, 1851–1857. [CrossRef] [PubMed]

8.   Mintz, G.S.; Garcia-Garcia, H.M.; Nicholls, S.J.; Weissman, N.J.; Bruining, N.; Crowe, T.; Tardif, J.C.; Serruys, P.W. Clinical experts consensus document on standards of acquisition, measurement and reporting of intravascular ultrasound regression/progression studies. *EuroIntervention* **2011**, *6*, 1123–1130. [CrossRef] [PubMed]

9.   Sanchez, O.D.; Sakakura, K.; Otsuka, F.; Yahagi, K.; Virmani, R.; Joner, M. Expectations and limitations in contemporary intravascular imaging: Lessons learned from pathology. *Expert Rev Cardiovasc. Ther.* **2014**, *12*, 601–611. [CrossRef] [PubMed]

10.   Abran, M.; Cloutier, G.; Cardinal, M.H.R.; Chayer, B.; Tardif, J.C.; Lesage, F. Development of a photoacoustic ultrasound and fluorescence imaging catheter for the study of atherosclerotic plaque. *IEEE Trans. Biomed. Circuits Syst.* **2014**, *8*, 696–703. [CrossRef] [PubMed]

11.   Dixon, A.J.; Hossack, J. Intravascular near-infrared fluorescence catheter with ultrasound guidance and blood attenuation correction. *J. Biomed. Opt.* **2013**, *18*. [CrossRef] [PubMed]

12.   Mallas, G.; Brooks, D.H.; Rosenthal, A.; Nudelman, R.N.; Mauskapf, A.; Jaffer, F.A.; Ntziachristos, V. Improving quantification of intravascular fluorescence imaging using structural information. *Phys. Med. Biol.* **2012**, *57*, 6395–6406. [CrossRef] [PubMed]

13.   Bec, J.; Xie, H.; Yankelevich, D.R.; Zhou, F.; Sun, Y.; Ghata, N.; Aldredge, R.; Marcu, L. Design construction and validation of a rotary multifunctional intravascular diagnostic catheter combining multispectral fluorescence lifetime imaging and intravascular ultrasound. *J. Biomed. Opt.* **2011**, *4*, 319–333. [CrossRef] [PubMed]

14.   Jaffer, F.A.; Calfon, M.A.; Rosenthal, A.; Mallas, G.; Razansky, R.N.; Mauskapf, A.; Weissleder, R.; Libby, P.; Ntziachristos, V. Two-dimensional intravascular near-infrared fluorescence molecular imaging of inflammation in atherosclerosis and stent-induced vascular injury. *J. Am. Coll. Cardiol.* **2011**, *57*, 2516–2526. [CrossRef] [PubMed]

15.   Jaffer, F.A.; Vinegoni, C.; John, M.C.; Aikawa, E.; Gold, H.K.; Finn, A.V.; Ntziachristos, V.; Libby, P.; Weissleder, R. Real-time catheter molecular sensing of inflammation in proteolytically active atherosclerosis. *Circulation* **2008**, *118*, 1802–1809. [CrossRef] [PubMed]

16.   Nahrendorf, M.; Jaffer, F.A.; Kelly, K.A.; Sosnovik, D.E.; Aikawa, E.; Libby, P.; Weissleder, R. Noninvasive vascular cell adhesion molecule-1 imaging identifies inflammatory activation of cells in atherosclerosis. *Circulation* **2006**, *114*, 1504–1511. [CrossRef] [PubMed]

17.   Rouleau, L.; Berti, R.; Ng, V.W.K.; Matteau-Pelletier, C.; Lam, T.; Saboural, P.; Kakkar, A.K.; Lesage, F.; Rhéaume, E.; Tardif, J.C. VCAM-1-targeting gold nanoshell probe for photoacoustic imaging of atherosclerotic plaque in mice. *Contrast Med. Mol. Imaging* **2013**, *8*, 27–39. [CrossRef] [PubMed]

18.   De Vries, B.M.W.; Hillebrands, J.; van Dam, G.M.; Tio, R.A.; de Jong, J.S.; Slart, R.H.J.A.; Zeebregts, C.J. Images in cardiovascular medicine. Multispectral near-infrared fluorescence molecular imaging of matrix metalloproteinases in a human carotid plaque using a matrix-degrading metalloproteinase-sensitive activatable fluorescent probe. *Circulation* **2009**, *119*, e534–e536. [CrossRef] [PubMed]

19.   Abran, M.; Stähli, B.E.; Merlet, N.; Mihalache-Avram, T.; Mecteau, M.; Rhéaume, E.; Busseuil, D.; Tardif, J.C.; Lesage, F. Validating a bimodal intravascular ultrasound (IVUS) and near-infrared fluorescence (NIRF) catheter for atherosclerotic plaque detection in rabbits. *Biomed. Opt. Express* **2015**, *6*, 3989–3999. [CrossRef] [PubMed]

20.   Wang, H.; Zhu, J.; Akkin, T. Serial optical coherence scanner for large-scale brain imaging at microscopic resolution. *NeuroImage* **2014**, *84*, 1007–1017. [CrossRef] [PubMed]

21.   Castonguay, A.; Avti, P.K.; Moeini, M.; Pouliot, P.; Tabatabaei, M.S.; Bélanger, S.; Lesage, F. Investigating the correlation between white matter and microvasculature in aging using large scale optical coherence tomography and confocal fluorescence imaging combined with tissue sectioning. *Proc. SPIE* **2015**, *9328*. [CrossRef]

22.   Pande, A.N.; Kohler, R.H.; Aikawa, E.; Weissleder, R.; Jaffer, F.A. Detection of macrophage activity in atherosclerosis in vivo using multichannel, high-resolution laser scanning fluorescence microscopy. *J. Biomed. Opt.* **2006**, *11*. [CrossRef] [PubMed]

23.   Preibisch, S.; Saalfeld, S. Fast stitching of large 3d biological datasets. In Proceedings of the 2nd ImageJ User and Developer Conference, Luxembourg, 7–8 November 2008.

24.   Faber, D.; van der Meer, F.; Aalders, M.; van Leeuwen, T. Quantitative measurement of attenuation coefficients of weakly scattering media using optical coherence tomography. *Opt. Express* **2004**, *12*, 4353–4365. [CrossRef] [PubMed]

11

Coronary CT Angiography in Managing Atherosclerosis

Joachim Eckert *, Marco Schmidt, Annett Magedanz, Thomas Voigtländer and Axel Schmermund

Cardioangiologisches Centrum Bethanien, Im Prüfling 23, D-60389 Frankfurt, Germany;
m.schmidt@ccb.de (M.S.); a.magedanz@ccb.de (A.M.); t.voigtlaender@ccb.de (T.V.);
a.schmermund@ccb.de (A.S.)
* Correspondence: j.eckert@ccb.de;

Academic Editor: Michael Henein

Abstract: Invasive coronary angiography (ICA) was the only method to image coronary arteries for a long time and is still the gold-standard. Technology of noninvasive imaging by coronary computed-tomography angiography (CCTA) has experienced remarkable progress during the last two decades. It is possible to visualize atherosclerotic lesions in the vessel wall in contrast to "lumenography" performed by ICA. Coronary artery disease can be ruled out by CCTA with excellent accuracy. The degree of stenoses is, however, often overestimated which impairs specificity. Atherosclerotic lesions can be characterized as calcified, non-calcified and partially calcified. Calcified plaques are usually quantified using the Agatston-Score. Higher scores are correlated with worse cardiovascular outcome and increased risk of cardiac events. For non-calcified or partially calcified plaques different angiographic findings like positive remodelling, a large necrotic core or spotty calcification more frequently lead to myocardial infarctions. CCTA is an important tool with increasing clinical value for ruling out coronary artery disease or relevant stenoses as well as for advanced risk stratification.

Keywords: atherosclerosis; coronary plaques; coronary computed-tomography angiography (CCTA); coronary calcium; cardiac events

1. Background

Recent developments of CT scanners have improved accuracy especially regarding the visualization of the coronary arteries. A better spatial and temporal resolution makes it possible to scan the heart and the coronary arteries free of motion and to detect vascular plaques and stenoses. Still, heart rates below 60–65/min are preferable to achieve high quality images with a low radiation exposure using prospective ECG (electrocardiographic)-gating. Common nomenclature distinguishes between different types of plaque: calcified, noncalcified and predominant calcified or predominant noncalcified [1]. Calcified plaques are visualized and quantified by CT scans without injection of contrast agent (calcium scanning). For detecting different types of plaque as well as determining possible coronary stenoses, intravenous contrast agent must be injected prior to the scan (CT-angiography, CTA).

2. Coronary Plaque Morphology and Pathophysiology

On the basis of the CT images, coronary plaques are classified as calcified and noncalcified or as "mixed" plaques containing both aspects. Pathophysiologically, subendothelial lipoprotein retention triggers inflammatory responses via macrophages and T-cells with chronic maladaptive progression of atherosclerotic lesions [2]. Looking at plaques on a cellular basis, early atherosclerotic changes can be classified into 3 types [3] which reflect microscopic changes like accumulation of macrophages (type I) and which are already seen in infant arteries. Later, fatty streaks, foam cells and deposits of lipid inside smooth-muscle cells can be found (type II). These lesions tend to start to develop in puberty. Type III lesions mark the border where these microscopic changes become visible to the eye. Macroscopic changes begin, and the so-called "atheroma" is formed. Advanced lesions can again be classified into 3 types (types IV–VI) [4]. Type IV lesions encompass the lipid core which is called atheroma. As soon as fibrous tissue grows the lesion is classified type V ("fibroatheroma"). If a thrombus or hemorrhage develops on the atheroma or fibroatheroma the lesion is regarded "complicated" (type VI) and, hence, patients can become symptomatic. Lesions IV and V can be asymptomatic due to maintenance of the vessel diameter. Glagov *et al.* first described adaptive changes of arterial size in the course of plaque formation [5]. The entire vessel grows with increasing plaque volume so that the lumen diameter is maintained. Furthermore, a frequent pathology seen in myocardial infarctions due to plaque rupture is the thin cap fibroatheroma (TCFA), which is characterized by a necrotic core covered by a fibrous cap measuring <65 μm [6]. Even though the classifications cannot be directly compared, the TCFA corresponds to a subgroup of the Stary type V lesion. Speckled calcification can be visualized in the majority of ruptured plaques. TCFA seems to be the precursor lesion of plaque rupture. It is frequently associated with expansive remodeling. These changes cannot be detected in invasive angiography because the vessel wall is invisible and only the lumen, which may appear normal, is displayed. Coronary CT-angiography (CCTA) may fill this diagnostic gap, since changes of the vessel wall can directly be visualized.

3. Coronary Calcification

Coronary artery calcification (CAC) is a frequent pathology seen in CT scans (Figure 1). The amount of calcium is quantified using the Agatston-Score [7]. It is correlated with the extent of atherosclerotic plaque burden [8]. In most patients presenting with acute coronary syndromes or sustaining sudden cardiac death, calcifications in the coronary artery wall can be detected [9,10]. A high amount of calcium, however, does not necessarily correlate with angiographic luminal stenoses, nor is there a fixed relationship with vulnerability of plaques [11]. *Vice versa*, a lack of coronary calcium makes stenotic lesions unlikely, but it is not possible to definitely rule out coronary stenoses [12,13].

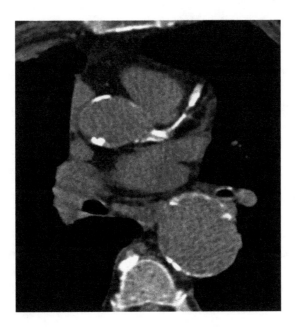

Figure 1. Native calcium scan with severe calcification of left main, left anterior descending (LAD) and the aorta.

There are still debates on the mechanisms of coronary artery calcification. Studies could show that calcification is not a mere passive response to injury but an active process similar to bone formation [14,15]. This process already starts in the second decade of life [16]. Mostly, calcifications are part of atherosclerotic changes, share the same risk factors, and can predominantly be found in advanced lesions [17].

The amount of calcium is influenced by gender, ethnicity and age [18]. Different data exist concerning the possible individual modification of coronary calcium. Lifestyle changes and aggressive medical therapy (especially with "statins") might slow the progress of calcification [19,20]. Interestingly, recent data show that the progression of calcification is mainly driven by genetic conditions and to a minor extent by classical risk factors such as hypertension or LDL cholesterol [21,22]. It is, however, important that although progression of calcification seems to be inevitable this does not hold true for the clinical outcome and adverse cardiac events of patients on lifestyle changes or medication for risk-factor modification.

4. Clinical Implication and Prognosis of Coronary Artery Calcium

Studies have demonstrated that cardiovascular events are low and the overall prognosis is good in the absence of coronary calcifications [23]. Coronary calcium scoring in combination with assessment of the Framingham Score in asymptomatic people can improve risk stratification especially in individuals with risks between 10% and 19% in 10 years according to the Framingham Score [24]. High calcium scores are associated with future cardiovascular events and worse survival outcome. Cardiovascular risk increases proportionally to the amount of calcium and is highest with Agatston-Scores above 400. An annual progression of more than 15% enhances the risk of myocardial infarctions [17,19,25]. Patients after myocardial infarctions have higher CAC progressions than subjects who remained event-free [26]. Positive predictive values of CAC progression as a marker of risk are, however, low [17]. Repeated CAC scans can therefore not be recommended as a control of adequate medical therapies or lifestyle changes. Single calcium scores are recommended in asymptomatic persons with intermediate risk (Framingham risk score 10%–20%) as support for clinical decisions whether to start aggressive medical therapy. In high or low risk populations, CAC scoring does not necessarily add relevant information.

5. Coronary CT Angiography

For calcium scoring, a native CT scan is sufficient. To gain information on coronary stenoses and plaque morphology, contrast media (50–100 mL) must be injected and the scan timed in the phase of maximal contrast enhancement. In contrast to invasive coronary angiography (ICA), CCTA offers the advantage of visualizing the vessel wall. Thus, it is possible to detect atherosclerotic lesions despite a preserved vessel lumen as well as lesions causing a coronary stenosis (Figure 2), even in revascularized patients (Figures 3 and 4).

For clinical purposes, CCTA performs best in individuals who are at low to intermediate risk of coronary artery disease (CAD) [27]. For high-risk individuals, the diagnostic performance of CCTA is lower; patients frequently need ICA afterwards due to suspected high-grade stenoses in CCTA or severe calcifications.

Using the latest CT scanners (at least 2×128 slices), CCTA can be performed with a radiation exposure of <1 mSv. High pitch spiral mode with iterative reconstruction is able to visualize the whole heart in a single diastole with excellent image quality [28–30]. To obtain images with low radiation exposure and little motion artifacts, patients' heart rate should be <60–65/min. Beta blockers are often administered prior to the scan.

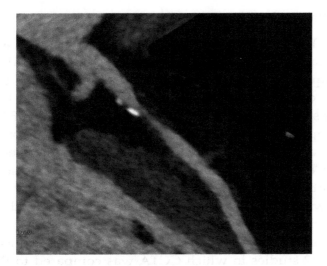

Figure 2. Predominantly noncalcified plaque with high-grade stenosis of LAD.

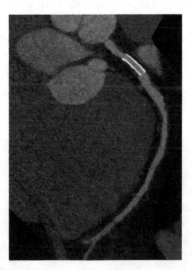

Figure 3. LAD after revascularization with a patent drug eluting stent showing a very good result 18 months after implantation.

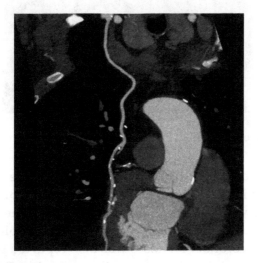

Figure 4. Patent right mammary artery bypass graft (free transplant with end-to-side anastomosis on left mammary artery) with anastomosis on obtuse marginal branch.

6. Imaging of Coronary Plaques and Stenoses

When performing CCTA in patients with intermediate risk for CAD, a substantial portion of the patients show coronary plaques (Figure 5). Hausleiter *et al.* assessed 161 patients of whom almost 30% had noncalcified plaques; most had both noncalcified and calcified plaques. In this group, 6% had plaques without any calcification [31]. Several studies compared the diagnostic accuracy of detecting coronary artery stenoses compared to invasive angiography [32], some additionally with intravascular ultrasonography (IVUS) [33–35]. Sensitivity for detection of plaques range above 90%, negative predictive values approach 100% in patients with low to intermediate probabilities of CAD. CCTA is a reliable method, especially for ruling out relevant plaques and stenoses in coronary arteries (Figure 6). One major limitation is a reduced ability to reliably quantify the degree of stenoses [36] which is the reason for lower positive predictive values and specificity due to the fact that stenoses tend to be overestimated in CCTA especially in calcified lesions. Specificity ranges between 64% and 87%, depending on patient characteristics such as obesity or calcification [32,35,37]. A recent meta-analysis comprised 42 studies in which CCTA was compared to IVUS for detection of any plaques. Sensitivity and specificity were 93% and 92%, respectively [34]. Furthermore, imaging artifacts can lead to misinterpretation. Most of the existing studies were, however, performed using 64-slice CCTA. Technology has remarkably improved in the last decade so that dual-source scanners with 2 × 128 slices and more are the technical standard at present. In a meta-analysis by Voros *et al.*, it could be demonstrated that sensitivity improves from 84% to 94% when images are obtained with 64-slice scanners compared to 16-slice scanners [38]. Still, different attenuation values inside the same plaques (fibrous, lipid-rich, necrotic and calcified) make the classification and reproducibility of lesions challenging.

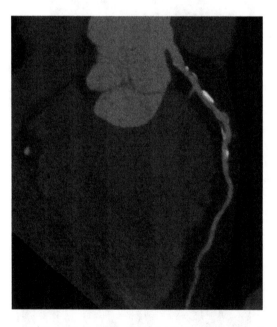

Figure 5. Calcified and noncalcified plaques in LAD.

Cheng *et al.* demonstrated that visual detection of plaque presence is reproducible [39]. Intraobserver, interobserver and interscan variability were excellent, but large differences in agreement existed regarding total plaque volume. The reason is probably the problem of quantifying small coronary plaques by CCTA due to technical limitations in spatial resolution. Moderate reproducibility of plaque burden and degree of coronary stenoses was also reported by Leber *et al.* using 64-slice CT scanners [36,40]. Interobserver variability depends on image quality. Pflederer *et al.* showed that in the left anterior descending coronary artery (LAD), where image quality was best, interobserver variability was significantly lower than in the left circumflex (LCX) or right coronary artery (RCA) (17% in LAD *versus* 32% RCA) [41].

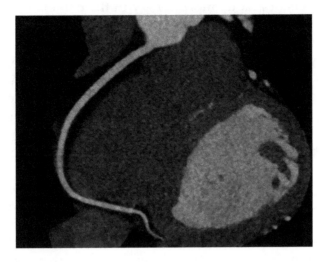

Figure 6. Normal right coronary artery.

A commonly used standardized score for quantification of coronary calcification is the Agatston-Score [7]. A standardized, reproducible tool for quantification of noncalcified plaques does not exist. One important reason for that is the limited spatial resolution of CCTA that makes small plaques difficult to detect. Furthermore, noncalcified plaques can show a wide range of attenuation values due to differences in morphology. An automated quantification using a special software to assess minimal lumen area, plaque burden, percentage luminal stenosis and degree of remodeling was used by Boogers *et al.* in 51 patients [42]. Plaque quantification was feasible and reproducible, and significant correlations could be demonstrated for all parameters. Minimal lumen area was, however, underestimated, and lumen area stenosis overestimated compared to IVUS, especially in calcified lesions.

Furthermore, CCTA is a helpful planning tool for revascularization of chronic total coronary occlusions (CTO). Rolf *et al.* could show that CCTA prior to percutaneous coronary intervention (PCI) could significantly improve success rates of the intervention in 30 patients [43]. Three-dimensional images derived from CCTA guided the advance of the guide wire during the intervention and could thus lead to a success rate of 90% *versus* 63% in the control group without CT. Another study with 100 patients could demonstrate significantly fewer complications, such as coronary perforations, but no improvement in success [44]. Severe coronary calcification seems to be an independent predictor of failure of revascularization of a CTO lesion [45].

7. Qualitative Plaque Characterization

IVUS is considered the gold standard for *in vivo* plaque quantification and characterization [46]. Normal intimal thickness of healthy young subjects measures 0.15 mm [47], below the spatial resolution of CCTA, which is 0.24–0.3 mm for the latest generation of CT scanners. The vessel wall becomes thickened in atherosclerotic lesions which makes it a diagnostic target for non invasive CT evaluation.

Attenuation values inside noncalcified plaques vary according to histological findings. Fibrotic tissue is associated with higher CT density whereas a necrotic core is negatively correlated to density, although with a wide range of overlap [33,48]. Contrast flow rates and concentration inside the vessel as well as microcalcifications often seen around the necrotic core affect density measurements [49,50]. Furthermore, slice thickness and convolution kernels hamper reproducibility of density measurements. Dual-energy CT might enhance the differentiation between the necrotic core and fibrous tissue, however, with a loss of temporal resolution [51].

Atherosclerotic lesions can lead to acute coronary events and death. The morphological characterization of plaques being prone to complications is of eminent interest, and some studies have been reported on aspects of plaque morphology in the context of acute coronary syndromes. Characteristics of ruptured plaques include expansive remodeling, a large necrotic core, thin cap fibroatheroma (TCFA) and macrophage infiltration [52]. Motoyama *et al.* demonstrated that in patients with acute coronary syndromes ACS, CT can identify plaques showing expansive remodeling, low atheroma attenuation values, and spotty calcifications [53]. In another study, 1059 patients underwent CCTA; 45 of these patients showed expansive remodeling and low attenuation plaques [54]. Twenty-two percent of the patients harboring both pathologies developed myocardial infarction in the follow-up period. On the other hand, only four of 820 patients with neither sign had a cardiac event. Hoffmann *et al.* suggested that culprit lesions tend to have greater noncalcified areas, whereas largely calcified plaques indicate more stability [55].

A special pathology in atherosclerotic lesions is the so-called "napkin-ring-sign" which has a high specificity and positive predictive value for advanced lesions [56]; it can be visualized by using CCTA. The napkin-ring-sign is characterized by a plaque core with low attenuation surrounded by a rim-like area of higher attenuation, potentially representing TCFA. Recently, Otsuka *et al.* could demonstrate that the presence of the napkin-ring-sign is strongly associated with acute coronary syndromes [57].

Another interesting approach of detecting vulnerable plaques might be ^{18}F-sodium fluoride and ^{18}F-FDG uptake diagnosed by PET-CT. Dweck *et al.* demonstrated that ^{18}F-NaF uptake was significantly higher in individuals with coronary atherosclerosis (defined by calcium score > 0) in contrast to subjects without (calcium score 0) [58]. Uptake of ^{18}F-NaF seems to be related to inflammation and active calcification with similarities to bone metabolism. Recently, evaluation of patients with myocardial infarction could show that >90% of the patients had increased uptakes in the culprit lesions [59]. In other plaques with increased uptake, high-risk factors such as expansive remodelling, microcalcifications, and a larger necrotic core could be seen on IVUS. It has yet to be demonstrated that increased uptake will translate into future cardiac events.

8. Hemodynamic Relevance of Angiographic Stenoses

Frequently, intermediate stenoses (30%–70%) of coronary arteries are detected on CCTA and it is not evident if these lesions cause ischemia. For intermediate stenoses diagnosed on invasive angiography it is recommended to perform Fractional Flow Reserve (FFR) measurements to assess the functional relevance. De Bruyne *et al.* demonstrated that patients having lesions with FFR of less than 0.8 benefit from revascularization whereas stenoses with FFR of more than 0.8 should be treated conservatively with medical therapy alone [60]. An FFR < 0.8 is thus considered to cause ischemia. Sensitivity for diagnosing high grade stenoses on CCTA is excellent; specificity is, however, poor due to false positive results because of overestimation of stenoses [61]. There was a weak correlation between significant coronary lesions on CCTA and ICA combined with FFR < 0.75; diagnostic accuracy was only 49%. Relying solely on the visual aspect might lead to unnecessary revascularizations and be potentially harmful. Hence, the concept of measuring FFR(CT) noninvasively by CCTA was perceived during the last years. Min *et al.* could show in a multicenter trial that diagnostic accuracy for FFR(CT) was superior to CCTA alone although specificity was still poor [62]. FFR(CT) measurements seem to be reproducible [63], and can be calculated from the normal CCTA dataset without additional image acquisition by using special equations of fluid dynamics [64].

9. CCTA in the Emergency Department

CCTA can be used to rule out relevant CAD in the emergency department for patients presenting with symptoms such as angina without signs of myocardial infarction (ST(segment)-elevation on ECG, positive cardiac enzymes). Frequently, patients presenting with chest pain are admitted to hospital, or stay in the emergency department for many hours. One trial showed a significant reduction of time to diagnosis from 15 h in the control group to 3.4 h in the CCTA group [65]. Both approaches were safe, but CCTA appeared cost effective, and patients who had a CT scan required less subsequent diagnostic workup for recurrent chest pain symptoms.

The ROMICAT-Trial described an excellent sensitivity (100%) of diagnosing CAD in patients presenting with chest pain at low to intermediate pretest probability [66]. Fifty percent of all patients had no CAD at all. Patients were followed-up for two years regarding major adverse cardiac events (MACE) [67]. Patients with no CAD in CCTA had no risk for MACE in the following two years whereas risk was 4.6% in nonobstructive CAD and 30.3% in obstructive CAD. A limitation was that almost 10% of patients were lost to follow-up.

CCTA seems to be a useful diagnostic tool with good safety in the early triage of patients in the emergency department.

10. Prognostic Data of CCTA

As for CAC many studies evaluated the prognostic implication of CCTA in symptomatic patients (Figure 7). Al-Mallah *et al.* followed up 8627 patients with suspected CAD concerning outcomes of death and myocardial infarction [68]. CCTA results added discriminatory power to the Agatston-Score regarding outcomes. This additional value was highest in patients with moderate calcium scores (Agatston 1–100). There is strong evidence supported by many trials that individuals without any signs of CAD in CCTA have an excellent prognosis [69–73]. Rates of MACE approached 0% in the years of follow-up in the studies. CCTA has not only incremental value over Calcium-Scoring but also over routine risk factors of cardiovascular disease [71,74–76].

On the other hand, individuals with signs of CAD on the images can be stratified regarding the risk of cardiovascular events according to different findings. Ahmadi *et al.* examined 3499 symptomatic patients of which 1102 had nonobstructive CAD; these patients were followed-up for 10 years [74]. Among the patients with plaques, event-free survival was best for patients with calcified plaques (98.6%) and decreased in mixed plaques (96.7%) and further decreased in non-calcified plaques (90.4%). Mortality rose proportionally to the amount of diseased vessels (1-, 2- or 3-vessel disease). Hou *et al.* did a follow-up on 5007 patients for myocardial infarction, death or coronary revascularization (MACE) [76]. MACE occurred in 0.8% with no plaque, 3.7% with nonobstructive disease, 27.6% with 1-vessel, 35.5% with 2-vessel and 57.7% with 3-vessel-disease.

No standardized score—such as the Agatston-Score for calcified plaques—exists for quantifying non-calcified plaques. Such a score which comprises the numbers of coronary segments with different morphology and amount of plaque is only used in studies [68,75]. In these, cardiac events are related to higher scores.

To conclude, rates of cardiovascular risk and MACE go hand in hand with the amount of plaque in the coronary arteries. Plaque morphology may play an important role, but it cannot be diagnosed on native calcium scans. A non-negligible number of individuals have non-calcified plaques in the absence of calcium, ranging from 4% to 25% according to selection of study population [68,78]. These patients might benefit most from CCTA for risk stratification over CAC although no data exist to prove that, and therefore CCTA is not recommended for that purpose.

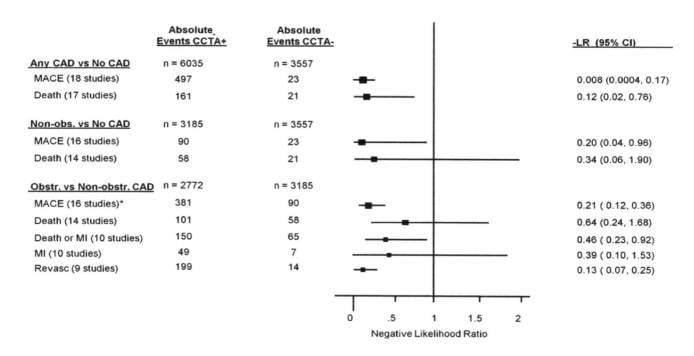

Figure 7. Pooled lifetime risk (LR) for major adverse cardiac events (MACE), death, death or myocardial infarctions (MI), MI and revascularization stratified by Coronary CT Angiography (CCTA) findings. Reproduced from [77] with permission from Hulten, *J. Am. Coll. Cardiol.*; published by Elsevier, 2011.

11. Summary and Future Directions

CCTA is a very reliable diagnostic tool for proving and ruling out obstructive CAD. Still, and in spite of remarkable improvements in image quality due to progress in technology, there are factors such as severe obesity or calcifications that impede diagnostic accuracy. Studies have demonstrated that the type and amount of plaque are related to cardiac events independently of the remaining lumen diameter. Important prognostic implications have been proven especially for calcium scoring. Different types of plaque can be visualized by CCTA, and high-risk lesions being prone to acute coronary syndromes have been described. This ability of CCTA may be able to provide important prognostic information, particularly compared with ICA. However, it remains to be demonstrated whether specific treatment of morphological high-risk plaques on CCTA will translate into fewer future cardiac events and improvements in prognosis.

References

1.   Leipsic, J.; Abbara, S.; Achenbach, S.; Cury, R.; Earls, J.P.; Mancini, G.J.; Nieman, K.; Pontone, G.; Raff, G.L. SCCT guidelines for the interpretation and reporting of coronary CT angiography: A report of the Society of Cardiovascular Computed Tomography Guidelines Committee. *J. Cardiovasc. Comput. Tomogr.* **2014**, *8*, 342–358. [CrossRef] [PubMed]

2.   Tabas, I.; Williams, K.J.; Borén, J. Subendothelial lipoprotein retention as the initiating process in atherosclerosis: Update and therapeutic implications. *Circulation* **2007**, *116*, 1832–1844. [CrossRef] [PubMed]

3.   Stary, H.C.; Chandler, A.B.; Glagov, S.; Guyton, J.R.; Insull, W.; Rosenfeld, M.E.; Schaffer, S.A.; Schwartz, C.J.; Wagner, W.D.; Wissler, R.W. A definition of initial, fatty streak, and intermediate lesions of atherosclerosis: A report from the Committee on Vascular Lesions of the Council on Arteriosclerosis, American Heart Association. *Arterioscler. Thromb. Vasc. Biol.* **1994**, *14*, 840–856. [CrossRef]

4.   Stary, H.C.; Chandler, A.B.; Dinsmore, R.E.; Fuster, V.; Glagov, S.; Insull, W.; Rosenfeld, M.E.; Schwartz, C.J.; Wagner, W.D.; Wissler, R.W. A definition of advanced types of atherosclerotic lesions and a histological classification of atherosclerosis: A report from the Committee on Vascular Lesions of the Council on Arteriosclerosis, American Heart Association. *Circulation* **1995**, *92*, 1355–1374. [CrossRef] [PubMed]

5.   Glagov, S.; Weisenberg, E.; Zarins, C.K.; Stankunavicius, R.; Kolettis, G.J. Compensatory enlargement of human atherosclerotic coronary arteries. *N. Engl. J. Med.* **1987**, *316*, 1371–1375. [CrossRef] [PubMed]

6.   Virmani, R.; Burke, A.P.; Farb, A.; Kolodgie, F.D. Pathology of the vulnerable plaque. *J. Am. Coll. Cardiol.* **2006**, *47*, C13–C18. [CrossRef] [PubMed]

7.   Agatston, A.S.; Janowitz, W.R.; Hildner, F.J.; Zusmer, N.R.; Viamonte, M., Jr.; Detrano, R. Quantification of coronary artery calcium using ultrafast computed tomography. *J. Am. Coll. Cardiol.* **1990**, *15*, 827–832. [CrossRef]

8.   O'Rourke, R.A.; Brundage, B.H.; Froelicher, V.F.; Greenland, P.; Grundy, S.M.; Hachamovitch, R.; Pohost, G.M.; Shaw, L.J.; Weintraub, W.S.; Winters, W.L.; *et al.* American college of cardiology/American heart association expert consensus document on electron-beam computed tomography for the diagnosis and prognosis of coronary artery disease committee members. *J. Am. Coll. Cardiol.* **2000**, *36*, 326–340. [CrossRef] [PubMed]

9.   Pohle, K.; Ropers, D.; Mäffert, R.; Geitner, P.; Moshage, W.; Regenfus, M.; Kusus, M.; Daniel, W.G.; Achenbach, S. Coronary calcifications in young patients with first, unheralded myocardial infarction: A risk factor matched analysis by electron beam tomography. *Heart* **2003**, *89*, 625–628. [CrossRef] [PubMed]

10. Schmermund, A.; Schwartz, R.S.; Adamzik, M.; Sangiorgi, G.; Pfeifer, E.A.; Rumberger, J.A.; Burke, A.P.; Farb, A.; Virmani, R. Coronary atherosclerosis in unheralded sudden coronary death under age 50: Histo-pathologic comparison with "healthy" subjects dying out of hospital. *Atherosclerosis* **2001**, *155*, 499–508. [CrossRef] [PubMed]

11. Davies, M.J. The composition of coronary-artery plaques. *N. Engl. J. Med.* **1997**, *336*, 1312–1314. [CrossRef] [PubMed]

12. Marwan, M.; Ropers, D.; Pflederer, T.; Daniel, W.G.; Achenbach, S. Clinical characteristics of patients with obstructive coronary lesions in the absence of coronary calcification: An evaluation by coronary CT angiography. *Heart* **2009**, *95*, 1056–1060. [CrossRef]

13. Gottlieb, I.; Miller, J.M.; Arbab-Zadeh, A.; Dewey, M.; Clouse, M.E.; Sara, L.; Niinuma, H.; Bush, D.E.; Paul, N.; Vavere, A.L.; *et al.* The absence of coronary calcification does not exclude obstructive coronary artery disease or the need for revascularization in patients referred for conventional coronary angiography. *J. Am. Coll. Cardiol.* **2010**, *55*, 627–634. [CrossRef] [PubMed]

14. Boström, K.; Watson, K.E.; Horn, S.; Wortham, C.; Herman, I.M.; Demer, L.L. Bone morphogenetic protein expression in human atherosclerotic lesions. *J. Clin. Investig.* **1993**, *91*, 1800–1809. [CrossRef] [PubMed]

15. Jeziorska, M.; McCollum, C.; Wooley, D.E. Observations on bone formation and remodelling in advanced atherosclerotic lesions of human carotid arteries. *Virchows Arch.* **1998**, *433*, 559–565. [CrossRef] [PubMed]

16. Stary, H.C. The sequence of cell and matrix changes in atherosclerotic lesions of coronary arteries in the first forty years of life. *Eur. Heart J.* **1990**, *11* (Suppl. E), 3–19. [CrossRef]

17. Greenland, P.; Bonow, R.O.; Brundage, B.H.; Budoff, M.J.; Eisenberg, M.J.; Grundy, S.M.; Lauer, M.S.; Post, W.S.; Raggi, P.; Redberg, R.F.; *et al.* ACCF/AHA 2007 clinical expert consensus document on coronary artery calcium scoring by computed tomography in global cardiovascular risk assessment and in evaluation of patients with chest pain. *J. Am. Coll. Cardiol.* **2007**, *49*, 378–402. [CrossRef] [PubMed]

18. McClelland, R.L.; Chung, H.; Detrano, R.; Post, W.; Kronmal, R.A. Distribution of coronary artery calcium by race, gender, and age: Results from the Multi-Ethnic Study of Atherosclerosis (MESA). *Circulation* **2006**, *113*, 30–37. [CrossRef] [PubMed]

19. Raggi, P.; Cooil, B.; Ratti, C.; Callister, T.Q.; Budoff, M. Progression of coronary artery calcium and occurrence of myocardial infarction in patients with and without diabetes mellitus. *Hypertension* **2005**, *46*, 238–243. [CrossRef] [PubMed]

20. Goh, V.K.; Lau, C.P.; Mohlenkamp, S.; Rumberger, J.A.; Achenbach, S.; Budoff, M.J. Outcome of coronary plaque burden: A 10-year follow-up of aggressive medical management. *Cardiovasc. Ultrasound* **2010**, *8*, 5. [CrossRef] [PubMed]

21. Cassidy-Bushrow, A.E.; Bielak, L.F.; Sheedy, P.F.; Turner, S.T.; Kullo, I.J.; Lin, X.; Peyser, P.A. Coronary artery calcification progression is heritable. *Circulation* **2007**, *116*, 25–31. [CrossRef] [PubMed]

22. Erbel, R.; Lehmann, N.; Churzidse, S.; Rauwolf, M.; Mahabadi, A.A.; Möhlenkamp, S.; Moebus, S.; Bauer, M.; Kälsch, H.; Budde, T.; *et al.* Heinz Nixdorf Recall study investigators progression of coronary artery calcification seems to be inevitable, but predictable—Results of the Heinz Nixdorf Recall (HNR) study. *Eur. Heart J.* **2014**, *35*, 2960–2971. [CrossRef] [PubMed]

23. Sarwar, A.; Shaw, L.J.; Shapiro, M.D.; Blankstein, R.; Hoffmann, U.; Hoffman, U.; Cury, R.C.; Abbara, S.;

Brady, T.J.; Budoff, M.J.; *et al.* Diagnostic and prognostic value of absence of coronary artery calcification. *JACC Cardiovasc. Imaging* **2009**, *2*, 675–688. [CrossRef] [PubMed]

24. Greenland, P.; LaBree, L.; Azen, S.P.; Doherty, T.M.; Detrano, R.C. Coronary artery calcium score combined with Framingham score for risk prediction in asymptomatic individuals. *JAMA* **2004**, *291*, 210–215. [CrossRef] [PubMed]

25. Budoff, M.J.; Hokanson, J.E.; Nasir, K.; Shaw, L.J.; Kinney, G.L.; Chow, D.; Demoss, D.; Nuguri, V.; Nabavi, V.; Ratakonda, R.; *et al.* Progression of coronary artery calcium predicts all-cause mortality. *JACC Cardiovasc. Imaging* **2010**, *3*, 1229–1236. [CrossRef] [PubMed]

26. Raggi, P.; Callister, T.Q.; Shaw, L.J. Progression of coronary artery calcium and risk of first myocardial infarction in patients receiving cholesterol-lowering therapy. *Arterioscler. Thromb. Vasc. Biol.* **2004**, *24*, 1272–1277. [CrossRef] [PubMed]

27. Meijboom, W.B.; van Mieghem, C.A.G.; Mollet, N.R.; Pugliese, F.; Weustink, A.C.; van Pelt, N.; Cademartiri, F.; Nieman, K.; Boersma, E.; de Jaegere, P.; *et al.* 64-Slice computed tomography coronary angiography in patients with high, intermediate, or low pretest probability of significant coronary artery disease. *J. Am. Coll. Cardiol.* **2007**, *50*, 1469–1475. [CrossRef] [PubMed]

28. Achenbach, S.; Goroll, T.; Seltmann, M.; Pflederer, T.; Anders, K.; Ropers, D.; Daniel, W.G.; Uder, M.; Lell, M.; Marwan, M. Detection of coronary artery stenoses by low-dose, prospectively ECG-triggered, high-pitch spiral coronary CT angiography. *JACC Cardiovasc. Imaging* **2011**, *4*, 328–337. [CrossRef] [PubMed]

29. Kröpil, P.; Rojas, C.A.; Ghoshhajra, B.; Lanzman, R.S.; Miese, F.R.; Scherer, A.; Kalra, M.; Abbara, S. Prospectively ECG-triggered high-pitch spiral acquisition for cardiac CT angiography in routine clinical practice: Initial results. *J. Thorac. Imaging* **2012**, *27*, 194–201. [CrossRef] [PubMed]

30. Yin, W.H.; Lu, B.; Hou, Z.H.; Li, N.; Han, L.; Wu, Y.J.; Niu, H.X.; Silverman, J.R.; Nicola De Cecco, C.; Schoepf, U.J. Detection of coronary artery stenosis with sub-milliSievert radiation dose by prospectively ECG-triggered high-pitch spiral CT angiography and iterative reconstruction. *Eur. Radiol.* **2013**, *23*, 2927–2933. [CrossRef] [PubMed]

31. Hausleiter, J.; Meyer, T.; Hadamitzky, M.; Kastrati, A.; Martinoff, S.; Schömig, A. Prevalence of noncalcified coronary plaques by 64-slice computed tomography in patients with an intermediate risk for significant coronary artery disease. *J. Am. Coll. Cardiol.* **2006**, *48*, 312–318. [CrossRef] [PubMed]

32. Budoff, M.J.; Dowe, D.; Jollis, J.G.; Gitter, M.; Sutherland, J.; Halamert, E.; Scherer, M.; Bellinger, R.; Martin, A.; Benton, R.; *et al.* Diagnostic performance of 64-multidetector row coronary computed tomographic angiography for evaluation of coronary artery stenosis in individuals without known coronary artery disease: results from the prospective multicenter ACCURACY (Assessment by Coronary Computed Tomographic Angiography of Individuals Undergoing Invasive Coronary Angiography) trial. *J. Am. Coll. Cardiol.* **2008**, *52*, 1724–1732. [CrossRef] [PubMed]

33. Choi, B.J.; Kang, D.K.; Tahk, S.J.; Choi, S.Y.; Yoon, M.H.; Lim, H.S.; Kang, S.J.; Yang, H.M.; Park, J.S.; Zheng, M.; *et al.* Comparison of 64-slice multidetector computed tomography with spectral analysis of intravascular ultrasound backscatter signals for characterizations of noncalcified coronary arterial plaques. *Am. J. Cardiol.* **2008**, *102*, 988–993. [CrossRef] [PubMed]

34. Fischer, C.; Hulten, E.; Belur, P.; Smith, R.; Voros, S.; Villines, T.C. Coronary CT angiography *versus* intravascular ultrasound for estimation of coronary stenosis and atherosclerotic plaque burden: A meta-analysis. *J. Cardiovasc. Comput. Tomogr.* **2013**, *7*, 256–266. [CrossRef] [PubMed]

35. Meijboom, W.B.; Meijs, M.F.L.; Schuijf, J.D.; Cramer, M.J.; Mollet, N.R.; van Mieghem, C.A.G.; Nieman, K.; van Werkhoven, J.M.; Pundziute, G.; Weustink, A.C.; *et al.* Diagnostic accuracy of 64-slice computed tomography coronary angiography: A prospective, multicenter, multivendor study. *J. Am. Coll. Cardiol.* **2008**, *52*, 2135–2144. [CrossRef] [PubMed]

36. Leber, A.W.; Knez, A.; von Ziegler, F.; Becker, A.; Nikolaou, K.; Paul, S.; Wintersperger, B.; Reiser, M.; Becker, C.R.; Steinbeck, G.; *et al.* Quantification of obstructive and nonobstructive coronary lesions by 64-slice computed tomography: A comparative study with quantitative coronary angiography and intravascular ultrasound. *J. Am. Coll. Cardiol.* **2005**, *46*, 147–154. [CrossRef] [PubMed]

37. Alkadhi, H.; Scheffel, H.; Desbiolles, L.; Gaemperli, O.; Stolzmann, P.; Plass, A.; Goerres, G.W.; Luescher, T.F.; Genoni, M.; Marincek, B.; *et al.* Dual-source computed tomography coronary angiography: Influence of obesity, calcium load, and heart rate on diagnostic accuracy. *Eur. Heart J.* **2008**, *29*, 766–776. [CrossRef] [PubMed]

38. Voros, S.; Rinehart, S.; Qian, Z.; Joshi, P.; Vazquez, G.; Fischer, C.; Belur, P.; Hulten, E.; Villines, T.C. Coronary atherosclerosis imaging by coronary CT angiography: Current status, correlation with intravascular interrogation and meta-analysis. *JACC Cardiovasc. Imaging* **2011**, *4*, 537–548. [CrossRef] [PubMed]

39. Cheng, V.Y.; Nakazato, R.; Dey, D.; Gurudevan, S.; Tabak, J.; Budoff, M.J.; Karlsberg, R.P.; Min, J.; Berman, D.S. Reproducibility of coronary artery plaque volume and composition quantification by 64-detector row coronary computed tomographic angiography: An intraobserver, interobserver, and interscan variability study. *J. Cardiovasc. Comput. Tomogr.* **2009**, *3*, 312–320. [CrossRef] [PubMed]

40. Leber, A.W.; Becker, A.; Knez, A.; von Ziegler, F.; Sirol, M.; Nikolaou, K.; Ohnesorge, B.; Fayad, Z.A.; Becker, C.R.; Reiser, M.; *et al.* Accuracy of 64-slice computed tomography to classify and quantify plaque volumes in the proximal coronary system: A comparative study using intravascular ultrasound. *J. Am. Coll. Cardiol.* **2006**, *47*, 672–677. [CrossRef] [PubMed]

41. Pflederer, T.; Schmid, M.; Ropers, D.; Ropers, U.; Komatsu, S.; Daniel, W. G.; Achenbach, S. Interobserver variability of 64-slice computed tomography for the quantification of non-calcified coronary atherosclerotic plaque. *Rofo* **2007**, *179*, 953–957. [CrossRef] [PubMed]

42. Boogers, M.J.; Broersen, A.; van Velzen, J.E.; de Graaf, F.R.; El-Naggar, H.M.; Kitslaar, P.H.; Dijkstra, J.; Delgado, V.; Boersma, E.; de Roos, A.; *et al.* Automated quantification of coronary plaque with computed tomography: Comparison with intravascular ultrasound using a dedicated registration algorithm for fusion-based quantification. *Eur. Heart J.* **2012**, *33*, 1007–1016. [CrossRef] [PubMed]

43. Rolf, A.; Werner, G.S.; Schuhbäck, A.; Rixe, J.; Möllmann, H.; Nef, H.M.; Gundermann, C.; Liebetrau, C.; Krombach, G.A.; Hamm, C.W.; *et al.* Preprocedural coronary CT angiography significantly improves success rates of PCI for chronic total occlusion. *Int. J. Cardiovasc. Imaging* **2013**, *29*, 1819–1827. [CrossRef] [PubMed]

44. Ueno, K.; Kawamura, A.; Onizuka, T.; Kawakami, T.; Nagatomo, Y.; Hayashida, K.; Yuasa, S.; Maekawa, Y.; Anzai, T.; Jinzaki, M.; *et al.* Effect of preoperative evaluation by multidetector computed tomography in percutaneous coronary interventions of chronic total occlusions. *Int. J. Cardiol.* **2012**, *156*, 76–79. [CrossRef] [PubMed]

45. Soon, K.H.; Cox, N.; Wong, A.; Chaitowitz, I.; Macgregor, L.; Santos, P.T.; Selvanayagam, J.B.; Farouque, H.M.O.; Rametta, S.; Bell, K.W.; *et al.* CT coronary angiography predicts the outcome of percutaneous coronary intervention of chronic total occlusion. *J. Interv. Cardiol.* **2007**, *20*, 359–366. [CrossRef] [PubMed]

46. Mintz, G.S.; Nissen, S.E.; Anderson, W.D.; Bailey, S.R.; Erbel, R.; Fitzgerald, P.J.; Pinto, F.J.; Rosenfield, K.; Siegel, R.J.; Tuzcu, E.M.; *et al.* American college of cardiology clinical expert consensus document on standards for acquisition, measurement and reporting of Intravascular Ultrasound Studies (IVUS): A report of the American college of cardiology task force on clinical expert consensus documents. *J. Am. Coll. Cardiol.* **2001**, *37*, 1478–1492. [CrossRef] [PubMed]

47. Nissen, S.E.; Yock, P. Intravascular ultrasound: Novel pathophysiological insights and current clinical applications. *Circulation* **2001**, *103*, 604–616. [CrossRef] [PubMed]

48. Marwan, M.; Taher, M.A.; El Meniawy, K.; Awadallah, H.; Pflederer, T.; Schuhbäck, A.; Ropers, D.; Daniel, W.G.; Achenbach, S. *In vivo* CT detection of lipid-rich coronary artery atherosclerotic plaques using quantitative histogram analysis: A head to head comparison with IVUS. *Atherosclerosis* **2011**, *215*, 110–115. [CrossRef] [PubMed]

49. Schroeder, S.; Flohr, T.; Kopp, A.F.; Meisner, C.; Kuettner, A.; Herdeg, C.; Baumbach, A.; Ohnesorge, B. Accuracy of density measurements within plaques located in artificial coronary arteries by X-ray multislice CT: Results of a phantom study. *J. Comput. Assist. Tomogr.* **2001**, *25*, 900–906. [CrossRef] [PubMed]

50. Cademartiri, F.; Mollet, N.R.; Runza, G.; Bruining, N.; Hamers, R.; Somers, P.; Knaapen, M.; Verheye, S.; Midiri, M.; Krestin, G.P.; *et al.* Influence of intracoronary attenuation on coronary plaque measurements using multislice computed tomography: Observations in an ex vivo model of coronary computed tomography angiography. *Eur. Radiol.* **2005**, *15*, 1426–1431. [CrossRef] [PubMed]

51. Obaid, D.R.; Calvert, P.A.; Gopalan, D.; Parker, R.A.; West, N.E.J.; Goddard, M.; Rudd, J.H.F.; Bennett, M.R. Dual-energy computed tomography imaging to determine atherosclerotic plaque composition: A prospective study with tissue validation. *J. Cardiovasc. Comput. Tomogr.* **2014**, *8*, 230–237. [CrossRef] [PubMed]

52. Narula, J.; Finn, A.V.; Demaria, A.N. Picking plaques that pop . . . . *J. Am. Coll. Cardiol.* **2005**, *45*, 1970–1973. [CrossRef]

53. Motoyama, S.; Kondo, T.; Sarai, M.; Sugiura, A.; Harigaya, H.; Sato, T.; Inoue, K.; Okumura, M.; Ishii, J.; Anno, H.; *et al.* Multislice computed tomographic characteristics of coronary lesions in acute coronary syndromes. *J. Am. Coll. Cardiol.* **2007**, *50*, 319–326. [CrossRef] [PubMed]

54. Motoyama, S.; Sarai, M.; Harigaya, H.; Anno, H.; Inoue, K.; Hara, T.; Naruse, H.; Ishii, J.; Hishida, H.; Wong, N.D.; *et al.* Computed tomographic angiography characteristics of atherosclerotic plaques subsequently resulting in acute coronary syndrome. *J. Am. Coll. Cardiol.* **2009**, *54*, 49–57. [CrossRef]

55. Hoffmann, U.; Moselewski, F.; Nieman, K.; Jang, I.K.; Ferencik, M.; Rahman, A.M.; Cury, R.C.; Abbara, S.; Joneidi-Jafari, H.; Achenbach, S.; *et al.* Noninvasive assessment of plaque morphology and composition in culprit and stable lesions in acute coronary syndrome and stable lesions in stable angina by multidetector computed tomography. *J. Am. Coll. Cardiol.* **2006**, *47*, 1655–1662. [CrossRef] [PubMed]

56. Maurovich-Horvat, P.; Schlett, C.L.; Alkadhi, H.; Nakano, M.; Otsuka, F.; Stolzmann, P.; Scheffel, H.; Ferencik, M.; Kriegel, M.F.; Seifarth, H.; *et al.* The napkin-ring sign indicates advanced atherosclerotic lesions in coronary CT angiography. *JACC Cardiovasc. Imaging* **2012**, *5*, 1243–1252. [CrossRef] [PubMed]

57. Otsuka, K.; Fukuda, S.; Tanaka, A.; Nakanishi, K.; Taguchi, H.; Yoshikawa, J.; Shimada, K.; Yoshiyama, M. Napkin-ring sign on coronary CT angiography for the prediction of acute coronary syndrome. *JACC Cardiovasc. Imaging* **2013**, *6*, 448–457. [CrossRef] [PubMed]

58. Dweck, M.R.; Chow, M.W.L.; Joshi, N.V.; Williams, M.C.; Jones, C.; Fletcher, A.M.; Richardson, H.; White, A.; McKillop, G.; van Beek, E.J.R.; *et al.* Coronary arterial ^{18}F-sodium fluoride uptake: A novel marker of plaque biology. *J. Am. Coll. Cardiol.* **2012**, *59*, 1539–1548. [CrossRef] [PubMed]

59. Joshi, N.V.; Vesey, A.T.; Williams, M.C.; Shah, A.S.V.; Calvert, P.A.; Craighead, F.H.M.; Yeoh, S.E.; Wallace, W.; Salter, D.; Fletcher, A.M.; *et al.* ^{18}F-fluoride positron emission tomography for identification of ruptured and high-risk coronary atherosclerotic plaques: A prospective clinical trial. *Lancet* **2014**, *383*, 705–713. [CrossRef] [PubMed]

60. De Bruyne, B.; Fearon, W.F.; Pijls, N.H.J.; Barbato, E.; Tonino, P.; Piroth, Z.; Jagic, N.; Mobius-Winckler, S.; Rioufol, G.; Witt, N.; *et al.* Fractional flow reserve-guided PCI for stable coronary artery disease. *N. Engl. J. Med.* **2014**, *371*, 1208–1217. [CrossRef] [PubMed]

61. Meijboom, W.B.; van Mieghem, C.A.G.; van Pelt, N.; Weustink, A.; Pugliese, F.; Mollet, N.R.; Boersma, E.; Regar, E.; van Geuns, R.J.; de Jaegere, P.J.; *et al.* Comprehensive assessment of coronary artery stenoses: Computed tomography coronary angiography *versus* conventional coronary angiography and correlation with fractional flow reserve in patients with stable angina. *J. Am. Coll. Cardiol.* **2008**, *52*, 636–643. [CrossRef] [PubMed]

62. Min, J.K.; Leipsic, J.; Pencina, M.J.; Berman, D.S.; Koo, B.K.; van Mieghem, C.; Erglis, A.; Lin, F.Y.; Dunning, A.M.; Apruzzese, P.; *et al.* Diagnostic accuracy of fractional flow reserve from anatomic CT angiography. *JAMA* **2012**, *308*, 1237–1245. [CrossRef] [PubMed]

63. Gaur, S.; Bezerra, H.G.; Lassen, J.F.; Christiansen, E.H.; Tanaka, K.; Jensen, J.M.; Oldroyd, K.G.; Leipsic, J.; Achenbach, S.; Kaltoft, A.K.; *et al.* Fractional flow reserve derived from coronary CT angiography: Variation of repeated analyses. *J. Cardiovasc. Comput. Tomogr.* **2014**, *8*, 307–314. [CrossRef] [PubMed]

64. Taylor, C.A.; Fonte, T.A.; Min, J.K. Computational fluid dynamics applied to cardiac computed tomography for noninvasive quantification of fractional flow reserve: Scientific basis. *J. Am. Coll. Cardiol.* **2013**, *61*, 2233–2241. [CrossRef] [PubMed]

65. Goldstein, J.A.; Gallagher, M.J.; O'Neill, W.W.; Ross, M.A.; O'Neil, B.J.; Raff, G.L. A randomized controlled trial of multi-slice coronary computed tomography for evaluation of acute chest pain. *J. Am. Coll. Cardiol.* **2007**, *49*, 863–871. [CrossRef] [PubMed]

66. Hoffmann, U.; Bamberg, F.; Chae, C.U.; Nichols, J.H.; Rogers, I.S.; Seneviratne, S.K.; Truong, Q.A.; Cury, R.C.; Abbara, S.; Shapiro, M.D.; *et al.* Coronary computed tomography angiography for early triage of patients with acute chest pain: The ROMICAT (Rule Out Myocardial Infarction using Computer Assisted Tomography) trial. *J. Am. Coll. Cardiol.* **2009**, *53*, 1642–1650. [CrossRef] [PubMed]

67. Schlett, C.L.; Banerji, D.; Siegel, E.; Bamberg, F.; Lehman, S.J.; Ferencik, M.; Brady, T.J.; Nagurney, J.T.; Hoffmann, U.; Truong, Q.A. Prognostic value of CT angiography for major adverse cardiac events in patients with acute chest pain from the emergency department: 2-Year outcomes of the ROMICAT trial. *JACC Cardiovasc. Imaging* **2011**, *4*, 481–491. [CrossRef] [PubMed]

68. Al-Mallah, M.H.; Qureshi, W.; Lin, F.Y.; Achenbach, S.; Berman, D.S.; Budoff, M.J.; Callister, T.Q.; Chang, H.J.; Cademartiri, F.; Chinnaiyan, K.; *et al.* Does coronary CT angiography improve risk stratification over

coronary calcium scoring in symptomatic patients with suspected coronary artery disease? Results from the prospective multicenter international CONFIRM registry. *Eur. Heart J. Cardiovasc. Imaging* **2014**, *15*, 267–274. [CrossRef] [PubMed]

69. Andreini, D.; Pontone, G.; Mushtaq, S.; Bartorelli, A.L.; Bertella, E.; Antonioli, L.; Formenti, A.; Cortinovis, S.; Veglia, F.; Annoni, A.; *et al.* A long-term prognostic value of coronary CT angiography in suspected coronary artery disease. *JACC Cardiovasc. Imaging* **2012**, *5*, 690–701. [CrossRef] [PubMed]

70. Hadamitzky, M.; Täubert, S.; Deseive, S.; Byrne, R.A.; Martinoff, S.; Schömig, A.; Hausleiter, J. Prognostic value of coronary computed tomography angiography during 5 years of follow-up in patients with suspected coronary artery disease. *Eur. Heart J.* **2013**, *34*, 3277–3285. [CrossRef] [PubMed]

71. Hadamitzky, M.; Freissmuth, B.; Meyer, T.; Hein, F.; Kastrati, A.; Martinoff, S.; Schömig, A.; Hausleiter, J. Prognostic value of coronary computed tomographic angiography for prediction of cardiac events in patients with suspected coronary artery disease. *JACC Cardiovasc. Imaging* **2009**, *2*, 404–411. [CrossRef] [PubMed]

72. Min, J.K.; Shaw, L.J.; Devereux, R.B.; Okin, P.M.; Weinsaft, J.W.; Russo, D.J.; Lippolis, N.J.; Berman, D.S.; Callister, T.Q. Prognostic value of multidetector coronary computed tomographic angiography for prediction of all-cause mortality. *J. Am. Coll. Cardiol.* **2007**, *50*, 1161–1170. [CrossRef] [PubMed]

73. Pundziute, G.; Schuijf, J.D.; Jukema, J.W.; Boersma, E.; de Roos, A.; van der Wall, E.E.; Bax, J.J. Prognostic value of multislice computed tomography coronary angiography in patients with known or suspected coronary artery disease. *J. Am. Coll. Cardiol.* **2007**, *49*, 62–70. [CrossRef] [PubMed]

74. Ahmadi, N.; Nabavi, V.; Hajsadeghi, F.; Flores, F.; French, W.J.; Mao, S.S.; Shavelle, D.; Ebrahimi, R.; Budoff, M. Mortality incidence of patients with non-obstructive coronary artery disease diagnosed by computed tomography angiography. *Am. J. Cardiol.* **2011**, *107*, 10–16. [CrossRef] [PubMed]

75. Chow, B.J.W.; Wells, G.A.; Chen, L.; Yam, Y.; Galiwango, P.; Abraham, A.; Sheth, T.; Dennie, C.; Beanlands, R.S.; Ruddy, T.D. Prognostic value of 64-slice cardiac computed tomography severity of coronary artery disease, coronary atherosclerosis, and left ventricular ejection fraction. *J. Am. Coll. Cardiol.* **2010**, *55*, 1017–1028. [CrossRef] [PubMed]

76. Hou, Z.; Lu, B.; Gao, Y.; Jiang, S.; Wang, Y.; Li, W.; Budoff, M.J. Prognostic value of coronary CT angiography and calcium score for major adverse cardiac events in outpatients. *JACC Cardiovasc. Imaging* **2012**, *5*, 990–999. [CrossRef] [PubMed]

77. Hulten, E.A.; Carbonaro, S.; Petrillo, S.P.; Mitchell, J.D.; Villines, T.C. Prognostic value of cardiac computed tomography angiography: A systematic review and meta-analysis. *J. Am. Coll. Cardiol.* **2011**, *57*, 1237–1247. [CrossRef] [PubMed]

78. Choi, E.K.; Choi, S.I.; Rivera, J.J.; Nasir, K.; Chang, S.A.; Chun, E.J.; Kim, H.K.; Choi, D.J.; Blumenthal, R.S.; Chang, H.J. Coronary computed tomography angiography as a screening tool for the detection of occult coronary artery disease in asymptomatic individuals. *J. Am. Coll. Cardiol.* **2008**, *52*, 357–365. [CrossRef] [PubMed]

12

The Clinical Value of High-Intensity Signals on the Coronary Atherosclerotic Plaques: Noncontrast T1-Weighted Magnetic Resonance Imaging

Shoichi Ehara *, Kenji Matsumoto and Kenei Shimada

Department of Cardiovascular Medicine, Osaka City University Graduate School of Medicine, Osaka 545-8585, Japan; matsumoto1110@hotmail.co.jp (K.M.); shimadak@med.osaka-cu.ac.jp (K.S.)
* Correspondence: ehara@med.osaka-cu.ac.jp;

Academic Editor: Michael Henein

Abstract: Over the past several decades, significant progress has been made in the pathohistological assessment of vulnerable plaques and in invasive intravascular imaging techniques. However, the assessment of plaque morphology by invasive modalities is of limited value for the detection of subclinical coronary atherosclerosis and the subsequent prediction or prevention of acute cardiovascular events. Recently, magnetic resonance (MR) imaging technology has reached a sufficient level of spatial resolution, which allowed the plaque visualization of large and static arteries such as the carotids and aorta. However, coronary wall imaging by MR is still challenging due to the small size of coronary arteries, cardiac and respiratory motion, and the low contrast-to-noise ratio between the coronary artery wall and the surrounding structures. Following the introduction of carotid plaque imaging with noncontrast T1-weighted imaging (T1WI), some investigators have reported that coronary artery high-intensity signals on T1WI are associated with vulnerable plaque morphology and an increased risk of future cardiac events. Although there are several limitations and issues that need to be resolved, this novel MR technique for coronary plaque imaging could influence treatment strategies for atherothrombotic disease and may be useful for understanding the pathophysiological mechanisms of atherothrombotic plaque formation.

Keywords: acute coronary syndrome; atherosclerosis; magnetic resonance imaging; plaque; thrombosis; intraplaque hemorrhage

1. Introduction

Acute myocardial infarction or sudden cardiac death frequently occurs as the first symptom of coronary diseases, without prodromal angina [1]. Therefore, the prediction or prevention of acute cardiovascular events has become a crucial clinical issue.

The degree of luminal narrowing is used as a marker for high risk plaques [2], but it is widely recognized that plaque composition is likely to be much more clinically significant than luminal narrowing because the arterial lumen is often preserved by positive arterial remodeling [3]. Therefore, the direct evaluation of the arterial wall is an important goal in cardiovascular imaging. From the 1990s onward, pathohistological studies have demonstrated that plaque rupture or erosion of the endothelial surface with subsequent thrombus formation is the most important mechanisms in acute coronary syndromes (ACSs) [4–6]. A large lipid-pool, thin-cap fibroatheroma (TCFA), macrophage accumulation, and intraplaque hemorrhage have been identified as the key features of rupture-prone plaques [7]. Over the past several decades, significant progress has been made in the assessment of vulnerable plaques using invasive intravascular imaging, such as intravascular ultrasound (IVUS) [8–10], coronary angioscopy [11,12], or optimal coherence tomography (OCT) [13–15]. Those vulnerable features in the coronary artery have been confirmed not only in patients who died from the disease but also in patients who survived an ACS. However, the assessment of plaque morphology by invasive modalities is of limited value for the detection of subclinical coronary atherosclerosis and the subsequent prediction or prevention of acute cardiovascular events.

Hence, there is widespread interest in alternative non-invasive modalities, such as magnetic resonance (MR) imaging or computed tomography (CT), to directly visualize the arterial wall and characterize plaque composition. MR imaging is an attractive option because it is performed with magnetic fields and it is a safe and completely non-invasive technique with excellent soft tissue contrast capable of differentiating the plaque components on the basis of their biophysical and biochemical parameters.

In this review, we focus on the accumulated data on vulnerable plaque imaging using MR techniques, and we also introduce the results from our recent studies.

2. The Beginning of Coronary Artery Plaque Imaging Based on High-Intensity Signal on Noncontrast T1-Weighted Imaging

With any imaging technique, its most important qualities are the spatial resolution required to visualize the lesion components and good contrast between the various components of the lesions. Recently, MR imaging technology has reached a sufficient level of spatial resolution, which allowed the plaque visualization of large and static arteries such as the carotids and aorta [16–20]. The advent of carotid plaque characterization with noncontrast T1-weighted imaging (T1WI) in MR has facilitated plaque imaging based on the presence of a high-intensity signal (HIS) within the thrombus or intraplaque hemorrhage caused by methemoglobin T1 shortening [6–21].

However, coronary wall imaging by MR is still challenging due to the small size of coronary arteries, cardiac and respiratory motion, and the low contrast-to-noise ratio between the coronary artery wall and the surrounding structures. Despite these challenges, coronary wall imaging by MR has been successfully applied in patients using breathhold [22,23] or respiratory gating (i.e., free-breathing) techniques [24–28]. It has been demonstrated that MR can measure coronary vessel area, wall thickness, plaque burden, or arterial remodeling [23]. However, the use of MR to identify plaque components in coronary arteries has been limited.

Some investigators have reported that coronary artery HISs on T1WI are associated with a vulnerable plaque morphology [24–26,28] and an increased risk of future cardiac events [27]. These coronary plaque images have been obtained while the patients were breathing freely, by using a three-dimensional T1WI, inversion-recovery, gradient-echo technique with fat-suppression. Kawasaki et al. proposed the calculation "the ratio between the signal intensities of coronary plaque and cardiac muscle (PMR)", which was defined as the highest signal intensity of the coronary plaque divided by the signal intensity of the left ventricular muscle near the coronary plaque [24]. Areas with a PMR >1.0 were defined as HIS in this report. They reported that the typical coronary HIS on T1WI was associated with a high frequency of IVUS-derived low attenuation and positive remodeling, remarkably low CT density, and transient slow-flow phenomena during percutaneous coronary intervention (PCI) [24]. These features seemed to represent vulnerable plaques. Jansen et al. reported that the HIS on T1WI correctly corresponded to the intracoronary thrombus detected by invasive coronary angiography in patients with acute myocardial infarction within 72 h after the initial onset of symptoms [25]. In our study involving a small number of patients, we demonstrated a direct association between coronary HISs on T1WI and the presence of intracoronary thrombus as detected through OCT (Figure 1) [26].

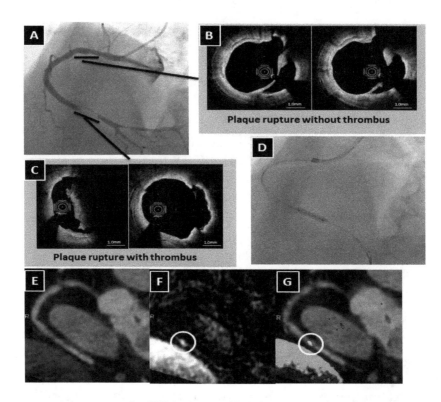

Figure 1. A representative case of a HIS lesion on T1WI associated with an intraluminal thrombus. (**A**) Coronary angiography revealing an intracoronary thrombus identified by the presence of intraluminal filling defects surrounded by contrast agents in the distal right coronary artery (RCA) and an ulceration in the proximal RCA; (**B**) The OCT examination showing a plaque rupture without a thrombus in the proximal RCA; (**C**) In contrast, the culprit lesion in the distal RCA with a plaque rupture with a large intracoronary thrombus; (**D**) Thrombus aspiration and plain old balloon angioplasty (POBA) performed on the culprit lesion; (**E**) Two days later after POBA, whole-heart coronary MR angiography revealing no significant stenosis in the distal RCA; (**F**) Coronary T1WI demonstrating intraluminal HIS on the culprit lesion (circle). However, there is no HIS at the ulceration of the proximal RCA; (**G**) Fused image showing intraluminal HIS in the area corresponding to the culprit lesion (circle). R in panels **E–G** indicates right side.

3. What Appears as High-intensity Signal on T1-Weighted Imaging in the Coronary Artery? What Is the Best PMR Cutoff Value?

There are two highly controversial topics related to HIS in the coronary artery. First, what appears as a HIS on T1WI in the coronary artery? At this stage, the precise characterization of HISs is not known, because no comparisons with histopathological data have been performed in the coronary artery studies; comparative studies have been done on the carotid artery. Therefore, indirect comparisons have been performed by using a surrogate marker mostly derived from other imaging modalities, such as IVUS or OCT. Recently, Teruo Noguchi et al. reported that coronary artery HISs on T1WI were associated with future cardiac events in patients with mildly atherosclerotic lesions that had not yet caused an acute coronary event or induced cardiac ischemia [27]. It seems unlikely that HISs localized within the vessel wall are associated with thrombus in the subclinical population. We investigated the relationship between localization of HISs on T1WI and plaque morphology detected on OCT in patients with either stable or unstable angina [28]. Areas with a PMR $\leqslant$ 1.0 were classified as non-HISs. HISs with a PMR > 1.0 were then classified into two types, according to the localization of HIS, using cross-sectional coronary T1WI. Areas that were localized within the coronary wall when the lumen was identified were defined as intrawall HISs, whereas areas that occupied the lumen when the lumen was not identified were defined as intraluminal HISs. The multivariate analysis revealed that intraluminal HISs were associated with thrombus and intimal vasculature assessed by OCT. In contrast, macrophage accumulation and the absence of calcification were independent factors associated with intrawall HISs (Figure 2). The plaque morphology of the culprit lesions in ACS patients varies from thrombosis with or without plaque rupture to sudden luminal narrowing caused by intraplaque hemorrhage. When previous data are taken together with our findings, one can speculate that coronary intrawall HISs on T1WI may indicate intraplaque hemorrhage associated with inflammation. Some observations have indicated that hemorrhage components appear as signal-poor OCT regions that must be distinguished from lipid necrotic pools. Regrettably, the current imaging techniques, including OCT, do not allow a definitive discrimination between hemorrhage and lipid components, and that is a major issue that will require additional validation studies using histopathological materials from coronary, rather than carotid arteries. In addition, we found that in intrawall HIS lesions the presence of lipid-rich plaques was more frequent than in non-HIS lesions, although these differences were not statistically significant when analyzed by multivariate analysis [28]. Do lipid-rich plaques generate HIS? Although this MR technique uses a fat-suppressed sequence, perivascular fat, which is mainly composed of triglycerides, has a different appearance on MR than the lipids in atherosclerotic plaques. The plaque lipids consist primarily of unesterified cholesterol and cholesterol esters [29]. Therefore, it is not known whether the lipids within the atherosclerotic plaques were successfully suppressed. There is increasing evidence that multiple vulnerable plaques with lipid are present within the whole coronary tree in patients who experience an ACS, even though it may be a single localized culprit lesion that caused the acute cardiovascular event [30]. However, most lipid pools do not generate HISs except at the culprit lesion (Figure 3). The proportion, age, and volume of methemoglobin based on the presence of vulnerable complex plaques may determine the PMR values.

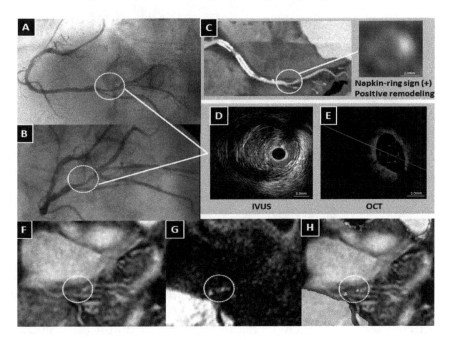

Figure 2. A representative case of an intrawall HIS lesion on T1WI compared with plaque morphology on CT, IVUS and OCT. (**A,B**) Coronary angiography revealing severe coronary stenosis (circle) in the distal right coronary artery (RCA); (**C**) Coronary CT angiography showing the napkin-ring sign and positive arterial remodeling; (**D**) The IVUS image showing a low attenuation plaque; (**E**) The OCT examination showing a signal-poor region with irregular high- or low-backscattering borders without thrombus; (**F**) Whole-heart coronary MR angiography showing significant stenosis in the distal RCA (circle); (**G**) Coronary T1WI demonstrating intrawall HIS (circle); (**H**) Fused image showing intrawall HIS (circle) in the area corresponding to the severe stenosis.

The second controversial topic is the fact that several MR studies used different PMR cutoff values to detect HIS, so there is no consensus on which cutoff is best for risk stratification.

Recently, two studies by Noguchi et al. demonstrated that the optimal PMR cutoff values for predicting future cardiac events and myocardial injury during elective PCI, defined as an increase in serum troponin T levels, were of 1.4 and 1.3, respectively [27,31]. At this stage, it is not known which PMR cutoff value is best or whether there is a need to determine the cutoff values. In our unpublished data, the PMR increased in proportion to the accumulation of the number vulnerable plaque features, such as intraluminal thrombus, lipid-rich plaque, plaque rupture, macrophage accumulation, and intimal vasculature. HISs with a higher PMR are likely to represent more vulnerable plaques. Future studies are needed to clarify the significance of PMR values on T1WI.

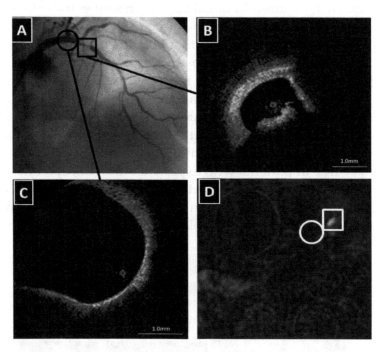

Figure 3. The culprit lesion in the proximal left anterior descending coronary artery (LAD). (**A**) Coronary angiography revealing severe coronary stenosis in the proximal LAD (square) and no significant stenosis in the left main coronary artery (LMCA) (circle); (**B**) The OCT examination showing intracoronary thrombus in the proximal LAD; (**C**) There is a lipid-rich plaque in the LMCA (circle); (**D**) Coronary T1WI demonstrating HIS in the area corresponding to the culprit lesion of the proximal LAD (square). However, no HIS in the LMCA with the lipid-rich plaque is found (circle).

4. The Clinical Implication of High-Intensity Signal in Coronary Atherosclerotic Plaques

What is the clinical implication of detecting HIS on noncontrast T1WI in MR in coronary atherosclerotic plaques? One of the goals of researchers is to investigate whether the presence of HIS on T1WI in subclinical coronary atherosclerosis is associated with the subsequent development of acute cardiovascular events. Noguchi et al. demonstrated that a PMR cutoff value of 1.4 was best for identifying vulnerable coronary plaques associated with future cardiac events, including nonfatal ST-segment elevation myocardial infarction, high-sensitivity cardiac troponin T-positive unstable angina pectoris or non-ST-segment elevation myocardial infarction, and ischemia-driven PCI due to progressive angina pectoris [27]. Moreover, their stratified analysis using PMR values of 1.0 and 1.4 revealed that the incidence of cardiac events was well differentiated: 25.8% for PMR $\geq$ 1.4, 8.4% for PMR 1.0–1.4, and 1.1% for PMR < 1.0. Interestingly, of the segments with plaques with PMRs $\geq$ 1.4, 17% were associated with coronary events, which developed in 51% of the segments in the first 12 months.

Moreover, some studies have demonstrated that the presence of HIS on noncontrast T1WI has the potential to predict a PCI-related myocardial injury, which is associated with worse short-term and long-term clinical outcomes [31–33]. Although the etiology of PCI-related myocardial injury is a multifactorial phenomenon, the predominant mechanism involves the distal embolization of atheromatous or thrombotic materials, and results from the mechanical fragmentation of the culprit plaque during PCI [34]. Asaumi et al. examined the relationship between HISs on T1WI and PCI-related myocardial injury, which is manifested by the elevation of cardiac troponin, in patients undergoing elective PCI [31]. They reported that the optimal PMR cutoff value for predicting PCI-related myocardial injury was 1.3, and the sensitivity and specificity were 67% and 86%, respectively. Hoshi et al. also reported that in patients with stable angina pectoris undergoing elective PCI, the PMR cutoff value of 1.44 predicted PCI-related myocardial injury, and the sensitivity and specificity were 78% and 82%, respectively [32]. In our study, which employed distal protection devices, we investigated predictors of the filter no-reflow (FNR) phenomenon during PCI by using multimodality, such as HIS on T1WI, plaque composition by using OCT, and serum biomarkers, in patients with either stable or unstable angina [33]. Our multivariate analysis revealed that only the presence of HISs with PMR > 1.85 remained an independent predictor of the FNR phenomenon, and the sensitivity and specificity were 65% and 93%, respectively. It is unclear why there are differences in PMR cutoff values for predicting cardiac events. In our study involving patients with unstable angina pectoris, FNR occurred at a high rate (40%) compared with the rate of PCI-related myocardial injury (26%) reported in a previous study [31]. HISs with a higher PMR are likely to represent more vulnerable plaques, and thus the occurrence of FNR might be more closely associated with vulnerable plaque morphology and plaque volume with a higher PMR than that of PCI-related myocardial injury assessed by troponin. The differences in study population or outcomes might be associated to the different PMR cutoff values.

A noninvasive imaging technique capable of identifying not only the presence of a thrombus or hemorrhage but also its stage of development would be invaluable. It has already been established that cerebral hemorrhage staging can be accurately assessed by MR using multicontrast images. Despite the existence of well-defined criteria for staging cerebral hemorrhages, few reports are available regarding the staging of an intraluminal thrombus or intraplaque hemorrhages. Recently, Tan et al. revealed that MR imaging was a precise and reproducible method for distinguishing an acute ipsilateral recurrent deep vein thrombosis from an at least six-month-old chronic residual thrombus in the leg veins, when recurrence was not suspected [35]. Moreover, Chu et al. have shown that multicontrast MR images can detect and classify a carotid intraplaque hemorrhage into three stages: fresh (<1 week), recent (1–6 weeks), and old (>6 weeks) [36]. If HIS on T1WI can be shown to be limited to a fixed term, its presence could be used to accurately identify recent plaque thrombosis or hemorrhage. This information may have several novel clinical implications in the field of PCI, including the prediction or prevention of no-flow phenomena or the aging of a chronic total occlusion. The precise assessment of recent plaque thrombosis or hemorrhage in the coronary occlusion site may influence procedural success rates for chronic total occlusions. Furthermore, although ACS patients with the high-risk should be considered for early invasive intervention, the differential diagnosis and treatment of the remaining patients is challenging in emergency triage. A noninvasive thrombus-detection technique would be useful for further risk stratification and for obtaining prognostic information in patients with coronary artery disease.

Finally, the extent of intraplaque hemorrhage corresponded positively to the size of necrotic core, and the development of hemorrhage resulted in plaque volume expansion and subsequent plaque rupture [37]. If coronary intrawall HISs on T1WI represent intraplaque hemorrhage, early identification of patents with hemorrhage may prove invaluable in optimizing management to minimize future cardiovascular events. Noguchi et al. reported that statin therapy reduced the PMR values, as well as low-density lipoprotein cholesterol and high-sensitivity C-reactive protein levels in patients with coronary artery disease [38]. If statin therapy not only modifies plaque morphology and makes it more stable, but also accelerates the degradation of methemoglobin, that could be invaluable for treatment strategies for atherosclerosis.

5. Limitations and Issues to Be Resolved in the Future

Several limitations should be mentioned in this study field. First, the major issue is that there was no evidence based on pathohistological findings. Therefore, the previous results should be interpreted with caution. Second, when an inversion-recovery gradient-echo sequence is used for the T1WI, issues with spatial resolution and partial volume effect could provide artifacts that look like HIS. This MR technique overcomes many of the difficulties associated with conventional techniques that generate a signal based on flowing blood. With T1WI, signal generation does not rely on flowing blood because it uses a non-slice-selective inversion recovery pulse for the black-blood method. Therefore, the image interpretation requires only the detection of a high signal, beyond the high-resolution display of vessel walls [21]. Although theoretically the T1WI technique is unaffected by blood flow, it is not known whether this supposition applies to actual clinical images. There is a possibility that the HIS might result from a gap in a null point. Future studies are needed to verify whether flow disturbance cause artifact like a HIS. Third, contrast agents such as gadopentic acid (Gd-DTPA), attached to specific imaging probes targeted to biochemical and cellular markers of atherosclerotic plaque vulnerability, may be useful for plaque characterization [39]. Finally, previous coronary plaque imaging studies on MR used only a single-contrast sequence as T1WI [24–28,31–33,38]. The multi-contrast high-resolution protocol is ideal since they generate a wide range of contrast for the individual plaque characterization. However, the acquisition of multi-contrast images is time-consuming, especially in conjunction with the need for high spatial resolution.

6. Conclusions

To determine which plaque features pose a higher risk for future cardiovascular events, we need a noninvasive imaging tool that can identify high-risk plaque features. MR imaging has the potential to identify thrombus and distinguish intraplaque hemorrhage from other plaque components. Because this MR technique has a very short history and no comparisons with histopathological data or multicenter randomized trials have been carried out, many more studies will be needed before this method could be considered to be applied in the clinical arena. Although there are several limitations and issues that need to be resolved, this novel MR technique for coronary plaque imaging could influence treatment strategies for atherothrombotic disease and may be useful for understanding the pathophysiological mechanisms of atherothrombotic plaque formation.

Author Contributions: Shoichi Ehara was the primary author of the text, and conceived the report; Kenji Matsumoto performed patient recruitment, data collection, and analysis including statistics; Kenei Shimada supervised the interpretation of the clinical results.

Abbreviations

The following abbreviations are used in this manuscript:

ACS	acute coronary syndrome
TCFA	thin-cap fibroatheroma
IVUS	intravascular ultrasound
OCT	optical coherence tomography
MR	magnetic resonance
CT	computed tomography
T1WI	T1-weighted imaging
HIS	high-intensity signal
PMR	the ratio between the signal intensities of coronary plaque and cardiac muscle
PCI	percutaneous coronary intervention
FNR	filter no-reflow

References

1. Braunwald, E. Acute myocardial infarction—The value of being prepared. *N. Engl. J. Med.* **1996**, *334*, 51–52. [CrossRef] [PubMed]

2. Stone, G.W.; Maehara, A.; Lansky, A.J.; de Bruyne, B.; Cristea, E.; Mintz, G.S.; Mehran, R.; McPherson, J.; Farhat, N.; Marso, S.P.; et al. A prospective natural-history study of coronary atherosclerosis. *N. Engl. J. Med.* **2011**, *364*, 226–235. [CrossRef] [PubMed]

3. Glagov, S.; Weisenberg, E.; Zarins, C.K.; Stankunavicius, R.; Kolettis, G.J. Compensatory enlargement of human atherosclerotic coronary arteries. *N. Engl. J. Med.* **1987**, *316*, 1371–1375. [CrossRef] [PubMed]

4. Van der Wal, A.C.; Becker, A.E.; van der Loos, C.M.; Das, P.K. Site of intimal rupture or erosion of thrombosed coronary atherosclerotic plaques is characterized by an inflammatory process irrespective of the dominant plaque morphology. *Circulation* **1994**, *89*, 36–44. [CrossRef] [PubMed]

5. Arbustini, E.; dal Bello, B.; Morbini, P.; Burke, A.P.; Bocciarelli, M.; Specchia, G.; Virmani, R. Plaque erosion is a major substrate for coronary thrombosis in acute myocardial infarction. *Heart* **1999**, *82*, 269–272. [CrossRef] [PubMed]

6. Virmani, R.; Kolodgie, F.D.; Burke, A.P.; Farb, A.; Schwartz, S.M. Lessons from sudden coronary death: A comprehensive morphological classification scheme for atherosclerotic lesions. *Arterioscler. Thromb. Vasc. Biol.* **2000**, *20*, 1262–1275. [CrossRef] [PubMed]

7. Finn, A.V.; Nakano, M.; Narula, J.; Kolodgie, F.D.; Virmani, R. Concept of vulnerable/unstable plaque. *Arterioscler. Thromb. Vasc. Biol.* **2010**, *30*, 1282–1292. [CrossRef] [PubMed]

8. Schoenhagen, P.; Ziada, K.M.; Kapadia, S.R.; Crowe, T.D.; Nissen, SE.; Tuzcu, E.M. Extent and direction of arterial remodeling in stable versus unstable coronary syndromes: An intravascular ultrasound study. *Circulation* **2000**, *101*, 598–603. [CrossRef] [PubMed]

9. Ehara, S.; Kobayashi, Y.; Yoshiyama, M.; Shimada, K.; Shimada, Y.; Fukuda, D.; Nakamura, Y.; Yamashita, H.; Yamagishi, H.; Takeuchi, K.; et al. Spotty calcification typifies the culprit plaque in patients with acute myocardial infarction: An intravascular ultrasound study. *Circulation* **2004**, *110*, 3424–3429. [CrossRef] [PubMed]

10. Fujii, K.; Carlier, S.G.; Mintz, G.S.; Takebayashi, H.; Yasuda, T.; Costa, R.A.; Moussa, I.; Dangas, G.; Meran, R.; Lansky, A.J.; et al. Intravascular ultrasound study of patterns of calcium in ruptured coronary plaques. *Am. J. Cardiol.* **2005**, *96*, 352–357. [CrossRef] [PubMed]

11. Okamatsu, K.; Takano, M.; Sakai, S.; Ishibashi, F.; Uemura, R.; Takano, T.; Mizuno, K. Elevated troponin T levels and lesion characteristics in non-ST-elevation acute coronary syndromes. *Circulation* **2004**, *109*, 465–470. [CrossRef] [PubMed]

12. Ohtani, T.; Ueda, Y.; Mizote, I.; Oyabu, J.; Okada, K.; Hirayama, A.; Kodama, K. Number of yellow plaques detected in a coronary artery is associated with future risk of acute coronary syndrome: Detection of vulnerable patients by angioscopy. *J. Am. Coll. Cardiol.* **2006**, *47*, 2194–2200. [CrossRef] [PubMed]

13. Kubo, T.; Imanishi, T.; Takarada, S.; Kuroi, A.; Ueno, S.; Yamano, T.; Tanimoto, T.; Matsuo, Y.; Masho, T.; Kitabata, H.; et al. Assessment of culprit lesion morphology in acute myocardial infarction: Ability of optical coherence tomography compared with intravascular ultrasound and coronary angioscopy. *J. Am. Coll. Cardiol.* **2007**, *50*, 933–939. [CrossRef] [PubMed]

14. Mizukoshi, M.; Imanishi, T.; Tanaka, A.; Kubo, T.; Liu, Y.; Takarada, S.; Kitabata, H.; Tanimoto, T.; Komukai, K.; Ishibashi, K.; et al. Clinical classification and plaque morphology determined by optical coherence tomography in unstable angina pectoris. *Am. J. Cardiol.* **2010**, *106*, 323–328. [CrossRef] [PubMed]

15. Sinclair, H.; Bourantas, C.; Bagnall, A.; Mintz, G.S.; Kunadian, V. OCT for the identification of vulnerable plaque in acute coronary syndrome. *J. Am. Coll. Cardiol.* **2015**, *8*, 198–209. [CrossRef] [PubMed]

16. Hatsukami, T.S.; Ross, R.; Polissar, N.L.; Yuan, C. Visualization of fibrous cap thickness and rupture in human atherosclerotic carotid plaque in vivo with high-resolution magnetic resonance imaging. *Circulation* **2000**, *102*, 959–964. [CrossRef] [PubMed]

17. Yuan, C.; Mitsumori, L.M.; Beach, K.W.; Maravilla, K.R. Carotid atherosclerotic plaque: Noninvasive MR characterization and identification of vulnerable lesions. *Radiology* **2001**, *221*, 285–289. [CrossRef] [PubMed]

18. Cai, J.M.; Hatsukami, T.S.; Ferguson, M.S.; Small, R.; Polissar, N.L.; Yuan, C. Classification of human carotid atherosclerotic lesions with in vivo multicontrast magnetic resonance imaging. *Circulation* **2002**, *106*, 1368–1373. [CrossRef] [PubMed]

19. Moody, A.R.; Murphy, R.E.; Morgan, P.S.; Martel, A.L.; Delay, G.S.; Allder, S.; MacSweeney, S.T.; Tennant, W.G.; Gladman, J.; Lowe, J.; et al. Characterization of complicated carotid plaque with magnetic resonance direct thrombus imaging in patients with cerebral ischemia. *Circulation* **2003**, *107*, 3047–3052. [CrossRef] [PubMed]

20. Murphy, R.E.; Moody, A.R.; Morgan, P.S.; Martel, A.L.; Delay, G.S.; Allder, S.; MacSweeney, S.T.; Tennant, W.G.; Gladman, J.; Lowe, J.; et al. Prevalence of complicated carotid atheroma as detected by magnetic resonance direct thrombus imaging in patients with suspected carotid artery stenosis and previous acute cerebral ischemia. *Circulation* **2003**, *107*, 3053–3058. [CrossRef] [PubMed]

21. Kelly, J.; Hunt, B.J.; Moody, A. Magnetic resonance direct thrombus imaging: A novel technique for imaging venous thromboemboli. *Thromb. Haemost.* **2003**, *89*, 773–782. [PubMed]

22. Fayad, Z.A.; Fuster, V.; Fallon, J.T.; Jayasundera, T.; Worthley, S.G.; Helft, G.; Aguinaldo, J.G.; Badimon, J.J.; Sharma, S.K. Noninvasive in vivo human coronary artery lumen and wall imaging using black-blood magnetic resonance imaging. *Circulation* **2000**, *102*, 506–510. [CrossRef] [PubMed]

23. Terashima, M.; Nguyen, P.K.; Rubin, G.D.; Meyer, C.H.; Shimakawa, A.; Nishimura, D.G.; Ehara, S.; Iribarren, C.; Courtney, B.K.; Go, A.S.; et al. Right coronary wall CMR in the older asymptomatic advance cohort: positive remodeling and associations with type 2 diabetes and coronary calcium. *J. Cardiovasc. Magn. Reson.* **2010**, *12*, 1. [CrossRef] [PubMed]

24. Kawasaki, T.; Koga, S.; Koga, N.; Noguchi, T.; Tanaka, H.; Koga, H.; Serikawa, T.; Orita, Y.; Ikeda, S.; Mito, T.; et al. Characterization of hyperintense plaque with noncontrast T(1)-weighted cardiac magnetic resonance coronary plaque imaging: Comparison with multislice computed tomography and intravascular ultrasound. *J. Am. Coll. Cardiol.* **2009**, *2*, 720–728. [CrossRef] [PubMed]

25. Jansen, C.H.; Perera, D.; Makowski, M.R.; Wiethoff, A.J.; Phinikaridou, A.; Razavi, R.M.; Marber, M.S.; Greil, G.F.; Nagel, E.; Maintz, D.; et al. Detection of intracoronary thrombus by magnetic resonance imaging in patients with acute myocardial infarction. *Circulation* **2011**, *124*, 416–424. [CrossRef] [PubMed]

26. Ehara, S.; Hasegawa, T.; Nakata, S.; Matsumoto, K.; Nishimura, S.; Iguchi, T.; Kataoka, T.; Yoshikawa, J.; Yoshiyama, M. Hyperintense plaque identified by magnetic resonance imaging relates to intracoronary thrombus as detected by optical coherence tomography in patients with angina pectoris. *Eur. Heart J.* **2012**, *13*, 394–399. [CrossRef] [PubMed]

27. Noguchi, T.; Kawasaki, T.; Tanaka, A.; Yasuda, S.; Goto, Y.; Ishihara, M.; Nishimura, K.; Miyamoto, Y.; Node, K.; Koga, N. High-intensity signals in coronary plaques on non-contrast T1-weighted magnetic resonance imaging as a novel determinant of coronary events. *J. Am. Coll. Cardiol.* **2014**, *63*, 989–999. [CrossRef] [PubMed]

28. Matsumoto, K.; Ehara, S.; Hasegawa, T.; Sakaguchi, M.; Otsuka, K.; Yoshikawa, J.; Shimada, K. Localization of coronary high-intensity signals on T1-weighted MR imaging: Relation to plaque morphology and clinical severity of angina pectoris. *J. Am. Coll. Cardiol.* **2015**, *8*, 1143–1152. [CrossRef] [PubMed]

29. Quick, H.H.; Debatin, J.F.; Ladd, M.E. MR imaging of the vessel wall. *Eur. Radiol.* **2002**, *12*, 889–900. [CrossRef] [PubMed]

30. Kubo, T.; Imanishi, T.; Kashiwagi, M.; Ikejima, H.; Tsujioka, H.; Kuroi, A.; Ishibashi, K.; Komukai, K.; Tanimoto, T.; Ino, Y.; et al. Multiple coronary lesion instability in patients with acute myocardial infarction as determined by optical coherence tomography. *Am. J. Cardiol.* **2010**, *105*, 318–322. [CrossRef] [PubMed]

31. Asaumi, Y.; Noguchi, T.; Morita, Y.; Fujiwara, R.; Kanaya, T.; Matsuyama, TA.; Kawasaki, T.; Fujino, M.; Yamane, T.; Nagai, T.; et al. High-intensity plaques on noncontrast T1-weighted imaging as a predictor of periprocedural myocardial injury. *J. Am. Coll. Cardiol.* **2015**, *8*, 741–743. [CrossRef] [PubMed]

32. Hoshi, T.; Sato, A.; Akiyama, D.; Hiraya, D.; Sakai, S.; Shindo, M.; Mori, K.; Minami, M.; Aonuma, K. Coronary high-intensity plaque on T1-weighted magnetic resonance imaging and its association with myocardial injury after percutaneous coronary intervention. *Eur. Heart J.* **2015**, *36*, 1913–1922. [CrossRef] [PubMed]

33. Matsumoto, K.; Ehara, S.; Hasegawa, T.; Otsuka, K.; Yoshikawa, J.; Shimada, K. Prediction of the filter no-reflow phenomenon in patients with angina pectoris by using multimodality: Magnetic resonance imaging, optical coherence tomography, and serum biomarkers. *J. Cardiol.* **2016**, *67*, 430–436. [CrossRef] [PubMed]

34. Kaul, S. The "no reflow" phenomenon following acute myocardial infarction: Mechanisms and treatment options. *J. Cardiol.* **2014**, *64*, 77–85. [CrossRef] [PubMed]

35. Tan, M.; Mol, G.C.; van Rooden, C.J.; Klok, F.A.; Westerbeek, R.E.; del Sol, A.I.; van de Ree, M.A.; de Roos, A.; Huisman, M.V. Magnetic resonance direct thrombus imaging differentiates acute recurrent ipsilateral deep vein thrombosis from residual thrombosis. *Blood* **2014**, *124*, 623–627. [CrossRef] [PubMed]

36. Chu, B.; Kampschulte, A.; Ferguson, M.S.; Kerwin, W.S.; Yarnykh, V.L.; O'Brien, K.D.; Polissar, N.L.; Hatsukami, T.S.; Yuan, C. Hemorrhage in the atherosclerotic carotid plaque: A high-resolution MRI study. *Stroke* **2004**, *35*, 1079–1084. [CrossRef] [PubMed]

37. Sun, J.; Underhill, H.R.; Hippe, D.S.; Xue, Y.; Yuan, C.; Hatsukami, T.S. Sustained acceleration in carotid atherosclerotic plaque progression with intraplaque hemorrhage: A long-term time course study. *J. Am. Coll. Cardiol.* **2012**, *5*, 798–804. [CrossRef] [PubMed]

38. Noguchi, T.; Tanaka, A.; Kawasaki, T.; Goto, Y.; Morita, Y.; Asaumi, Y.; Nakao, K.; Fujiwara, R.; Nishimura, K.; Miyamoto, Y.; et al. Effect of intensive statin therapy on coronary high-intensity plaques detected by noncontrast T1-weighted imaging. *J. Am. Coll. Cardiol.* **2015**, *66*, 245–256. [CrossRef] [PubMed]

39. Briley-Saebo, K.C.; Shaw, P.X.; Mulder, W.J.; Choi, S.H.; Vucic, E.; Aguinaldo, J.G.; Witztum, J.L.; Fuster, V.; Tsimikas, S.; Fayad, Z.A. Targeted molecular probes for imaging atherosclerotic lesions with magnetic resonance using antibodies that recognize oxidation-specific epitopes. *Circulation* **2008**, *117*, 3206–3215. [CrossRef] [PubMed]

13

Ultrasound Assessment of Carotid Plaque Echogenicity Response to Statin Therapy

Pranvera Ibrahimi, Fisnik Jashari *, Gani Bajraktari, Per Wester and Michael Y. Henein

Department of Public Health and Clinical Medicine, Umeå University, Umeå 901 87, Sweden;
pranvera.ibrahimi@medicin.umu.se (P.I.); ganibajraktari@yahoo.co.uk (G.B.); per.wester@medicin.umu.se (P.W.);
michael.henein@medicin.umu.se (M.Y.H.)
* Correspondence: fisnik.jashari@medicin.umu.se;

Academic Editor: William Chi-shing Cho

Abstract: Objective: To evaluate in a systematic review and meta-analysis model the effect of statin therapy on carotid plaque echogenicity assessed by ultrasound. Methods: We have systematically searched electronic databases (PubMed, MEDLINE, EMBASE and Cochrane Center Register) up to April, 2015, for studies evaluating the effect of statins on plaque echogenicity. Two researchers independently determined the eligibility of studies evaluating the effect of statin therapy on carotid plaque echogenicity that used ultrasound and grey scale median (GSM) or integrated back scatter (IBS). Results: Nine out of 580 identified studies including 566 patients' carotid artery data were meta-analyzed for a mean follow up of 7.2 months. A consistent increase in the echogenicity of carotid artery plaques, after statin therapy, was reported. Pooled weighted mean difference % (WMD) on plaque echogenicity after statin therapy was 29% (95% CI 22%–36%), $p < 0.001$, $I^2 = 92.1\%$. In a meta-regression analysis using % mean changes of LDL, HDL and hsCRP as moderators, it was shown that the effects of statins on plaque echogenicity were related to changes in hsCRP, but not to LDL and HDL changes from the baseline. The effect of statins on the plaque was progressive; it showed significance after the first month of treatment, and the echogenicity continued to increase in the following six and 12 months. Conclusions: Statin therapy is associated with a favorable increase of carotid plaque echogenicity. This effect seems to be dependent on the period of treatment and hsCRP change from the baseline, independent of changes in LDL and HDL.

Keywords: carotid atherosclerosis; plaque echogenicity; ultrasound; statins

1. Introduction

Carotid atherosclerosis is an important cause of ischemic stroke, the risk of which is mainly related to the degree of stenosis [1]. Adding the evaluation of carotid plaque echogenicity features, on the other hand, it was found to better risk stratify patients beyond the degree of stenosis. Treatment of carotid atherosclerosis with statins has proven effective in reducing such stroke risk, universally considered to be caused by vulnerable plaques [2].

Many imaging techniques are currently used to identify vulnerable plaque features. The most feasible one with less radiation remains carotid ultrasound, which can accurately identify the presence of the plaque and determine its echogenicity, as well as the degree of stenosis. Vulnerable plaques are known for their high lipid and hemorrhage content, in contrast to stable plaques, which are predominately rich in fibrous tissue and calcification [3,4]. Furthermore, such detailed plaque composition has been found to correlate with the textural features (echogenicity) obtained by ultrasound imaging. This can easily be assessed using off-line plaque image analysis techniques, such as grey scale median (GSM) and integrated backscatter (IBS), with plaques rich in lipid and hemorrhagic content appearing echolucent (low GSM or IBS) and those with fibrous or calcific content appearing echogenic (high GSM or IBS) [5,6].

The effect of statins treatment on plaque regression and change in its features is well documented in the literature, but a consensus analysis is lacking. Such an effect has been reported using various imaging modalities, other than US [7], not only in carotid disease, but also in coronary and aortic disease [8]. The aim of this study was to determine, in a systematic and meta-analysis model, the response of plaque features' "echogenicity" to statin therapy in patients with carotid artery disease.

2. Results

2.1. Study Selection

We identified 576 studies in total after systematic searching in PubMed (Figure 1). No additional studies were found in MEDLINE, EMBASE or in the Cochrane Center Register. After reading the titles and abstracts of the papers, we first depicted 12 studies that evaluated the effects of statins on plaque echogenicity. Of these studies, three were excluded, two measured the effect of statins on the carotid artery wall (intima-media) echogenicity [9,10] and one was a case report [11]. The remaining nine studies [12–20] were included in the final qualitative analysis (Figure 1, Tables 1 and 2). Out of the nine studies, two studies analyzed two groups of patients separately, and we have included both groups in the meta-analysis. In addition, we have used meta-regression and subgroup analysis to determine the effect of % changes in LDL, HDL, hsCRP, the period of treatment and baseline patients' characteristics on echogenicity change. Statins effect on LDL, HDL and hsCRP were also evaluated (Supplementary Material).

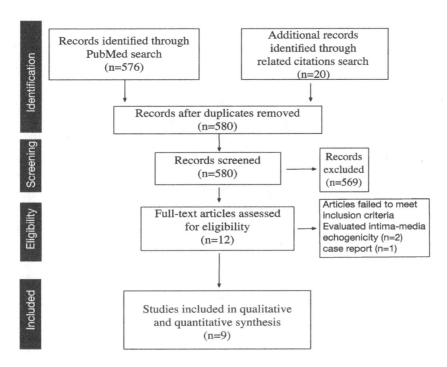

Figure 1. Study selection.

2.2. Qualitative Assessment and Study Characteristics

2.2.1. Effect of Statins on Plaque Features

All nine studies included were prospective; five were prospective open-label, and four of them were randomized controlled trials [8–11]. Atorvastatin was the most commonly used [13,15,17,18], followed by simvastatin [13], pravastatin and pitavastatin [12,14] and rosuvastatin [20]. In three studies, the statin dosage was fixed [14,16,19], and in the remaining six, it was ranged [12,13,15,17,18,20]. The mean follow up of patients was 7.2 months (1–12). Studies included in this review used different methods to quantify plaque echogenicity. The grey scale median (GSM) was used in five studies to evaluate plaque echogenicity, and integrated backscatter (IBS) analysis was used in the remaining four. In one study, patients were divided into two groups based on the statin dose (intensive *vs.* moderate) [18] and, in the other one, based on treatment strategy (statins + carotid artery stenting (CAS) *vs.* statin alone) [17]. In seven studies [12–14,16–18,20], controls were commenced on a set diet, and in one study [15], patients on statins were compared with those on placebo. The diet type applied in the controls was mentioned in two studies [12,19], which used the Adult Treatment Panel-III lipid-lowering diet. There was only one study that used more than one type of statin in the treated group [13].

In all nine studies presented in this meta-analysis, there was a significant increase of plaque echogenicity after statin therapy. In the compared high (atorvastatin 80 mg/d) and low (atorvastatin 20 mg/d) statin therapy, the GSM was significantly increased more in the group receiving aggressive statin therapy.

In six studies, other ultrasound-derived measurements were evaluated, including: intima-media thickness [12,16,20], plaque thickness [13,19], plaque volume [16] and degree of stenosis [12]. Except for one study that found a decrease in plaque thickness after statin therapy [13], there was no other change, of the above-mentioned measures, observed after statin therapy.

2.2.2. Effect of Statins on Blood Lipids and Inflammatory Markers

All studies measured LDL and HDL cholesterol levels, and in all, there was a significant decrease in LDL with statin therapy; in only two [12,14] did the HDL cholesterol significantly increase. However, only one study has evaluated the change of plaque echogenicity after adjusting for LDL cholesterol and its changes from baseline, which concluded that statins' effect on plaque echogenicity was independent of the fall in LDL cholesterol [19].

The included studies used different blood-derived markers of atherosclerosis, such as: high sensitivity CRP (hsCRP) [12–18,20], vasogenic endothelial growth factor (VEGF) [14], interleukins (IL) IL-6 and IL-18 [13], osteopontin (OPN) [15,17,18], osteoprotegerin (OPG) [15,17,18] and tumor necrosis factor-alpha (TNF-α) [14]. Except for IL-6, which was not affected [13], the other markers, hsCRP, VEGF, IL-18, OPN, OPG and TNF-α, were significantly decreased in patients treated with statins compared to controls. Even at only one month after statin therapy, the levels of hsCRP, VEGF and TNF-α decreased significantly [14]. In the study that compared aggressive (atorvastatin 80 mg/d) and modest (atorvastatin 10 mg/d) statin therapy, OPN and OPG levels were lower in patients receiving aggressive statin therapy; however, hsCRP was not different between groups [18].

Table 1. Studies included in meta-analysis.

Author/Year	Population (*n*)	Mean Age ± SD	Gender (Male)	Hypercholesterolemic	Carotid Stenosis	Echogenicity Measured	Minor Score
1. Watanabe et al., 2005 [12]	30	69.9 ± 8.8	63%	No	Moderate	IBS	RT
2. Yamagami et al., 2008 [13]	41	63.4 ± 8.3	24%	Yes	Moderate	IBS	RT
3. Nakamura et al., 2008 [14]	33	60 ± 9	25%	Yes	Moderate	IBS	RT
4. Kadoglou et al., 2008 [15]	113	63.6 ± 9.9	67%	Yes	Moderate symptomatic	GSM	20
5. Yamada et al., 2009 [16]	40	71 ± 8	90%	No	30%–60%	IBS	RT
6. Kadoglou et al., 2009 [17]	67 + 46	66.7 ± 7.3	40%	No	>40%	GSM	20
7. Kadoglou et al., 2010 [18]	66 + 65	64.9 ± 10	46%	Yes	30%–60%	GSM	24
8. Della-Morte et al., 2011 [19]	40	>45	NA	Yes	NA	GSM	15
9. Nohara et al., 2013 [20]	25	63.9 ± 8.1	50%	Yes	NA	GSM	20

GSM, grey scale median; IBS, integrated back scatter; RT, randomized trial; SD, standard deviation.

Table 2. Studies characteristics and statins effect on plaque echogenicity and LDL, HDL and hsCRP level on the blood.

Author/Year	Study Design	Statin/Dose	Follow-up (Months)	% Change Echogenicity	% Change LDL	% Change HDL	% Change hsCRP
1. Watanabe et al., 2005 [12]	Randomized case-control trial	Pravastatin	6	14.1 ± 3.3	24.5 ± 6.4	10.2 ± 6.0	45.0 ± 58.3
3. Yamagami et al., 2008 [13]	Randomized case-control trial	Simvastatin 10 mg	1	10.6 ± 4.3	34.2 ± 18.4	0	43.0 ± 119.8
2. Nakamura et al., 2008 [14]	Randomized case-control trial	Pitavastatin 4 mg	12	32.1 ± 5.9	37.8 ± 12.4	9.3 ± 2.0	43.7 ± 51.5
4. Kadoglou et al., 2008 [15]	Open-label prospective trial	Atorvastatin	6	36.0 ± 15.2	41.7 ± 19.9	4.5 ± 2.4	58.9 ± 34.0
5. Yamada et al., 2009 [16]	Randomized case-control trial	Simvastatin	6	17.0 ± 5.9	44.0 ± 23.9	0	42.1 ± 94.6
6a. Kadoglou et al., 2009 [17]	Open-label prospective trial	Atorvastatin	6	36.8 ± 9.8	38.6 ± 20.0	13.4 ± 6.6	78.3 ± 74.9
6b. Kadoglou et al., 2009 [17]	Open-label prospective trial	Atorvastatin + CAS	6	48.4 ± 18.6	33.3 ± 15.0	4.4 ± 2.2	52.1 ± 39.5
7a. Kadoglou et al., 2010 [18]	Randomized case-control trial	Atorvastatin 10–20 mg	12	32.6 ± 11.7	64.5 ± 23.6	5.5 ± 2.6	52.9 ± 55.2
7b. Kadoglou et al., 2010 [18]	Randomized case-control trial	Atorvastatin 80 mg	12	51.4 ± 18.4	54.2 ± 37.2	10.3 ± 6.0	65.0 ± 80.0
8. Della-Morte et al., 2011 [19]	Prospective pilot study	NA	1	21.9 ± 4.8	51.4 ± 31.0	2.0 ± 1.1	NA
9. Nohara et al., 2013 [20]	Prospective open label, blinded-endpoint	Rosuvastatin	12	16.9 ± 33.1	50.1 ± 22.9	8.1 ± 3.6	NA

CAS, carotid artery stenting.

2.3. Meta-Analysis Results

All nine studies met the inclusion criteria to be included in the meta-analysis. Two of the studies have divided patients into two groups. The first one [18] had two groups on different statin dosage (atorvastatin 10 vs. 80 mg), and the other study [17] had two groups on statin therapy; one of them underwent CAS in addition. In total, 566 patients' carotid artery data were meta-analyzed for a mean follow up of 7.2 months. A consistent increase in the echogenicity of carotid artery plaques, after statin therapy, was found. Pooled weighted mean difference % (WMD) on plaque echogenicity after statin therapy was 29% (95% CI: 22%–36%), $p < 0.001$, $I^2 = 92.1\%$ (Figure 2). In these studies, evaluating the effect of statins on plaque echogenicity was the main objective; in addition, their effect on LDL, HDL and hsCRP level was also evaluated. LDL was significantly decreased after statins therapy; the pooled weighted mean difference % (WMD) was −40.8% (95% CI, −48.9%––32.8%), $p < 0.001$, $I^2 = 81.2\%$ (Supplemental Figure S1). Furthermore, HDL and hsCRP were increased and decreased after statin therapy, respectively (Supplemental Figures S2 and S3).

In a meta-regression analysis, mean changes % of LDL, HDL and hsCRP from baseline were used as moderators to evaluate their association with changes in plaque echogenicity. The increase in plaque echogenicity with statins therapy was independent of LDL ($\beta = 0.32$ (−0.28–0.94), $p < 0.29$) (Figure 3a) and HDL cholesterol ($\beta = 0.91$ (−0.01–3.55), $p = 0.051$) (Figure 3b), but it was related to hsCRP changes from the baseline ($\beta = 1.01$ (0.49–1.52), $p < 0.001$) (Figure 3c).

Patients were divided into subgroups and analyzed based on treatment period. Although the increase of plaque echogenicity was significant even after the first month of treatment, this increase was more evident in the following six and 12 months (Figure 4). Mean difference % was 16.2% (5.2%–27.2%) vs. 30.4% (18.2%–42.3%) vs. 35.4% (26.3%–44.4%), $p = 0.03$, between 1, 6 and 12 months of treatment, respectively. In addition, we have analyzed separately studies based on baseline cholesterolemia status (hypercholesterolemic vs. non-hypercholesterolemic), and it seems that the effects of statins on carotid plaque echogenicity is independent of cholesterol levels at baseline, since it was similarly increased in both groups (Figure 5).

Study name	%Difference in means	Standard error	Variance	Lower limit	Upper limit	Z-Value	p-Value	%Difference in means and 95% CI
Watanabe 2005	14.10	0.85	0.73	12.43	15.77	16.55	0.00	
Yamagami 2008	10.63	0.97	0.95	8.72	12.54	10.93	0.00	
Nakamura 2008	32.10	1.47	2.15	29.22	34.98	21.88	0.00	
Kadaglou 2008	36.00	2.18	4.76	31.72	40.28	16.49	0.00	
Yamada 2009	17.00	1.87	3.48	13.34	20.66	9.11	0.00	
Kadaglou 2009*	48.44	3.89	15.12	40.82	56.06	12.46	0.00	
Kadaglou 2009**	36.80	1.70	2.90	33.46	40.14	21.60	0.00	
Kadaglou 2010^	32.60	1.98	3.92	28.72	36.48	16.47	0.00	
Kadaglou 2010^^	51.40	3.13	9.77	45.27	57.53	16.45	0.00	
Della-Morte 2011	21.90	1.08	1.18	19.77	24.03	20.19	0.00	
Nohara 2013	16.93	9.37	87.75	-1.43	35.29	1.81	0.07	
	29.02	3.56	12.68	22.04	36.00	8.15	0.00	

-57.60 -28.80 0.00 28.80 57.60

Echogenicity decreased   Echogenicity increased

Figure 2. Effects of statin on plaque echogenicity. Note: Kadaglou 2009 [17] has divided and analyzed patients in two groups: the first group (*) was on statin, but underwent contralateral carotid artery stenting (CAS), and the second group (**) was treated only with statins. Kadaglou 2010 [18] has divided and analyzed patients into two groups: the first group (^) received atorvastatin 10–20 mg, and the second group (^^) atorvastatin 80 mg.

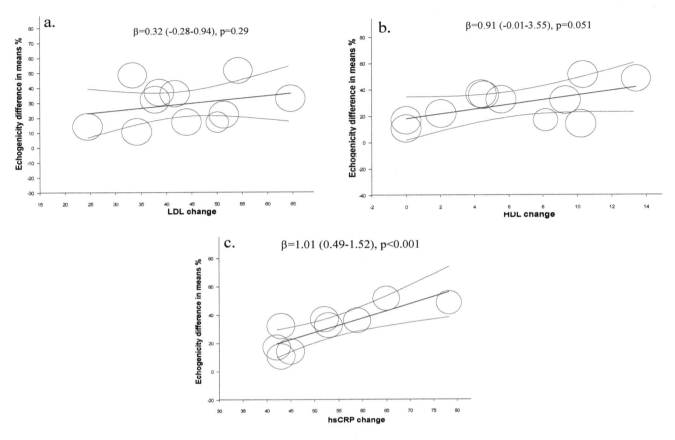

Figure 3. Meta-regression. Regression of LDL (**a**), HDL (**b**) and hsCRP (**c**) changes on plaque echogenicity after statin therapy.

Study name	Treatment period	% Difference in means	Standard error	Variance	Lower limit	Upper limit	Z-Value	p-Value	% Difference in means and 95% CI
Yamagami 2008	1 m	10.6	1.0	0.9	8.7	12.5	10.9	0.0	
Della-Morte 2011	1 m	21.9	1.1	1.2	19.8	24.0	20.2	0.0	
		16.3	5.6	31.8	5.2	27.3	2.9	0.0	
Watanabe 2005	6 m	14.1	0.9	0.7	12.4	15.8	16.5	0.0	
Kadaglou 2008	6 m	36.0	2.2	4.8	31.7	40.3	16.5	0.0	
Yamada 2009	6 m	17.0	1.9	3.5	13.3	20.7	9.1	0.0	
Kadaglou 2009*	6 m	48.4	3.9	15.1	40.8	56.1	12.5	0.0	
Kadaglou 2009**	6 m	36.8	1.7	2.9	33.5	40.1	21.6	0.0	
		30.2	6.2	38.1	18.1	42.3	4.9	0.0	
Nakamura 2008	12 m	32.1	1.5	2.2	29.2	35.0	21.9	0.0	
Kadaglou 2010^	12 m	32.6	2.0	3.9	28.7	36.5	16.5	0.0	
Kadaglou 2010^^	12 m	51.4	3.1	9.8	45.3	57.5	16.4	0.0	
Nohara 2013	12 m	16.9	9.4	87.8	-1.4	35.3	1.8	0.1	
		35.4	4.6	21.3	26.4	44.5	7.7	0.0	
		28.3	3.1	9.6	22.3	34.4	9.2	0.0	

-57.60　-28.80　0.00　28.80　57.60
Echogenicity decreased　　Echogenicity increased

Figure 4. Analysis of studies based on treatment period in months. The effect of statins on plaque echogenicity was obvious from the first month after treatment, and the effect was progressive on the following six and 12 months (m). (*) was on statin, but underwent contralateral carotid artery stenting (CAS), and (**) was treated only with statins. (^) received atorvastatin 10–20 mg, and (^^) atorvastatin 80 mg.

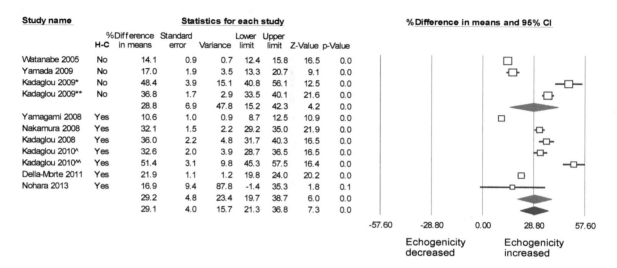

Study name		Statistics for each study								%Difference in means and 95% CI
	H–C	%Difference in means	Standard error	Variance	Lower limit	Upper limit	Z-Value	p-Value		
Watanabe 2005	No	14.1	0.9	0.7	12.4	15.8	16.5	0.0		
Yamada 2009	No	17.0	1.9	3.5	13.3	20.7	9.1	0.0		
Kadaglou 2009*	No	48.4	3.9	15.1	40.8	56.1	12.5	0.0		
Kadaglou 2009**	No	36.8	1.7	2.9	33.5	40.1	21.6	0.0		
		28.8	6.9	47.8	15.2	42.3	4.2	0.0		
Yamagami 2008	Yes	10.6	1.0	0.9	8.7	12.5	10.9	0.0		
Nakamura 2008	Yes	32.1	1.5	2.2	29.2	35.0	21.9	0.0		
Kadaglou 2008	Yes	36.0	2.2	4.8	31.7	40.3	16.5	0.0		
Kadaglou 2010^	Yes	32.6	2.0	3.9	28.7	36.5	16.5	0.0		
Kadaglou 2010^^	Yes	51.4	3.1	9.8	45.3	57.5	16.4	0.0		
Della-Morte 2011	Yes	21.9	1.1	1.2	19.8	24.0	20.2	0.0		
Nohara 2013	Yes	16.9	9.4	87.8	-1.4	35.3	1.8	0.1		
		29.2	4.8	23.4	19.7	38.7	6.0	0.0		
		29.1	4.0	15.7	21.3	36.8	7.3	0.0		

Figure 5. The effect of statins on plaque echogenicity was similar in hypercholesterolemic and non-hypercholesterolemic patients. H–C = hypercholesterolemia at baseline. (*) was on statin, but underwent contralateral carotid artery stenting (CAS), and (**) was treated only with statins. (^) received atorvastatin 10–20 mg, and (^^) atorvastatin 80 mg.

2.4. Assessment of Potential Publication Bias

No publication bias was noted in our analyses (Table 3).

Table 3. Heterogeneity and publication bias measures.

	Test of Heterogeneity	Publication Bias (Begg and Mazumdar Rank Correlation)		
	I^2	Kendell Tau	Test Statistic Z	p-Value
Echogenicity	92.1	0.34	1.41	0.16
LDL	81.2	−0.33	1.25	0.12
HDL	98.1	0.05	0.20	0.41
hsCRP	0	0	0	1.0

3. Discussion

Atherosclerosis is a long-lasting pathology with well-established stages starting with mild wall thickness and ending with complete fibrosis and calcification [1]. Along the course of the disease, plaques are formed mainly based on a lipid core, and they too are subject to structural and functional changes over time [21]. Increasing plaque area and volume while parts of it might be healing and developing fibrosis and spotty calcification characterize active plaque pathology. Soft plaques can easily be identified by various imaging techniques, including ultrasound, which has shown that echolucent plaques are the ones associated with potential complications [22,23], including even micro-emboli [24] and strokes [25].

Statins are well-established treatment for atherosclerosis and its complications. Their beneficial clinical effect, in the form of reduced events, e.g., stroke and coronary syndromes, is through lowering LDL-cholesterol levels [2] and their anti-inflammatory effect [26]; the two mechanisms result in volume reduction and plaque stabilization, as shown by increased plaque echogenicity. Our results support that pathway; however, in addition, they show that the increase in plaque echogenicity seem to be independent of the changes in intima-media thickness, plaque area or volume. These findings suggest that the statins-related increase in plaque echogenicity represents an early effect that could be used for monitoring individual patient's response to therapy. Indeed, evidence exists that the effect of statins on plaque volume appears later, after changes in echogenicity. This is not a unique feature of just carotid disease, but also coronary plaques, which have been shown to demonstrate quantitative regression in volume after 19 months of statins therapy [8]. In our meta-regression analysis, the effect of statins on plaque echogenicity was also independent of changes in LDL and HDL levels, but was related to changes of hsCRP levels. In addition, the increased echogenicity was higher in patients treated for a longer period, again irrespective of the cholesterol level at baseline.

Current data indicate that higher statins doses (atorvastatin 80 mg) have a more potent effect on increasing plaque echogenicity compared to smaller doses (atorvastatin 20 mg). These findings mirror those we previously showed in coronary artery disease, with higher statins doses resulting in a faster rate of coronary calcification compared to smaller doses [27]. Furthermore, the effect of statins duration on plaque features mirrors what we recently reported in the coronary circulation [28].

In addition to the beneficial clinical effect of statins on plaque features and potential stability, our analysis shows that ultrasound carotid imaging plays a pivotal role in early and potential continuous monitoring of such an effect. Atherosclerotic plaques can be detected and their features studied by CT and MRI scanning; however, the two techniques are known for their significant limitations, particularly radiation in the former and claustrophobia in the latter, adding to their higher cost compared with ultrasound. With carotid ultrasound free of those limitations, its accuracy in studying plaque echogenicity makes it emerge as a unique non-invasive image modality ideal for early identification of the disease and accurate monitoring of its progress and response to treatment. Ultrasound, on the other hand, has the limitation of being more time consuming with a potential inter-observer variability, particularly so when using plaque characterization methods that are, to some extent, superior to the conventionally-used intima-media thickness for early disease detection [29]. Finally, statins are usually well-tolerated medications with few adverse effects, including myopathy and elevation of liver enzymes. Rhabdomyolysis is a rare related complication [30]. Likewise, liver dysfunction is very rare, which was a reason for the FDA to remove the old recommendation of routine monitoring of liver enzymes [31]. As for diabetes mellitus, two comprehensive meta-analyses [32,33] have shown a slightly increased risk of diabetes development in subjects on statin therapy; however, the risk is low both in absolute terms and when compared with the reduction in cardiovascular events.

Study limitations: A systematic review based on relevant key words might have missed some relevant publications, but the search was checked by two investigators blinded to each other's means of search. We used only publications in the English language; other relevant ones in different languages might have been missed. Another limitation was the low number of patients included in studies and that different studies have used different statins of variable dosages. Patients were followed up for different periods of time, and in most studies, statins dosage was ranged, thus limiting us to assessing the dose effect on plaque echogenicity using the meta-regression analysis. This is the nature of searching various studies of different designs.

Clinical implications: Our results support the use of carotid ultrasound analysis of plaque features and echogenicity as a marker of plaque stability in response to statins therapy. These changes are independent of plaque area or volume, suggesting that they might reflect an early effect before anatomical response and plaque shrinking is detected. In addition, the effects of statins on the plaque were progressive and independent of baseline cholesterol levels. Applying this method in monitoring individuals at high risk for vascular events might support treatment adjustment for targeting better clinical outcome.

4. Experimental Section

4.1. Methods

The methodology for this study was based on the Preferred Reporting Items for Systematic Reviews and Meta-Analyses statement [34].

4.2. Information Search and Data Collection

Up to April, 2015, we systematically searched electronic databases (PubMed, MEDLINE, EMBASE and Cochrane Center Register) for studies evaluating the effect of statins on carotid plaque echogenicity. The search terms used were: "carotid atherosclerosis", "carotid plaque", "ultrasound" "statins", "HMG-CoA reductase inhibitors" and "lipid-lowering drugs", in various combinations. Two researchers (Pranvera Ibrahimi and Fisnik Jashari), independent of each other, performed the literature search, study selection and data extraction. There was no time, language or publication limit in the literature search. The selected reports were manually searched, and relevant publications, obtained from the reference lists, were retrieved.

4.3. Study Eligibility Criteria

Clinical studies that reported results on the effect of statin therapy on the plaque echogenicity (GSM, IBS) evaluated by duplex ultrasound were eligible. Specific inclusion criteria were: (1) observational, non-randomized or randomized studies that explored the effect on statin treatment either as primary or secondary cardiovascular disease prevention; (2) ultrasound of the carotid arteries before and at least once at a follow-up of at least one month; (3) English language articles; (4) studies with ≥ 15 subjects; and (5) ultrasound-based characterization of carotid artery plaque composition. All other studies that used different imaging techniques (e.g., MRI, CT, IVUS, PET) and those that used plaque features other than echogenicity (volume, degree of stenosis, ulceration, neovascularization) as a target for monitoring statin therapy were excluded. We have performed a quality score of the retrieved studies utilizing the methodological index for the non-randomized studies (MINORS) [35]. Studies that scored over 20 out of 24 (or 14 out of the 16 for those non-comparative, but rather solely observational) were considered of adequate quality. In the meta-analysis, we included studies that specified duration of the study and presented plaque echogenicity means and standard deviations prior to and during (or at the completion of) the intervention or the percent change in plaque echogenicity before and during intervention.

4.4. Statistical Analyses

For the plaque echogenicity analysis, the treatment effects of interest were the differences in the extent of changes in echogenicity (GSM or IBS), low-density lipoprotein cholesterol (LDL), high-density lipoprotein (HDL) and high sensitivity C-reactive protein (hsCRP) before and after treatment. Because of the significant variation in study size, length and follow-up, as well as patient's characteristics, we have used random-effects. Heterogeneity was measured using I^2 statistics. We performed analyses within each imaging group stratified by pre- *vs.* post-treatment. All analyses were conducted using Comprehensive Meta Analysis Version 3 software (Biostat inc., Englewood, NJ, USA).

5. Conclusions

Statins therapy is associated with a favorable increase of carotid plaque echogenicity, even after one month of treatment. This effect is independent of changes in plaque morphology and, furthermore, is more profound using higher doses of statins. Finally, the effect of statins seems to be related to the decrease of hsCRP from the baseline rather than dyslipidemia.

Author Contributions: Pranvera Ibrahimi conceived the study and wrote the manuscript. Pranvera Ibrahimi and Fisnik Jashari performed the literature search, study selection and data extraction and analysis. Gani Bajraktari, Per Wester and Michael Y. Henein critically revised the manuscript.

References

1. Ibrahimi, P.; Jashari, F.; Nicoll, R.; Bajraktari, G.; Wester, P.; Henein, M.Y. Coronary and carotid atherosclerosis: How useful is the imaging? *Atherosclerosis* **2013**, *231*, 323–333. [CrossRef] [PubMed]

2. Amarenco, P.; Labreuche, J.; Lavallee, P.; Touboul, P.J. Statins in stroke prevention and carotid atherosclerosis: Systematic review and up-to-date meta-analysis. *Stroke J. Cereb. Circ.* **2004**, *35*, 2902–2909. [CrossRef]

3. Martinez-Sanchez, P.; Serena, J.; Alexandrov, A.V.; Fuentes, B.; Fernandez-Dominguez, J.; Diez-Tejedor, E. Update on ultrasound techniques for the diagnosis of cerebral ischemia. *Cerebrovasc. Dis.* **2009**, *27*, 9–18. [PubMed]

4. Seeger, J.M.; Barratt, E.; Lawson, G.A.; Klingman, N. The relationship between carotid plaque composition and neurologic symptoms. *J. Surg. Res.* **1987**, *43*, 78–85. [CrossRef] [PubMed]

5. Gronholdt, M.L.; Nordestgaard, B.G.; Bentzon, J.; Wiebe, B.M.; Zhou, J.; Falk, E.; Sillesen, H. Macrophages are associated with lipid-rich carotid artery plaques, echolucency on B-mode imaging, and elevated plasma lipid levels. *J. Vasc. Surg.* **2002**, *35*, 137–145. [PubMed]

6. El-Barghouty, N.M.; Levine, T.; Ladva, S.; Flanagan, A.; Nicolaides, A. Histological verification of computerised carotid plaque characterisation. *Eur. J. Vasc. Endovasc. Surg.* **1996**, *11*, 414–416. [CrossRef] [PubMed]

7. Makris, G.C.; Lavida, A.; Nicolaides, A.N.; Geroulakos, G. The effect of statins on carotid plaque morphology: A LDL-associated action or one more pleiotropic effect of statins? *Atherosclerosis* **2010**, *213*, 8–20. [CrossRef] [PubMed]

8. Noyes, A.M.; Thompson, P.D. A systematic review of the time course of atherosclerotic plaque regression. *Atherosclerosis* **2014**, *234*, 75–84. [CrossRef] [PubMed]

9. Lind, L.P.S.; den Ruijter, H.M.; Palmer, M.K.; Grobbee, D.E.; Crouse, J.R., 3rd; O'Leary, D.H.; Evans, G.W.; Raichlen, J.S.; Bots, M.L. Effect of rosuvastatin on the echolucency of the common carotid intima-media in low-risk individuals: The METEOR trial. *J. Am. Soc. Echocardiogr.* **2012**, *25*, 1120–1127. [CrossRef] [PubMed]

10. Yamagishi, T.; Kato, M.; Koiwa, Y.; Omata, K.; Hasegawa, H.; Kanai, H. Evaluation of plaque stabilization by fluvastatin with carotid intima-medial elasticity measured by a transcutaneous ultrasonic-based tissue characterization system. *J. Atheroscler. Thromb.* **2009**, *16*, 662–673. [CrossRef] [PubMed]

11. Stivali, G.; Cerroni, F.; Bianco, P.; Fiaschetti, P.; Cianci, R. Images in cardiovascular medicine. Carotid plaque reduction after medical treatment. *Circulation* **2005**, *112*, e276–e277. [CrossRef] [PubMed]

12. Watanabe, K.; Sugiyama, S.; Kugiyama, K.; Honda, O.; Fukushima, H.; Koga, H.; Horibata, Y.; Hirai, T.; Sakamoto, T.; Yoshimura, M.; *et al.* Stabilization of carotid atheroma assessed by quantitative ultrasound analysis in nonhypercholesterolemic patients with coronary artery disease. *J. Am. Coll. Cardiol.* **2005**, *46*, 2022–2030. [CrossRef] [PubMed]

13. Yamagami, H.; Sakaguchi, M.; Furukado, S.; Hoshi, T.; Abe, Y.; Hougaku, H.; Hori, M.; Kitagawa, K. Statin therapy increases carotid plaque echogenicity in hypercholesterolemic patients. *Ultrasound Med. Biol.* **2008**, *34*, 1353–1359. [CrossRef] [PubMed]

14. Nakamura, T.; Obata, J.E.; Kitta, Y.; Takano, H.; Kobayashi, T.; Fujioka, D.; Saito, Y.; Kodama, Y.; Kawabata, K.; Mende, A.; *et al.* Rapid stabilization of vulnerable carotid plaque within 1 month of pitavastatin treatment in patients with acute coronary syndrome. *J. Cardiovasc. Pharmacol.* **2008**, *51*, 365–371. [CrossRef] [PubMed]

15. Kadoglou, N.P.; Gerasimidis, T.; Moumtzouoglou, A.; Kapelouzou, A.; Sailer, N.; Fotiadis, G.; Vitta, I.; Katinios, A.; Kougias, P.; Bandios, S.; *et al.* Intensive lipid-lowering therapy ameliorates novel calcification markers and GSM score in patients with carotid stenosis. *Eur. J. Vasc. Endovasc. Surg.* **2008**, *35*, 661–668. [CrossRef] [PubMed]

16. Yamada, K.; Yoshimura, S.; Kawasaki, M.; Enomoto, Y.; Asano, T.; Minatoguchi, S.; Iwama, T. Effects of atorvastatin on carotid atherosclerotic plaques: A randomized trial for quantitative tissue characterization of carotid atherosclerotic plaques with integrated backscatter ultrasound. *Cerebrovasc. Dis.* **2009**, *28*, 417–424. [CrossRef] [PubMed]

17. Kadoglou, N.P.; Gerasimidis, T.; Kapelouzou, A.; Moumtzouoglou, A.; Avgerinos, E.D.; Kakisis, J.D.; Karayannacos, P.E.; Liapis, C.D. Beneficial changes of serum calcification markers and contralateral carotid plaques echogenicity after combined carotid artery stenting plus intensive lipid-lowering therapy in patients with bilateral carotid stenosis. *Eur. J. Vasc. Endovasc. Surg.* **2010**, *39*, 258–265. [CrossRef] [PubMed]

18. Kadoglou, N.P.; Moumtzouoglou, A.; Kapelouzou, A.; Gerasimidis, T.; Liapis, C.D. Aggressive lipid-lowering is more effective than moderate lipid-lowering treatment in carotid plaque stabilization. *J. Vasc. Surg.* **2010**, *55*, 114–121. [CrossRef]

19. Della-Morte, D.; Moussa, I.; Elkind, M.S.; Sacco, R.L.; Rundek, T. The short-term effect of atorvastatin on carotid plaque morphology assessed by computer-assisted gray-scale densitometry: A pilot study. *Neurol. Res.* **2011**, *33*, 991–994. [CrossRef] [PubMed]

20. Nohara, R.; Daida, H.; Hata, M.; Kaku, K.; Kawamori, R.; Kishimoto, J.; Kurabayashi, M.; Masuda, I.; Sakuma, I.; Yamazaki, T.; *et al.* Effect of long-term intensive lipid-lowering therapy with rosuvastatin on progression of carotid intima-media thickness—Justification for atherosclerosis regression treatment (JART) extension study. *Circ. J.* **2013**, *77*, 1526–1533. [CrossRef] [PubMed]

21. Jashari, F.; Ibrahimi, P.; Nicoll, R.; Bajraktari, G.; Wester, P.; Henein, M.Y. Coronary and carotid atherosclerosis: Similarities and differences. *Atherosclerosis* **2013**, *227*, 193–200. [CrossRef] [PubMed]

22. Nicolaides, A.N.; Kyriacou, E.; Griffin, M.; Sabetai, M.; Thomas, D.J.; Tegos, T.; Geroulakos, G.; Labropoulos, N.; Doré, C.J.; Morris, T.P.; *et al.* Asymptomatic internal carotid artery stenosis and cerebrovascular risk stratification. *J. Vasc. Surg.* **2010**, *52*, 1486–1496. [CrossRef] [PubMed]

23. Ibrahimi, P.; Jashari, F.; Johansson, E.; Gronlund, C.; Bajraktari, G.; Wester, P.; Henein, M.Y. Vulnerable plaques in the contralateral carotid arteries in symptomatic patients: A detailed ultrasound analysis. *Atherosclerosis* **2014**, *235*, 526–531. [CrossRef] [PubMed]

24. Sztajzel, R.; Momjian-Mayor, I.; Comelli, M.; Momjian, S. Correlation of cerebrovascular symptoms and microembolic signals with the stratified gray-scale median analysis and color mapping of the carotid plaque. *Stroke J. Cereb. Circ.* **2006**, *37*, 824–829. [CrossRef]

25. Aburahma, A.F.; Thiele, S.P.; Wulu, J.T., Jr. Prospective controlled study of the natural history of asymptomatic 60% to 69% carotid stenosis according to ultrasonic plaque morphology. *J. Vasc. Surg.* **2002**, *36*, 437–442. [CrossRef] [PubMed]

26. Takemoto, M.; Liao, J.K. Pleiotropic effects of 3-hydroxy-3-methylglutaryl coenzyme a reductase inhibitors. *Arterioscler. Thromb. Vasc. Biol.* **2001**, *21*, 1712–1719. [CrossRef] [PubMed]

27. Schmermund, A.A.S.; Budde, T.; Buziashvili, Y.; Förster, A.; Friedrich, G.; Henein, M.; Kerkhoff, G.; Knollmann, F.; Kukharchuk, V.; Lahiri, A.; *et al.* Effect of intensive *versus* standard lipid-lowering treatment with atorvastatin on the progression of calcified coronary atherosclerosis over 12 months: A multicenter, randomized, double-blind trial. *Circulation* **2006**, *113*, 427–437. [CrossRef] [PubMed]

28. Henein, M.; Granåsen, G.; Wiklund, U.; Schmermund, A.; Guerci, A.; Erbel, R.; Raggi, P. High dose and long-term statin therapy accelerate coronary artery calcification. *Int. J. Cardiol.* **2015**, *184*, 581–586. [CrossRef] [PubMed]

29. Coll, B.; Feinstein, S.B. Carotid intima-media thickness measurements: Techniques and clinical relevance. *Curr. Atheroscler. Rep.* **2008**, *10*, 444–450. [CrossRef] [PubMed]

30. Silva, M.A.; Swanson, A.C.; Gandhi, P.J.; Tataronis, G.R. Statin-related adverse events: A meta-analysis. *Clin. Ther.* **2006**, *28*, 26–35. [CrossRef] [PubMed]

31. Jukema, J.W.; Cannon, C.P.; de Craen, A.J.; Westendorp, R.G.; Trompet, S. The controversies of statin therapy: Weighing the evidence. *J. Am. Coll. Cardiol.* **2012**, *60*, 875–881. [CrossRef] [PubMed]

32. Sattar, N.; Preiss, D.; Murray, H.M.; Welsh, P.; Buckley, B.M.; de Craen, A.J.; Seshasai, S.R.; McMurray, J.J.; Freeman, D.J.; Jukema, J.W.; *et al.* Statins and risk of incident diabetes: A collaborative meta-analysis of randomised statin trials. *Lancet* **2010**, *375*, 735–742. [CrossRef] [PubMed]

33. Preiss, D.; Seshasai, S.R.; Welsh, P.; Murphy, S.A.; Ho, J.E.; Waters, D.D.; DeMicco, D.A.; Barter, P.; Cannon, C.P.; Sabatine, M.S.; *et al.* Risk of incident diabetes with intensive-dose compared with moderate-dose statin therapy: A meta-analysis. *JAMA* **2011**, *305*, 2556–2564. [CrossRef] [PubMed]

34. Liberati, A.A.D.; Tetzlaff, J.; Mulrow, C.; Gøtzsche, P.C.; Ioannidis, J.P.; Clarke, M.; Devereaux, P.J.; Kleijnen, J.; Moher, D. The PRISMA statement for reporting systematic reviews and meta-analyses of studies that evaluate health care interventions: Explanation and elaboration. *PLoS Med.* **2009**, *6*, 1–28. [CrossRef]

35. Slim, K.; Nini, E.; Forestier, D.; Kwiatkowski, F.; Panis, Y.; Chipponi, J. Methodological index for non-randomized studies (*MINORS*): Development and validation of a new instrument. *ANZ J. Surg.* **2003**, *73*, 712–716. [CrossRef] [PubMed]

14

Mutant *LRP6* Impairs Endothelial Cell Functions Associated with Familial Normolipidemic Coronary Artery Disease

Jian Guo [1], Yang Li [1], Yi-Hong Ren [2], Zhijun Sun [2], Jie Dong [1], Han Yan [1], Yujun Xu [3], Dao Wen Wang [3], Gu-Yan Zheng [1], Jie Du [4] and Xiao-Li Tian [1,5,*]

[1] Department of Human Population Genetics, Institute of Molecular Medicine, Peking University, Beijing 100871, China; deidei@163.com (J.G.); ly1306386063@pku.edu.cn (Y.L.); djqiu@163.com (J.D.); yanhan@pku.edu.cn (H.Y.); zhengguyan@163.com (G.-Y.Z.)

[2] Department of Cardiovascular, PLA General Hospital, Beijing 100853, China; rainbowren301@163.com (Y.-H.R.); sunzj301@sohu.com (Z.S.)

[3] The Institute of Hypertension and Department of Internal Medicine, Tongji Hospital, Tongji Medical College, Huazhong University of Science and Technology, Wuhan 430074, China; xuyujun3506@163.com (Y.X.); dwwang@tjh.tjmu.edu.cn (D.W.W.)

[4] Beijing Anzhen Hospital, Capital Medical University, The Key Laboratory of Remodeling-Related Cardiovascular Diseases, Ministry of Education, Beijing Collaborative Innovation Center for Cardiovascular Disorders, Beijing Institute of Heart, Lung & Blood Vessel Disease, Beijing 100029, China; jiedubj@126.com

[5] Department of Human Population Genetics, Human Aging Research Institute and School of Life Science, Nanchang University, Nanchang 330031, China

* Correspondence: tianxiaoli@pku.edu.cn or tianxiaoli@ncu.edu.cn;

Academic Editor: Michael Henein

Abstract: Mutations in the genes low-density lipoprotein (LDL) receptor-related protein-6 (*LRP6*) and myocyte enhancer factor 2A (*MEF2A*) were reported in families with coronary artery disease (CAD). We intend to determine the mutational spectrum of these genes among hyperlipidemic and normolipidemic CAD families. Forty probands with early-onset CAD were recruited from 19 hyperlipidemic and 21 normolipidemic Chinese families. We sequenced all exons and intron-exon boundaries of *LRP6* and *MEF2A*, and found a novel heterozygous variant in *LRP6* from a proband with normolipidemic CAD. This variant led to a substitution of histidine to tyrosine (Y418H) in an evolutionarily conserved domain YWTD in exon 6 and was not found in 1025 unrelated healthy individuals. Co-segregated with CAD in the affected family, $LRP6_{Y418H}$ significantly debilitated the Wnt3a-associated signaling pathway, suppressed endothelial cell proliferation and migration, and decreased anti-apoptotic ability. However, it exhibited no influences on low-density lipoprotein cholesterol uptake. Thus, mutation Y418H in *LRP6* likely contributes to normolipidemic familial CAD via impairing endothelial cell functions and weakening the Wnt3a signaling pathway.

Keywords: LDL receptor-related protein-6 (*LRP6*); normolipidemic; coronary artery disease; familial; endothelial cell dysfunction

1. Introduction

Coronary artery disease (CAD), the most common cause of death, is characterized by the stenosis or occlusions of coronary arteries that are mostly caused by the progressive deposition of lipids and fibrous matrix (atherosclerotic plaques) in the arterial wall [1]. The key steps of atherosclerogenesis include dysfunction of the endothelium, lipoprotein deposition, recruitment of monocytes and lymphocytes, and proliferation of smooth muscle cells [2]. Endothelial cell survival, proliferation, and migration are critical to maintain the homeostasis and normal functions of endothelium [3].

The common form of CAD appears multi-factorial in etiology, involving an interaction between genetic and environmental factors [4,5]. Over the past decades, great efforts have been made to systematically search for genes or chromosomal loci associated with CAD at the genome level by family or population-based association studies, leading to the identification of numbers of susceptibility genes or loci [6–10]. In contrast, familial CAD is rare but highly penetrated, presenting a monogenic effect and Mendelian inheritance. Mutations in genes *MEF2A* and *LRP6* were previously identified as pathogenic or CAD-causing variants for familial CAD [11,12]. The detections of these loci or genes apparently increase our knowledge of understanding the molecular mechanism of CAD and may be helpful in improving the clinical treatment and drug discovery.

In addition to genetic influences, other risk factors for CAD are well established, such as elevated cholesterol, hypertension, obesity, and unhealthy lifestyles [13]. For example, hyperlipidemia, particularly the elevated level of low-density lipoprotein cholesterol (LDL-C), increases the risk for atherosclerosis which is fundamental to CAD [14–16]. In contrast, the high-density lipoprotein cholesterol (HDL-C) is inversely related with CAD [15–17]. Although hyperlipidemia is a significant risk factor for CAD, a considerable proportion of CAD patients are normolipidemic. It has been reported that only a third of CAD patients exhibit elevated cholesterol levels, especially LDL-C [18]. More than 40% and 60% of male CAD patients have normal ranges of serum LDL-C (<130 mg/dL, 3.4 mmol/L) and HDL-C levels (>35 mg/dL, 0.9 mmol/L) respectively [19]. Ultimately, how genetic determinants contribute differentially to hyperlipidemic and normolipidemic CAD remains largely unknown.

In this study, we recruited 40 Chinese Han families with early-onset hyperlipidemic or normolipidemic CAD, sequenced all exons and intron-exon boundaries of *LRP6* and *MEF2A*, two previously reported CAD genes, and characterized the functions of newly identified mutations.

2. Results

2.1. A Novel Mutation in LRP6 Was Identified in a Family with Normolipidemic CAD

DNA was extracted from the peripheral blood lymphocytes of 40 probands, including 19 hyperlipidemic and 21 normolipidemic CAD patients from northern China (Table S1). After amplifying the genomic DNA with primers, as shown in Tables S2 and S3, all exons and intron-exon boundaries of *LRP6* and *MEF2A* were sequenced. As a result, a novel heterozygous variant in exon 6 of *LRP6* was identified in a proband, belonging to a patient who was 41 years old and diagnosed with myocardial infarction without hyperlipidemia. This proband (subject II7) was from a family with three generations, involving 20 patients and non-affected first-order relatives (Figure 1A). Two of his three major coronary arteries showed at least 80% stenosis (Figure 1B), leading to percutaneous coronary intervention. The variant was located in a domain named YWTD (Tyr–Trp–Thr–Asp), causing a substitution of histidine to tyrosine (Y418H) (Figure 1C). The multiple alignments using a basic local alignment search tool (BLAST) in the NCBI database showed that this region was highly conserved from *Denio rerio* to *Homo sapiens* (Figure 1D). Y418H was predicted to be a probable damaging change with a score of 0.994 in Polyphen-2 (available online: http://genetics.bwh.harvard.edu/pph2/, Table S4). We sequenced exon 6 of *LRP6* in another 1025 unrelated healthy individuals and found no variants.

In the Y418H family, another four members were previously diagnosed with CAD or suffered from sudden cardiac death before age 50 (men) or 55 (women), and two of them have been deceased. In addition to CAD, the proband (subject II7) and his sister (subject II5) were diagnosed with hypertension and diabetes. The third generation is too young and has no clinical symptoms, and is thus not subjected to clinical diagnosis. We genotyped 17 individuals from this family and found that the Y418H variant was co-segregated with CAD phenotypes (Figure 1A). It was speculated that this mutation came from subject I2. Eleven family members were available for measurement of fasting glucose, total cholesterol (TC), triglycerides, LDL-C, and HDL-C (Table 1). For subject II3 (unaffected) and subject II5 (CAD), who had not taken lipid-lowering drugs during the past six months, blood lipid levels were similar. Additionally, despite the similar ages, the blood lipid levels of Y418H-carriers III7 and III8 were significantly different. These suggested that Y418H is not co-segregated with dyslipidemia and that this familial CAD is not linked to hyperlipidemia.

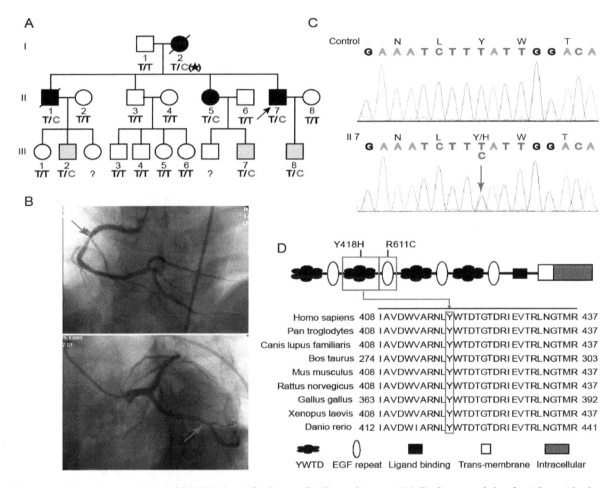

Figure 1. Novel mutation of *LRP6* identified in a CAD pedigree. (**A**) Pedigree of the family with the *LRP6* Y418H mutation. Numbered individuals correspond to those in Table 1. Circles represent females; Squares represent males; Proband is indicated by the arrow; Individuals with CAD are indicated by black symbols; Individuals without CAD are shown as unfilled symbols; Presymptomatic carriers are shown by symbols by gray symbols; Symbols with a slash through them indicate deceased subjects; Genotypes of the *LRP6* mutation were shown below the symbols who were willing to participate in the study; Filled stars indicates that the genotype of subject I2 was speculated; Individuals who were not available for studied are indicated with question mark; (**B**) Coronary angiogram of the proband. The red arrows indicates the stenosis; (**C**) DNA sequence analysis for a segment of *LRP6* exon 6 from a healthy control (**top**) and the proband (**below**). A red arrow points out a single base mutation in the proband, and it results in the substitution of histidine for tyrosine at codon 418; (**D**) Conservatism analysis by interspecies alignments. The mutation position is indicated with a red frame.

Although no other mutations in *LRP6* or *MEF2A* were found in the other 39 probands, we noticed several known single nucleotide polymorphisms (SNPs) included in the single nucleotide polymorphism database (dbSNP) during screening (data not shown). Nevertheless, we did not calculate their minor allele frequencies because of the limited number of samples.

Table 1. Clinical characteristic of members with CAD pedigree

ID	Age/Onset Age	Gender	BMI	SBP (mmHg)	DBP (mmHg)	Anti-HT Drug	Glucose mmol/L 3.9~6.1	Anti-D Drug	Triglyceride mmol/L 0.56~1.8	TC mmol/L 2.9~6.0	HDL-C mmol/L 0.8~1.8	LDL-C mmol/L 1.6~3.2	Anti-HL Drug	CAD Status
I1	86	male	23.9	140	80	no	NA	no	NA	NA	NA	NA	no	Unaffected
I2 *	65 †/NA	female	NA	NA	NA	NA	NA	NA	NA	NA	NA	NA	NA	CAD/Stroke
II1 *	49 †/49	male	NA	NA	NA	NA	NA	NA	NA	NA	NA	NA	NA	SCD
II3	58	male	25.0	140	80	no	6.06	no	1.80	5.46	1.31	3.53	no	Unaffected
II5 *	47/46	female	27.9	170	100	yes	8.08	yes	1.35	6.93	2.10	3.76	no	CAD
II7 *	44/41	male	25.4	135	80	yes	7.16	no	1.57	3.23	1.02	1.76	yes	CAD
III1	33	female	22.2	115	75	no	4.58	no	0.56	4.51	1.68	2.18	no	Unknown
III2 *	31	male	24.9	130	80	no	4.69	no	2.24	6.24	1.18	3.66	no	Unknown
III3	34	male	23.7	150	100	no	4.53	no	1.24	4.87	1.12	3.31	no	Unknown
III4	28	male	24.2	140	80	no	3.83	no	1.26	4.93	1.65	2.32	no	Unknown
III5	35	female	23.4	120	80	no	4.54	no	0.68	4.59	1.62	2.27	no	Unknown
III6	30	female	20.3	105	70	no	3.42	no	0.94	3.97	1.38	2.12	no	Unknown
III7 *	22	male	21.2	110	70	no	4.76	no	1.18	3.60	1.23	1.77	no	Unknown
III8 *	20	male	30.1	130	85	no	4.58	no	1.29	6.12	1.48	3.81	no	Unknown

ID corresponds to those in Figure 1; BMI: body mass index; SBP: systolic blood pressure; DBP: diastolic blood pressure; anti-H: anti-hypertension; anti-D: anti-diabetes; anti-HL: anti-hyperlipidemia; TC: total cholesterol; HDL-C: high density lipoprotein cholesterol; LDL-C: low density lipoprotein cholesterol; *: Y418H carrier; †: deceased; SCD: sudden cardiac death; NA: not available.

2.2. LRP6_{Y418H} Weakened the Wnt Signaling Pathway

As a receptor, *LRP6* activates the canonical Wnt-mediated signal pathway. To determine whether the mutation Y418H impaired Wnt signaling transduction, a comparative study was carried out among wild-type (*LRP6_{WT}*), mutant *LRP6* with Y418H (*LRP6_{Y418H}*) and mutant *LRP6* with a previously reported mutation R611C (*LRP6_{R611C}*) [12]. We transfected human umbilical vein endothelial cells (HUVEC) with the same amount of plasmids encoding LRP6_{WT}, LRP6_{R611C} or LRP6_{Y418H}, which were supported by RT-PCR (Figure 2A). Western blot showed that when an equal amount of protein was loaded, the distribution of mutant LRP6 protein in the cellular membrane faction was similar to wild type (Figure 2B–D). The luciferase reporter activity indicating the extent of Wnt signal activation was then measured. We found that the Wnt3a-induced signaling was decreased 20% and 30% for *LRP6_{R611C}* and *LRP6_{Y418H}* compared with *LRP6_{wt}*, respectively ($p < 0.05$) (Figure 2E). A more severe reduction was observed in the *LRP6_{Y418H}*- than in the *LRP6_{R611C}*-treated group ($p < 0.05$).

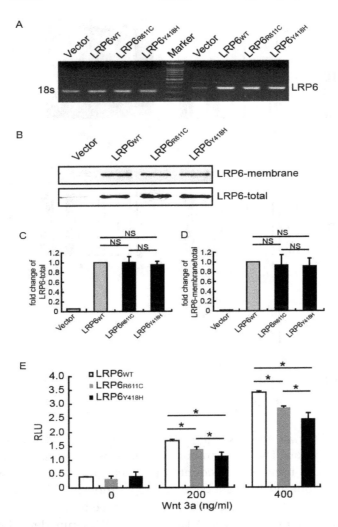

Figure 2. Effect of *LRP6_{Y418H}* and *LRP6_{R611C}* on Wnt signal transduction. (**A**) RT-PCR showed that there was no significant difference between the over-expression levels of LRP6_{WT}/LRP6_{R611C}/LRP6_{Y418H}; (**B**) Western blot showed no significant difference between total expression levels or membrane location of wild-type and mutant LRP6. Results were replicated three times and a representative figure was shown; (**C,D**) Statistical result of (**B**); (**E**) Luciferase assay was performed with different amount of Wnt3a. RLU: relative light units. Results were obtained with four independent transfections. Error bars, standard deviation. * indicate *p*-value for one-way ANOVA plus post-hoc test <0.05. NS, not significant in one-way ANOVA plus post-hoc test.

2.3. LRP6$_{Y418H}$ Impaired Endothelial Cell Functions

Endothelial cell dysfunction contributes to atherosclerogenesis. To investigate the possible mechanisms of atherosclerosis associated with *LRP6$_{Y418H}$*, we first screened the effect of this mutation on endothelial cell functions, including proliferation, migration, and anti-apoptosis, which were critical to maintaining the integrity of the endothelium. A significantly decreased proliferation and migration was observed in HUVEC over-expressing *LRP6$_{R611C}$* and *LRP6$_{Y418H}$* (all $p < 0.05$), and the effect of *LRP6$_{Y418H}$* was more profound than that of *LRP6$_{R611C}$* (Figure 3A,B as well as Supplementary Figure S1). The over-expression of *LRP6* (wild type and mutant) protected endothelial cells from the serum withdrawal-induced apoptosis, as shown by apoptotic DNA ladders (Figure 3C) and flow cytometric analyses (Figure 3D,E); the anti-apoptotic ability, however, was decreased in the cells infected by the mutant *LRP6* (*LRP6$_{R611C}$* and *LRP6$_{Y418H}$*). No significant difference was observed between the two mutations.

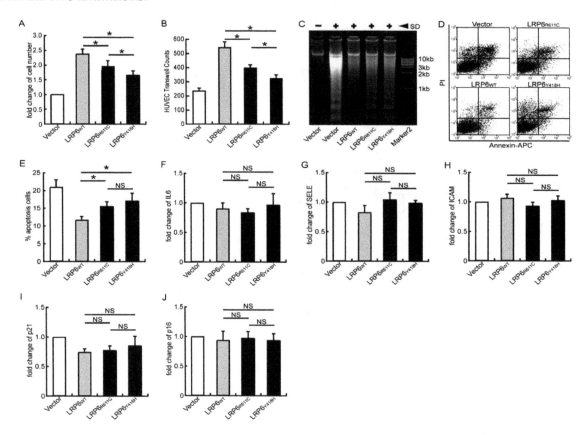

Figure 3. Effect of *LRP6$_{Y418H}$* and *LRP6$_{R611C}$* on endothelial cell functions; (**A**) Comparison of endothelial cells' proliferation. The same amount of cells was over-expressed with wild-type LRP6 or mutant. After 48 h, cell number was counted for each group. Results were calculated using eight random fields from four independent biological replications; (**B**) Comparison of endothelial cell migration. Results were calculated using six views from three independent replications of Boyden chamber assay; (**C**) Electrophorogram for DNA ladder assay. SD, serum depletion; (**D**) Scatter diagram from flow cytometry assay. Data were presented in 2D diagrams plotting PI against Annexin-APC. Compensation for background fluorescence was performed by measuring target signals of single color controls and negative controls. Two quadrants in the right-side diagram represent apoptotic cells; (**E**) Statistical result for proportion of apoptotic cells in each group. Three biological repeats were taken into calculation; (**F–J**) Relative mRNA level of markers for endothelial cell activation (*IL6*, *SELE*, and *ICAM*) and senescence (*P21* and *P16*). Three biological repeats were taken into calculation. Error bars, standard deviation. * indicate *p*-value for one-way ANOVA plus post-hoc test <0.05. NS, not significant.

We then assessed how the mutations influenced the inflammatory responses of endothelial cells and found no differences among the wild-type and two mutations in the mRNA expression of *IL6* (Figure 3F), *SELE* (Figure 3G), and *ICAM-1* (Figure 3H).

Finally, no differences were found in the mRNA expression of *P21* and *P16*, two markers for cell senescence, among all groups, suggesting senescence was not involved (Figure 3I,J).

2.4. The Influence of LRP6_{Y418H} on Cellular LDL-C Clearance

Compared with $LRP6_{wt}$, $LRP6_{R611C}$ has been shown to decrease cellular LDL-C clearance. We examined whether $LRP6_{Y418H}$ had a similar effect. After being incubated with LDL-C labeled by Dil (a red dye), cells transfected with $LRP6_{R611C}$ presented a reduced LDL uptake compared to the $LRP6_{wt}$ cells ($p < 0.05$) (Figure 4A,B), but no differences existed between $LRP6_{wt}$ and $LRP6_{Y418H}$.

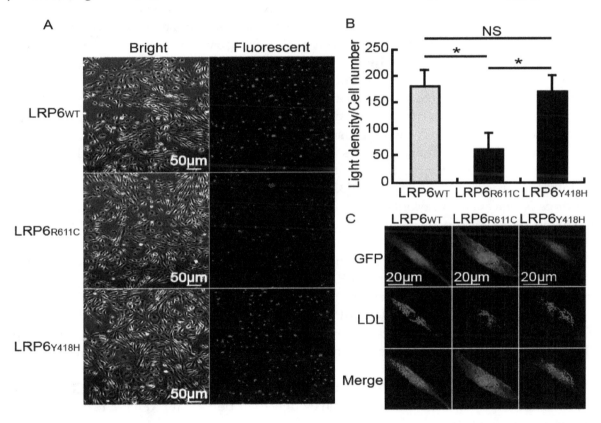

Figure 4. Effect of $LRP6_{Y418H}$ and $LRP6_{R611C}$ on LDL uptake in HUVEC. (**A**) An overview of the Dil-LDL uptake in HUVEC; Left, bright field; Right, Fluorescent field; (**B**) Quantitative results were calculated using six random views from three independent replications. Error bars, standard deviation. * indicate *p*-value for one-way ANOVA plus post-hoc test <0.05. NS, not significant; (**C**) Enlarged views for single cells. Top, GFP translated by IRES following *LRP6*; Middle, Dil-LDL; Bottom, merged data.

3. Discussion

Here we report a novel heterozygous mutation of LRP6 in a Chinese normolipidemic CAD family, which leads to a substitution of histidine to tyrosine (Y418H) in an evolutionarily conserved domain, YWTD. LRP6Y418H does not alter the lipid transportation; however, it weakens the Wnt signaling pathway and exhibits deleterious effects on the proliferation, migration, and survival of endothelial cells. Our study suggests that impaired endothelial functions caused by genetic mutation are critical in the pathogenesis of normolipidemic CAD.

Over the past decades, a large number of genetic studies have been performed to search for the genes or loci associated with CAD mostly with hyperlipidemia, but genetic knowledge on normolipidemic CAD remains limited [20]. Here, we identified a genetic variant (Y418H) of LRP6 in a

Chinese normolipidemic CAD family and provided several lines of evidence to show that this genetic variant was a possible defect for familial normolipidemic CAD. Genetically, Y418H occurred in an evolutionarily conserved YWTD domain, was co-segregated with CAD phenotypes in the family, and was not detected in 1025 healthy individuals in this study. In addition, we inspected this mutation in three other databases. Y418H was not found in the NHLBI GO Exome Sequencing Project (ESP) (6503 samples) and in the in-house control test (221 samples); however, there were two carriers in 1000GP (2504 samples), yielding an allele frequency of 0.0004 (Table S4). Due to the lack of diagnosis, we cannot rule out whether or not those carries are potential CAD patients occurring in Han Chinese South (CHS). It is very interesting to note that we have observed LRP6 mutations in sporadic Chinese CAD patients [21]. With the notion from the present study that *LRP6* can be a candidate gene for normolipidemic CAD, we checked the blood lipid levels and found that they were not elevated in their first clinic visits (Table S5). Differently, mutations in *LRP6* were screened out in American kindreds with early-onset hyperlipidemic CAD [22]. With the limited numbers of mutations found by far, it is difficult to make solid correlations between race, genotypes (positions of the mutations in *LRP6* gene) and phenotypes (normolipidemic or hyperlipidemic CAD). It appears clear that *LRP6* is a plausible candidate gene for both normolipidemic and hyperlipidemic CAD.

Functionally, Y418H is predicted to be a damaging allele with a Polyphen2 score of 0.994 that is higher than that of R611C. We demonstrated that LRP6Y418H weakened the ability in proliferation, migration, and survival of endothelial cells when exposed to stress. It is known that homeostasis or prompt renewal of endothelial cells is critical to maintain the integrity of the endothelium. Denuded by mechanical injuries, the endothelium can be amended by adjacent endothelial cells and endothelial progenitor cells as well [3,23–31]. This suggests that, in addition to endothelial progenitor cells, the survival, proliferation, and migration of endothelial cells localized in the zone adjacent to the injured region are important to maintain the homeostasis. The impaired or dysfunctional endothelium associated with LRP6Y418H should increase the susceptibility, together with other risk factors, such as hypertension and diabetes in the affected individuals, to develop atherosclerosis in coronary arteries. Finally, we showed that LRP6Y418H weakened the Wnt signaling pathway that had been reported to contribute to familial CAD [12]. The extracellular structure of the LRP6 protein is mainly composed of four beta propellers (BP) that contain six YWTD repeats which are separated by four EGF-like domains. It was reported that the four BPs have different functions, for example BP1 and BP2 are mainly responsible for the binding of Wnt and Wise [32,33]. Strikingly, most mutations in Supplementary Table S4 that were predicted to be seriously functionally damaged reside in the second propeller and EGF-like domain, suggesting the importance of the second YWTD-EGF structure and Wnt signal for CAD. This genetic and functional evidence supports that *LRP6* is a reasonable candidate gene for normolipidemic familial CAD.

Since R611C and Y418H were found in two CAD families, we compared clinical phenotypes and functions of the two mutant LRP6s. In clinical phenotypes, two families had some overlapping phenotypes: (1) some individuals in the families suffered from sudden cardiac death; and (2) the affected subjects (after age 40) had multiple CAD risk factors such as hypertension and diabetes. However, the blood lipid was dramatically different between the CAD patients in the two families: the Y418H family was normolipidemic while the R611C family was hyperlipidemic; high levels of LDL-C and triglycerides were co-segregated with CAD in the R611C family. Functionally distinct from Y418H, the R611C mutation was in the EGF-like domain and impaired the cellular LDL-C uptake. This was in agreement with a recent finding that the R611C mutation resulted in decreased LDL-C clearance [34] and reduced LRP6 activity in LRP6R611C mice that had elevated plasma LDL-C and TG levels and fatty liver [35]. Nonetheless, two mutations (Y418H and R611C) at the different positions of the *LRP6* gene can be linked to normolipidemic and hyperlipidemic CAD, two subtypes of familial CAD, suggestive of the importance of LRP6.

LRP6, a trans-membrane protein of the low-density lipoprotein receptor (LDLR) family, was identified based on its homology with the LDLR gene [36]. As a receptor of the canonical

Wnt signaling pathway, LRP6, together with LRP5 and Frizzled, activates β-catenin-TCF/LEF, and regulates downstream signaling which is important in the development and maintenance of the cardiovascular system [37]. For example, activation of this pathway induces the proliferation, migration, and survival of endothelial cells [38–40]. We in this study demonstrated that LRP6Y418H attenuated the Wnt3a-activated signaling pathway, decreased proliferation and mobility, and weakened the anti-apoptotic response of endothelial cells. Similarly, it has been shown that mutations of LRP6 found in sporadic CAD patients attenuated proliferation and migration of HUVEC as well as the Wnt signal [21]. LRP6R611C also attenuated the Wnt3a-activated signaling pathway [12]. These suggest that mutant LRP6 impairs endothelial cell functions, possibly through the attenuation of the Wnt-signaling pathway. However, how other risk factors, such as hypertension and diabetes, interact with the genetic defect in atherosclerogenesis needs to be further investigated.

Several limitations exist in this study: (1) the third generation of the studied pedigree is still young, and we cannot claim whether or not the mutation carriers in this generation are CAD patients; (2) LRP6 has a broad range of functions, and whether other signal pathways are involved in the pathogenic mechanism of this family cannot be excluded. For example, LRP6 is a co-receptor for multiple fibrogenic signaling pathways in pericytes and myofibroblasts [41]. It is not clear whether or not these pathways contribute to CAD associated with the LRP6 mutations; and (3) although Wang et al. identified *MEF2A* as a causal gene for CAD, we did not find any mutation in this gene during our first screening. Similar to our finding, Lieb et al. suggested the lack of association between the *MEF2A* gene and myocardial infarction [42]. However, limited by the modest sample number, we cannot rule out the role of *MEF2A* in CAD.

In conclusion, we identified a mutation (Y418H) in the YWTD domain of LRP6 that co-segregated with normolipidemic CAD in a Han Chinese family that impaired endothelial cell functions, implying that endothelial dysfunctions associated with a genetic mutation play an important role in normolipidemic CAD.

4. Materials and Methods

4.1. Study Subjects

We recruited 40 Chinese Han families with CAD that were ascertained through probands and included more than two early-onset CAD/ myocardial infarction (MI) patients (less than 50 years old for males or 55 years old for females). Blood pressure, glucose, hypertension, and diabetes mellitus were measured or defined [43]. Hyperlipidemia or normolipidemia were defined based on clinical diagnosis. 1025 unrelated Han Chinese controls were general healthy donors [44]. Written informed consent was obtained from all participants. The study was conducted in agreement with the principles outlined in the Declaration of Helsinki and approved by the Institutional Review Board, Institute of Molecular Medicine at Peking University.

4.2. Cell Culture

Primary human umbilical vein endothelial cells (HUVECs) were isolated from fresh human umbilical veins, cultured in complete Endothelial Cell Medium (ECM, ScienCell), and maintained at 37 °C in 5% CO_2. The informed consents were signed by babies' fathers. The study was conducted in agreement with the principles outlined in the Declaration of Helsinki and approved by the Institutional Review Board, Institute of Molecular Medicine at Peking University.

4.3. Mutational Screening

Human genomic DNA was isolated as described previously [44]. The exons of the target genes and their flanking exon-intron boundaries were amplified by PCR using specific primers listed in Tables S2 and S3. The amplified DNA fragments were purified and subjected to direct sequencing on ABI 3130XL according to the manual description of BigDye v3.1 kit.

4.4. Wnt Signaling Analysis

cDNA clone of LRP6 (pCR-XL-TOPO-LRP6) was purchased from FulenGen. cDNA sequence was validated by sequencing and inserted into pShuttle-IRES-hrGFP-1 vector. Mutations (Y418H and R611C, a previously reported mutation [12]) were introduced by PCR-based mutagenesis, respectively. The mutations were verified by DNA sequencing. HUVEC was electric transfected with equal amount of plasmids expressing wild-type (LRP6wt) and mutant LRP6 (LRP6R611C or LRP6Y418H), respectively. A Wnt pathway reporter system was utilized as previously described [12]. Briefly, plasmids encoding wild-type LRP6 or mutants, LEF-1, firefly luciferase, and renilla luciferase were introduced into cells by transfection. After 24 h, cells were lysed and luciferase reporter activity indicating the extent of Wnt signal activation was measured in accordance with the dual luciferase assay specifications (Promega, Hollow Road Madison, WI, USA).

4.5. Quantitative Real-Time PCR

Total RNA was extracted using Trizol reagent (Invitrogen, Waltham, MA, USA). Reverse transcription and quantitative real-time PCR were performed as previously described [45]. Information of specific primers is listed in Table S6. Results were normalized to 18S rRNA.

4.6. Western Blot Analysis of LRP6

Total and membrane protein were extracted using kit from Beyotime Biotechnology. Western blot was performed to detect the wild type and mutant LRP6 protein (primary antibody for LRP6: sc-25317, Santa Cruz, Dallas, TX, USA) based on the protocol previously reported [46]. GAPDH was used as a loading control.

4.7. HUVEC Proliferation, Migration, and Apoptosis Analysis

For overexpression wild-type LRP6 or mutants in HUVECs, infection was performed with adenovirus that constructed following manufacturer's protocol for AdEasy system (Stratagene, Santa Clara, CA, USA) [47]. We controlled the same over-expressional level among different groups by adjusting the amount of virus added. Proliferation was evaluated using MTT (Sigma, St. Louis, MO, USA) assay and actual cell number count, and migration was evaluated Boyden Chamber assay [48]. To avoiding the effect of proliferation, we controlled the migration time within 12 h. Apoptosis was presented by both DNA ladder gel electrophoresis [49] and FACS analysis (BD Biosciences Clontech Kit, San Jose, CA, USA).

4.8. Dil-LDL Uptake

HUVECs were placed in a six-well plate containing 20 µg/dL cholesterol and 2 µg/mL 25-hydroxycholesterol to down-regulate the endogenous LDLR (Supplementary Figure S2). After 24 h, 10 µg/mL Dil-LDL was added and incubated at 37 °C for six hours. Cells were washed three times with PBS containing 1% FBS and were fixed in 4% paraformaldehyde. Specimens were then examined by confocal microscope.

4.9. Statistic Analysis

Results are expressed as mean ± SD as indicated in the legends for measurement data. Comparisons were performed using one-way ANOVA with post-hoc in SPSS software. $p < 0.05$ was considered statistically significant.

Acknowledgments: We thank all the participants in our population study. This work was supported by the National Basic Research Program of the Chinese Ministry of Science and Technology (973 program) (Grant

No. 2013CB530700 and 2007CB512103); and the National Natural Science Foundation of China (NSFC Grant No. 81130003 and 81070262).

Author Contributions: Xiao-Li Tian supervised the study. Xiao-Li Tian, Yi-Hong Ren, Dao Wen Wang, Jie Du, Jian Guo and Yang Li participated in the study design. Yi-Hong Ren, Zhijun Sun and Yujun Xu performed sample collection and data management. Jian Guo and Yang Li conceived and designed the experiments; Jian Guo, Yang Li, Jie Dong, Han Yan, and Gu-Yan Zheng performed the experiments. Xiao-Li Tian, Jian Guo and Yang Li analyzed the data and wrote the manuscript. All authors read and contributed to the manuscript.

References

1. Watkins, H.; Farrall, M. Genetic susceptibility to coronary artery disease: From promise to progress. *Nat. Rev. Genet.* **2006**, *7*, 163–173. [CrossRef] [PubMed]

2. Hansson, G.K. Inflammation, atherosclerosis, and coronary artery disease. *N. Engl. J. Med.* **2005**, *352*, 1685–1695. [CrossRef] [PubMed]

3. Tian, X.L.; Li, Y. Endothelial cell senescence and age-related vascular diseases. *J. Genet. Genom.* **2014**, *41*, 485–495. [CrossRef] [PubMed]

4. Go, A.S.; Mozaffarian, D.; Roger, V.L.; Benjamin, E.J.; Berry, J.D.; Blaha, M.J.; Dai, S.; Ford, E.S.; Fox, C.S.; Franco, S.; et al. Heart disease and stroke statistics—2014 update: A report from the American Heart Association. *Circulation* **2014**, *129*. [CrossRef] [PubMed]

5. Ford, E.S.; Ajani, U.A.; Croft, J.B.; Critchley, J.A.; Labarthe, D.R.; Kottke, T.E.; Giles, W.H.; Capewell, S. Explaining the decrease in U.S. deaths from coronary disease, 1980–2000. *N. Engl. J. Med.* **2007**, *356*, 2388–2398. [CrossRef] [PubMed]

6. Schunkert, H.; Konig, I.R.; Kathiresan, S.; Reilly, M.P.; Assimes, T.L.; Holm, H.; Preuss, M.; Stewart, A.F.R.; Barbalic, M.; Gieger, C.; et al. Large-scale association analysis identifies 13 new susceptibility loci for coronary artery disease. *Nat. Genet.* **2011**, *43*, 333–338. [CrossRef] [PubMed]

7. Wang, F.; Xu, C.Q.; He, Q.; Cai, J.P.; Li, X.C.; Wang, D.; Xiong, X.; Liao, Y.H.; Zeng, Q.T.; Yang, Y.-Z.; et al. Genome-wide association identifies a susceptibility locus for coronary artery disease in the Chinese Han population. *Nat. Genet.* **2011**, *43*, 345–349. [CrossRef] [PubMed]

8. Lu, X.; Wang, L.; Chen, S.; He, L.; Yang, X.; Shi, Y.; Cheng, J.; Zhang, L.; Gu, C.C.; Huang, J.; et al. Genome-wide association study in Han Chinese identifies four new susceptibility loci for coronary artery disease. *Nat. Genet.* **2012**, *44*, 890–894. [CrossRef] [PubMed]

9. Lieb, W.; Vasan, R.S. Genetics of coronary artery disease. *Circulation* **2013**, *128*, 1131–1138. [CrossRef] [PubMed]

10. Roberts, R. Genetics of coronary artery disease. *Circ. Res.* **2014**, *114*, 1890–1903. [CrossRef] [PubMed]

11. Wang, L.; Fan, C.; Topol, S.E.; Topol, E.J.; Wang, Q. Mutation of MEF2A in an inherited disorder with features of coronary artery disease. *Science* **2003**, *302*, 1578–1581. [CrossRef] [PubMed]

12. Mani, A.; Radhakrishnan, J.; Wang, H.; Mani, A.; Mani, M.A.; Nelson-Williams, C.; Carew, K.S.; Mane, S.; Najmabadi, H.; Wu, D.; et al. *LRP6* mutation in a family with early coronary disease and metabolic risk factors. *Science* **2007**, *315*, 1278–1282. [CrossRef] [PubMed]

13. Kannel, W.B.; Dawber, T.R.; Kagan, A.; Revotskie, N.; Stokes, J., 3rd. Factors of risk in the development of coronary heart disease—Six year follow-up experience. The Framingham Study. *Ann. Intern. Med.* **1961**, *55*, 33–50. [CrossRef] [PubMed]

14. Thaker, A.M.; Frishman, W.H. Sortilin: The mechanistic link between genes, cholesterol, and coronary artery disease. *Cardiol. Rev.* **2014**, *22*, 91–96. [CrossRef] [PubMed]

15. Expert Panel on Detection, Evaluation, and Treatment of High Blood Cholesterol in Adults. Executive Summary of the Third Report of the National Cholesterol Education Program (NCEP) Expert Panel on Detection, Evaluation, and Treatment of High Blood Cholesterol in Adults (Adult Treatment Panel III). *J. Am. Med. Assoc.* **2001**, *285*, 2486–2497.

16. Grundy, S.M.; Cleeman, J.I.; Merz, C.N.; Brewer, H.B., Jr.; Clark, L.T.; Hunninghake, D.B.; Pasternak, R.C.; Smith, S.C.; Stone, N.J. Implications of recent clinical trials for the National Cholesterol Education Program Adult Treatment Panel III guidelines. *Circulation* **2004**, *110*, 227–239. [CrossRef] [PubMed]

17. Chernobelsky, A.; Ashen, M.D.; Blumenthal, R.S.; Coplan, N.L. High-density lipoprotein cholesterol: A potential therapeutic target for prevention of coronary artery disease. *Prev. Cardiol.* **2007**, *10*, 26–30. [CrossRef] [PubMed]

18. Ding, D.; Li, X.; Qiu, J.; Li, R.; Zhang, Y.; Su, D.; Li, Z.; Wang, M.; Lv, X.; Wang, D.; et al. Serum lipids, apolipoproteins, and mortality among coronary artery disease patients. *BioMed. Res. Int.* **2014**, *2014*, 709756. [CrossRef] [PubMed]

19. Rubins, H.B.; Robins, S.J.; Collins, D.; Iranmanesh, A.; Wilt, T.J.; Mann, D.; Mayo-Smith, M.; Faas, F.H.; Elam, M.B.; Rutan, G.H.; et al. Distribution of lipids in 8500 men with coronary artery disease. Department of Veterans Affairs HDL Intervention Trial Study Group. *Am. J. Cardiol.* **1995**, *75*, 1196–1201. [CrossRef]

20. Jguirim-Souissi, I.; Jelassi, A.; Hrira, Y.; Najah, M.; Slimani, A.; Addad, F.; Hassine, M.; Hamda, K.B.; Maatouk, F.; Rouis, M.; et al. +294T/C polymorphism in the PPAR-delta gene is associated with risk of coronary artery disease in normolipidemic Tunisians. *Genet. Mol. Res.* **2010**, *9*, 1326–1333. [CrossRef] [PubMed]

21. Xu, Y.; Gong, W.; Peng, J.; Wang, H.; Huang, J.; Ding, H.; Wang, D.W. Functional analysis *LRP6* novel mutations in patients with coronary artery disease. *PLoS ONE* **2014**, *9*, e84345. [CrossRef] [PubMed]

22. Singh, R.; Smith, E.; Fathzadeh, M.; Liu, W.; Go, G.W.; Subrahmanyan, L.; Faramarzi, S.; McKenna, W.; Mani, A. Rare nonconservative *LRP6* mutations are associated with metabolic syndrome. *Hum. Mutat.* **2013**, *34*, 1221–1225. [CrossRef] [PubMed]

23. Reidy, M.A.; Schwartz, S.M. Endothelial injury and regeneration. IV. Endotoxin: A nondenuding injury to aortic endothelium. *Lab. Investig.* **1983**, *48*, 25–34. [PubMed]

24. Caplan, B.A.; Schwartz, C.J. Increased endothelial cell turnover in areas of in vivo Evans Blue uptake in the pig aorta. *Atherosclerosis* **1973**, *17*, 401–417. [CrossRef]

25. Hansson, G.K.; Chao, S.; Schwartz, S.M.; Reidy, M.A. Aortic endothelial cell death and replication in normal and lipopolysaccharide-treated rats. *Am. J. Pathol.* **1985**, *121*, 123–127. [PubMed]

26. Langille, B.L.; Reidy, M.A.; Kline, R.L. Injury and repair of endothelium at sites of flow disturbances near abdominal aortic coarctations in rabbits. *Arteriosclerosis* **1986**, *6*, 146–154. [CrossRef] [PubMed]

27. Cines, D.B.; Pollak, E.S.; Buck, C.A.; Loscalzo, J.; Zimmerman, G.A.; McEver, R.P.; Pober, J.S.; Wick, T.M.; Konkle, B.A.; Schwartz, B.S.; et al. Endothelial cells in physiology and in the pathophysiology of vascular disorders. *Blood* **1998**, *91*, 3527–3561. [PubMed]

28. Walter, D.H.; Dimmeler, S. Endothelial progenitor cells: Regulation and contribution to adult neovascularization. *Herz* **2002**, *27*, 579–588. [CrossRef] [PubMed]

29. Iwakura, A.; Luedemann, C.; Shastry, S.; Hanley, A.; Kearney, M.; Aikawa, R.; Isner, J.M.; Asahara, T.; Losordo, D.W. Estrogen-mediated, endothelial nitric oxide synthase-dependent mobilization of bone marrow-derived endothelial progenitor cells contributes to reendothelialization after arterial injury. *Circulation* **2003**, *108*, 3115–3121. [CrossRef] [PubMed]

30. Werner, N.; Junk, S.; Laufs, U.; Link, A.; Walenta, K.; Bohm, M.; Nickenig, G. Intravenous transfusion of endothelial progenitor cells reduces neointima formation after vascular injury. *Circ. Res.* **2003**, *93*, e17–e24. [CrossRef] [PubMed]

31. Porto, I.; Leone, A.M.; De Maria, G.L.; Hamilton Craig, C.; Tritarelli, A.; Camaioni, C.; Natale, L.; Niccoli, G.; Biasucci, L.M.; Crea, F. Are endothelial progenitor cells mobilized by myocardial ischemia or myocardial necrosis? A cardiac magnetic resonance study. *Atherosclerosis* **2011**, *216*, 355–358. [CrossRef] [PubMed]

32. He, X.; Semenov, M.; Tamai, K.; Zeng, X. LDL receptor-related proteins 5 and 6 in Wnt/beta-catenin signaling: Arrows point the way. *Development* **2004**, *131*, 1663–1677. [CrossRef] [PubMed]

33. Cheng, Z.; Biechele, T.; Wei, Z.; Morrone, S.; Moon, R.T.; Wang, L.; Xu, W. Crystal structures of the extracellular domain of LRP6 and its complex with DKK1. *Nat. Struct. Mol. Biol.* **2011**, *18*, 1204–1210. [CrossRef] [PubMed]

34. Liu, W.; Mani, S.; Davis, N.R.; Sarrafzadegan, N.; Kavathas, P.B.; Mani, A. Mutation in EGFP domain of LDL receptor-related protein 6 impairs cellular LDL clearance. *Circ. Res.* **2008**, *103*, 1280–1288. [CrossRef] [PubMed]

35. Go, G.W.; Srivastava, R.; Hernandez-Ono, A.; Gang, G.; Smith, S.B.; Booth, C.J.; Ginsberg, H.N.; Mani, A. The combined hyperlipidemia caused by impaired Wnt-LRP6 signaling is reversed by Wnt3a rescue. *Cell Metab.* **2014**, *19*, 209–220. [CrossRef] [PubMed]

36. Brown, S.D.; Twells, R.C.; Hey, P.J.; Cox, R.D.; Levy, E.R.; Soderman, A.R.; Metzker, M.L.; Caskey, C.T.; Todd, J.A.; Hess, J.F. Isolation and characterization of *LRP6*, a novel member of the low density lipoprotein receptor gene family. *Biochem. Biophys. Res. Commun.* **1998**, *248*, 879–888. [CrossRef] [PubMed]

37. Bafico, A.; Liu, G.; Yaniv, A.; Gazit, A.; Aaronson, S.A. Novel mechanism of Wnt signalling inhibition mediated by Dickkopf-1 interaction with LRP6/Arrow. *Nat. Cell Biol.* **2001**, *3*, 683–686. [CrossRef] [PubMed]

38. Samarzija, I.; Sini, P.; Schlange, T.; Macdonald, G.; Hynes, N.E. Wnt3a regulates proliferation and migration of HUVEC via canonical and non-canonical Wnt signaling pathways. *Biochem. Biophys. Res. Commun.* **2009**, *386*, 449–454. [CrossRef] [PubMed]

39. Okumura, N.; Nakamura, T.; Kay, E.P.; Nakahara, M.; Kinoshita, S.; Koizumi, N. R-spondin1 regulates cell proliferation of corneal endothelial cells via the Wnt3a/β-catenin pathway. *Investig. Ophthalmol. Vis. Sci.* **2014**, *55*, 6861–6869. [CrossRef] [PubMed]

40. De Jesus Perez, V.A.; Alastalo, T.P.; Wu, J.C.; Axelrod, J.D.; Cooke, J.P.; Amieva, M.; Rabinovitch, M. Bone morphogenetic protein 2 induces pulmonary angiogenesis via Wnt-beta-catenin and Wnt-RhoA-Rac1 pathways. *J. Cell Biol.* **2009**, *184*, 83–99. [CrossRef] [PubMed]

41. Ren, S.; Johnson, B.G.; Kida, Y.; Ip, C.; Davidson, K.C.; Lin, S.L.; Kobayashi, A.; Lang, R.A.; Hadjantonakis, A.-K.; Moon, R.T.; et al. LRP-6 is a coreceptor for multiple fibrogenic signaling pathways in pericytes and myofibroblasts that are inhibited by DKK-1. *Proc. Natl. Acad. Sci. USA* **2013**, *110*, 1440–1445. [CrossRef] [PubMed]

42. Lieb, W.; Mayer, B.; Konig, I.R.; Borwitzky, I.; Gotz, A.; Kain, S.; Hengstenberg, C.; Linsel-Nitschke, P.; Fischer, M.; Döring, A.; et al. Lack of association between the *MEF2A* gene and myocardial infarction. *Circulation* **2008**, *117*, 185–191. [CrossRef] [PubMed]

43. Jiang, F.; Dong, Y.; Wu, C.; Yang, X.; Zhao, L.; Guo, J.; Li, Y.; Dong, J.; Zheng, G.-Y.; Cao, H.; et al. Fine mapping of chromosome 3q22.3 identifies two haplotype blocks in ESYT3 associated with coronary artery disease in female Han Chinese. *Atherosclerosis* **2011**, *218*, 397–403. [CrossRef] [PubMed]

44. Li, Y.; Wang, W.J.; Cao, H.; Lu, J.; Wu, C.; Hu, F.Y.; Guo, J.; Zhao, L.; Yang, F.; Zhang, Y.-X.; et al. Genetic association of *FOXO1A* and *FOXO3A* with longevity trait in Han Chinese populations. *Hum. Mol. Genet.* **2009**, *18*, 4897–4904. [CrossRef] [PubMed]

45. Yang, F.; Zhou, L.; Wang, Q.; You, X.; Li, Y.; Zhao, Y.; Han, X.; Chang, Z.; He, X.; Cheng, C.; et al. NEXN inhibits GATA4 and leads to atrial septal defects in mice and humans. *Cardiovasc. Res.* **2014**, *103*, 228–237. [CrossRef] [PubMed]

46. Tian, X.L.; Paul, M. Species-specific splicing and expression of angiotensin converting enzyme. *Biochem. Pharmacol.* **2003**, *66*, 1037–1044. [CrossRef]

47. Hu, F.Y.; Wu, C.; Li, Y.; Xu, K.; Wang, W.J.; Cao, H.; Tian, X.-L. AGGF1 is a novel anti-inflammatory factor associated with TNF-α-induced endothelial activation. *Cell Signal.* **2013**, *25*, 1645–1653. [CrossRef] [PubMed]

48. Yan, G.; Chen, S.; You, B.; Sun, J. Activation of sphingosine kinase-1 mediates induction of endothelial cell proliferation and angiogenesis by epoxyeicosatrienoic acids. *Cardiovasc. Res.* **2008**, *78*, 308–314. [CrossRef] [PubMed]

49. Matsuda, N.; Takano, Y.; Kageyama, S.; Hatakeyama, N.; Shakunaga, K.; Kitajima, I.; Yamazaki, M.; Hattori, Y. Silencing of caspase-8 and caspase-3 by RNA interference prevents vascular endothelial cell injury in mice with endotoxic shock. *Cardiovasc. Res.* **2007**, *76*, 132–140. [CrossRef] [PubMed]

15

Vasa Vasorum in Atherosclerosis and Clinical Significance

Junyan Xu [1,†], Xiaotong Lu [1,†] and Guo-Ping Shi [1,2,*]

[1] Second Clinical Medical College, Zhujiang Hospital and Southern Medical University, Guangzhou 510280, China; junyanxu_zj@126.com (J.X.); lxt0115@126.com (X.L.)

[2] Department of Medicine, Brigham and Women's Hospital and Harvard Medical School, Boston, MA 02115, USA

* Correspondence: gshi@rics.bwh.harvard.edu;

† These authors contributed equally to this work.

Academic Editor: Michael Henein

Abstract: Atherosclerosis is a chronic inflammatory disease that leads to several acute cardiovascular complications with poor prognosis. For decades, the role of the adventitial vasa vasorum (VV) in the initiation and progression of atherosclerosis has received broad attention. The presence of VV neovascularization precedes the apparent symptoms of clinical atherosclerosis. VV also mediates inflammatory cell infiltration, intimal thickening, intraplaque hemorrhage, and subsequent atherothrombosis that results in stroke or myocardial infarction. Intraplaque neovessels originating from VV can be immature and hence susceptible to leakage, and are thus regarded as the leading cause of intraplaque hemorrhage. Evidence supports VV as a new surrogate target of atherosclerosis evaluation and treatment. This review provides an overview into the relationship between VV and atherosclerosis, including the anatomy and function of VV, the stimuli of VV neovascularization, and the available underlying mechanisms that lead to poor prognosis. We also summarize translational researches on VV imaging modalities and potential therapies that target VV neovascularization or its stimuli.

Keywords: atherosclerosis; vasa vasorum; neovascularization; mechanism; imaging modality; angiogenic therapy

1. Introduction

Atherosclerosis is a systemic inflammatory disease that associates with several acute cardiovascular complications triggered by atherosclerotic plaque rupture, which primarily manifests as stroke and myocardial infarction. It remains the leading cause of morbidity and mortality worldwide [1]. Considering its poor prognosis, understanding the pathophysiology of atherosclerosis and exploring potential means to discover populations at risk as well as preventing its progression remain of significant importance. For decades, postmortem evaluations have concluded that the main characteristics of rupture-prone vulnerable plaques include a thin fibrous cap, high lipid content, increased numbers of inflammatory cells, and extensive adventitial and intimal neovascularization [2–5]. Though much emphasis has been placed on intimal accumulation of lipids and inflammatory cells, recent research suggests that the adventitia vasa vasorum (VV) also plays a critical role in transforming advanced but stable lesions into vulnerable plaques at risk for rupture.

VV are defined as small blood vessels that supply or drain the walls of larger arteries and veins, delivering nutrients and oxygen as well as removing systemic "waste" products [6]. The association between VV and atherosclerotic plaque formation was first reported in 1876 by Koster [7]. Later in the 1930s, the rich vascular channels surrounding and penetrating atherosclerotic lesions, namely VV, were suspected as the source of the plaque hemorrhages for the first time [8,9]. However, the role of VV in atherosclerosis did not attract sufficient attention until half a century later when it was hypothesized that the adventitial VV of coronary arteries allowed atherosclerotic plaques to develop beyond a critical thickness by supplying oxygen and nutrients to the core of the lesions [10]. Since then, numerous studies have demonstrated the relationship between VV neovascularization and atherogenic processes. Retrospective studies on autopsies derived from humans noted that VV density was significantly increased in plaques categorized as vulnerable and prone to rupture as was those in hypercholesterolemic animal models [11,12]. In humans, it was reported that more than 80% of VV neovascularization in coronary atherosclerotic plaques had weak integrity, resulting in leakage and subsequent plaque hemorrhage [13,14]. Increased VV also associated with intimal thickening and endothelial dysfunction in animal models, and these effects could be blocked with angiogenic inhibitors [15,16]. Growing evidence supports that vascular inflammation, a crucial factor in the process of atherosclerosis, is initiated in the adventitia, and extensive inflammatory cell infiltration has been observed in the adventitial neovascular network [17]. The critical role of VV in the process of atherosclerosis has been established and identified as an independent predictor of intraplaque hemorrhage and plaque rupture. As a consequence, imaging modalities were developed to visualize VV neovascularization in the early stage of atherosclerosis. Therapies targeted to VV have emerged as a new approach for the treatment of atherosclerosis.

2. Structure and Function of Vasa Vasorum

2.1. Structure

Human VV occurs as early as the first week of gestation under an X-ray microscope, and along with the lumen blood supplement, nourishes the vessel wall [18]. VV exists mainly in the adventitial and outer medial layers of the blood vessels with more than 29 medial lamellar units or 0.5 mm lumen diameters [19]. Normal vessels in mice and intramyocardial vessels in humans do not contain VV [6].

Three different types of VV have been identified in bovine aortic walls: the VV externae (VVE), the VV internae (VVI), and the venous VV (VVV). VVE originate from major branches and the VVI originate from the main lumen of the aorta. The VVV drain the arterial wall into companion veins [20]. Direct visualizations of VV in porcine coronary arteries confirmed the coexistence of VVE, VVI, and VVV [21]. VV are often used to refer to VVE in literature because more than 96% of the newly formed microvessels in atherosclerosis sprout from VV in the adventitia and only a small part extend from the vessel lumen [22,23].

High-resolution micro-computed tomography (micro-CT) displayed a more precise VV structure. This technique demonstrated that VV originate from the coronary artery branch and run longitudinally along the vessel wall (first-order VV) and branch to form a circumferential plexus around the main coronary lumen (second-order VV) (Figure 1). Normal hearts had significantly greater first-order than second-order VV density (ratio 3:2), while the second-order vessel density was twofold greater than the first in hypercholesterolemic hearts [12]. Furthermore, while VV branching architecture in non-diseased porcine vasculature showed a dichotomous tree structure similar to the vasculature of systemic circulation structure, VV in diseased arteries presented many more disorganized images [21].

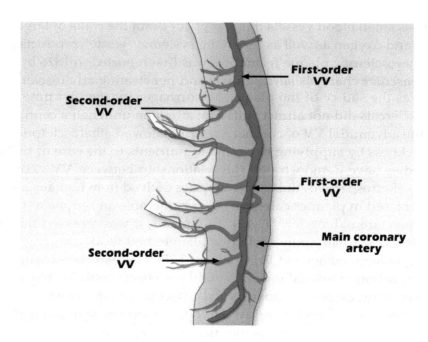

Figure 1. Scheme of first-order VV, second-order VV, and main coronary artery.

In atherosclerosis, previous work demonstrated that VV neovessels were immature, irregular, fragile, and prone to extravasation, particularly among those close to the atherosclerotic plaques [24,25]. Plaque neovessels showed poor coverage with mural cells and compromised structural integrity under electron microscopy, including abnormal endothelial cells (ECs), membrane blebs, intracytoplasmic vacuoles, open EC-EC junctions, and basement membrane (BM) detachment. When the mural cells are absent in either normal or atherosclerotic arteries, compromised structural integrity may cause leakage of the intraplaque microvessels [14]. Indeed, insufficient smooth muscle cell (SMC) coating in aberrant intraplaque vessels was observed in symptomatic patients when compared with asymptomatic patients [13].

2.2. Function

Rather than merely existing as a structural network, VV are recognized as functional end arteries that exist throughout the body [26,27]. Previous experiments demonstrate their ability to provide oxygen and nourishment to the outer third of the vascular media. Using probes to detect the diffusion of oxygen from the luminal or abluminal side of the canine femoral artery wall, the oxygen level was highest in the outer layers of the vessel wall and decreased as the probe gradually approached the lumen [28]. A more precise experiment by direct measurement of the oxygenation of the arterial wall showed the lowest level of oxygen tension of approximately 10 mmHg at about 300 μm from the lumen [29]. The varying oxygen levels between the inner and outer layers indicate that VV are the primary source of oxygen supply to the adventitia and outer media.

Along with their blood perfusion, the active exchange between VV and parent vessels meets the nutritional demands of the vessel wall and removes the "waste" products, either produced by intramural cells or introduced by diffusional transport through the luminal endothelium [6]. It is worth mentioning that VV also undertakes lipid transportation into the parent vessel wall in rabbit aorta [30], underlying a role of VV in progression of lipid core enlargement. It was also speculated that VV can regulate their own tone and vascular perfusion because the proximal VV form a regularly layered vascular structure of ECs, vascular smooth muscle cells (VSMCs), and surrounding connective tissue [31]. VV dissected from porcine and canine aorta are able to contract and dilate when exposed to endothelin-1 (ET-1) and several other vasodilators [32,33]. VV also participates in restoring the injured vessels [34] and thus are involved in several pathological conditions, including atherosclerosis, abdominal aortic aneurysm (AAA), and pulmonary artery hypertension. In fact, VV were described as "rich vascular channels surrounding and penetrating sclerotic lesions" via injecting India ink into the coronary artery wall, suggesting a role of VV in promoting atherogenesis [35]. Prior evidence suggests that VV neovascularization is a simple reaction that helps meet the demands of the intima and inner layers of the media in response to decreased oxygen concentration and malnourishment. This process gravitates towards preserving the integrity of atherosclerotic plaques. In advanced stages of atherosclerosis, however, the newly formed microvessels become important channels for various inflammatory cells and enable cellular migration to the intima, therefore becoming detrimental to the plaque integrity [36]. Plaques with a high density of neovessels are at a higher risk of hemorrhage, expansion, atherothrombosis, and rupture. As the channels conveying erythrocytes, lipids and inflammatory cells, VV neovessels seem to be multifaceted in atherosclerosis.

3. Stimuli of Vasa Vasorum Neovascularization

VV neovascularization is essential to atherogenesis. Metal cannulae-tied transparent visualization of human heart coronary arteries established an association of VV in atherosclerosis progression and associated sequelae [10]. High-fat diet-fed monkeys with atherosclerosis experienced blood flow from VV to the intima-media that was 10 times greater than monkeys on a normal diet. Reduced blood flow in VV directly associated with atherosclerosic lesion regression in monkeys [37]. Since these earlier pioneering studies, accumulating evidence has proven the role of VV neovascularization in both the initiation and progression of atherosclerosis, although many observations in VV neovascularization initiation and stimulation still remain incompletely understood. The extent and distribution of the ectopic neovascularization within the arterial wall depend on a number of physiological and pathological factors.

3.1. Hypoxia

Hypoxia and its role in the progression of VV neovascularization have been broadly studied in both cardiovascular and pulmonary arteries. Atherosclerosis, AAA, pulmonary artery hypertension, and many other systemic/pulmonary vascular diseases closely relate to hypoxia and its secondary complications [38,39]. Many factors contribute to the generation of a hypoxia environment.

Intimal thickening is an immediate element that causes hypoxia and the most prominent feature of atherosclerosis throughout the lesion initiation, progression, and ultimate rupture [40,41]. Insufficient arterial oxygen supply due to intimal thickening may shorten oxygen and nutrient diffusion distance between the deep layer of the intima and the luminal surface, resulting in regional hypoxia, ischemic injury of the inner arterial wall, and the eventual induction of VV neovascularization [42]. Increased intimal thickening and plaque growth will enhance the area and degree of hypoxia. Meanwhile, decreased oxygen supply and nourishment of the vessel wall can also originate from the changes VV undergo. As functional end arteries, VV are especially vulnerable to hypoxia [43]. An important consequence of the architecture of VV is that the blood supply cannot reach far enough from the adventitia into the media due to the pressure within the arterial wall, according to Lamé's Law [44]. Several risk factors affect VV blood flow and lesion hypoxia. Aging, compression, or hypertension inevitably increase the arterial vessel tensile force and interfere with VV blood circulation to the inner layers, leading to low oxygen concentration in VV capillaries [6]. Smoking or nicotine inhalation is another known risk factor that contracts the peripheral arteries, thereby reducing the peripheral blood flow as well as blood flow in VV. All these risk factors are common among patients with atherosclerosis. Therefore, poor blood supply from VV induces a hypoxia environment in the intima and part of the media. An increase of lesion oxygen consumption is another risk factor of hypoxia. An active metabolic process within the cholesterol-containing macrophages and foam cells in the lesions contribute to hypoxia by increasing oxygen consumption. Björnrheden et al. [45] demonstrated that oxygen consumption was increased in foam cells isolated from the aortic intima-media in atherosclerotic rabbits. Further experiments confirmed that hypoxia correlated with the presence of macrophages and angiogenesis in advanced human carotid plaques, suggesting that hypoxia depended more on the high metabolic demand of lesion inflammatory cells than the vessel wall thickness [46]. Therefore, impaired oxygen diffusion capacity due to intimal thickness, reduced VV blood circulation, and increased oxygen consumption in atherosclerosis together generate an oxygen-insufficient microenvironment.

As a compensatory reaction to the hypoxia, VV tend to sprout across the arterial wall toward the vessel lumen to support the inner layers, called lumenward, according to Zemplenyi *et al.* [42]. In balloon-injured arteries, in which the oxygen supply in the arterial wall is impaired, newly formed VV may compensate the shortage of oxygen supply [46,47]. Spatial VV contents were increased from the dense microvessel network in the adventitia and extended to plaques in the presence of atherosclerosis [48,49]. There was an inverse correlation between low VV contents and decreased oxygenation (*i.e.*, increased expression of hypoxia-inducible factor (HIF)-1α) and increased oxidative stress (*i.e.*, increased superoxide production) within the coronary vessels in atherosclerotic pigs [50]. Additionally, prior studies suggest the signaling pathway of hypoxia-induced angiogenesis is mediated partially via regulating the production of HIF and its downstream factors. HIF is a key regulator of atherosclerosis. It affects multiple pathological events in atherogenesis, including foam cell formation, cellular proliferation, plaque ulceration, lesion hemorrhage, and rupture [51]. HIF-1 is considered the most interrelated factor of the angiogenic process in atherosclerosis. It is a basic helix-loop-helix heterodimer containing HIF-1α and HIF-1β that activates the transcription of hypoxia-inducible genes, such as erythropoietin, vascular endothelial growth factor (VEGF), E26 transformation-specific-1 (Ets-1), heme oxygenase-1 (HO1), inducible nitric oxide synthase (iNOS), and the glycolytic enzyme aldolase A [52,53]. Among them, VEGF and Ets-1 are important regulators of hypoxia-induced angiogenesis via regulating the biology of ECs.

The VEGF family has potent mitogenic and promigratory actions specific for ECs, leading to the conversion to angiogenic phenotypes, which link tightly to neovessel development in both physiological and pathophysiological conditions [54]. VEGF-A is the major subtype of the VEGF family and plays a pivotal role in the induction of neovessels through binding and primarily activating the VEGF receptor type-2 (VEGFR-2, also called KDR or Flk-1) [55]. VEGF acts as a hypoxia-inducible factor [56]. In hypertensive rat aorta, the expressions of VEGF and HIF-1α change concurrently and associate with arterial VV formation. Such a relationship was also reported in atherosclerotic lesions [57]. VEGFR-3 is a receptor for VEGF-C and VEGF-D [58,59]. Although the current consensus is that VEGFR-3 is expressed restrictedly in lymphatic vessels and can induce lymphatic EC proliferation [60,61], an underlying relationship between VEGFR-3 and VV has also been proposed. Immunostaining demonstrated the existence of VEGFR-3 in the VV of the adult aorta and other fenestrated blood vessels in human tissues, such as bone marrow, splenic and hepatic sinusoids, kidney glomeruli, and endocrine glands [62]. In human aortas, VEGF-D is constitutively expressed in normal, fatty streak, and atherosclerotic lesions, as confirmed by both immunostainings and *in situ* hybridization. In atherosclerotic lesions, VEGFR-2 is expressed in SMCs and ECs from the intima, media, and adventitia, whereas VEGFR-3 mainly exists in ECs from the adventitia, which is rich in neovascularization. The VEGF-D/VEGFR-2 cascade was probably the prominent trigger in promoting atherosclerotic plaque neovascularization [63]. From a different study, immunostaining located VEGFR-2 to the luminal endothelium in human atherosclerotic lesions, whereas VEGFR-3 was expressed in SMCs from the media and adventitia, but not in the luminal endothelium [64]. Two studies showed different expression patterns of VEGFR-3 in human atherosclerosis lesions, suggesting that VEGFR-3 has functions other than neovascularization. In a mouse atherosclerosis model, transgenic expression of soluble VEGFR-3 or its mutant did not affect atherosclerotic lesion adventitial VV density, but nearly completely blocked the lymphoid vessel growth, leading to increased plasma cholesterol and triglyceride levels and enhanced atherosclerosis [65]. These studies suggest that VEGFR-3 contributes to atherosclerosis by interacting with VV in addition to lymphoid vessels.

Evidence shows that the Ets transcription factor regulates the expression of matrix metalloproteinase (*MMP*) genes, which are related to the essential steps in angiogenesis and tumor invasion (extracellular matrix degradation and vascular EC migration) [66]. Hypoxia induces Ets-1 expression via the activity of HIF-1 [53], likely via the hypoxia-responsive element (HRE) located at the Ets promoter. In addition to inducing protease expression, Ets-1 also influences angiogenesis by enhancing the transcription of hepatocyte growth factor (HGF) and VEGF, and forming an auto-loop of their upregulation [67]. It is speculated that the role of Ets-1 in atherosclerosis may have the same activities. Indeed, HIF-1, VEGF, and Ets-1 were all expressed in 29 human carotid plaques obtained from carotid endarterectomy [68]. Hypoxia-induced HIF-1a/VEGF/Ets-1 cascade was suggested as important for angiogenesis in human atherosclerosis. Nevertheless, the connections among these hypoxia-induced angiogenesic pathways still remain unclear. For example, in contrast to the studies discussed above, acidic fibroblast growth factor (FGF), basic fibroblast growth factor (bFGF), VEGF, and epidermal growth factor all induce the expression of Ets-1 mRNA in ECs [69,70], suggesting that multiple mechanisms can contribute to hypoxia-induced angiogenesis. Therefore, whether VEGF and Ets play an independent role in the process of VV neovascularization, or act synergistically with other growth factors, merits further investigation (Figure 2).

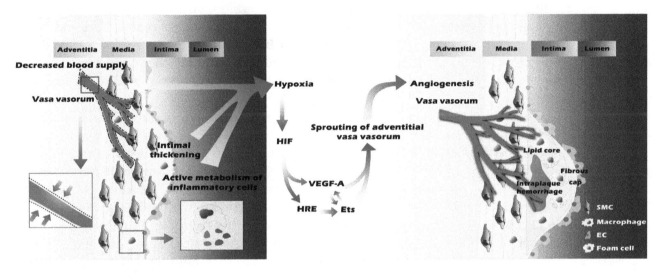

Figure 2. Intimal thickening, decreased blood supply (due to high pressure in parent vessel and the stimulated constriction of VV, represented by grey arrows in the left closed box) and active metabolism of inflammatory cells together contribute to hypoxia in atherosclerotic vessels (**left** panel). The oxygen-insufficient microenvironment in inner layers of vessel wall further induces angiogenesis through activating HIF, VEGF-A and Ets signaling pathways. As a result, the formation of intraplaque neovessels originating from VV leads to the progression of atherosclerotic plaques, including intraplaque hemorrhage, lipid core enlargement, inflammatory cell infiltration, and ultimate rupture (**right** panel).

3.2. Inflammation

Systemic atherosclerosis, parenchymal inflammation and VV neovascularization are inseparably linked. There are two main hypotheses for the initiation of vascular inflammation. The traditional concept of vascular inflammation includes "inside-out" responses centered on the monocyte adhesion and lipid oxidation hypotheses. However, growing evidence supports a new paradigm of an "outside-in" hypothesis, in which vascular inflammation is initiated in the adventitia and progresses inward toward the intima [17]. Although the initiation of vascular inflammation is still up for debate, VV neovascularization is no doubt triggered and perpetuated by inflammatory reactions within the vascular wall [71]. In fact, the role of inflammation in neovessel formation was proposed decades ago [72]. VV neovascularization occurs most prevalently at the sites of the intima that contain chronic inflammatory cell infiltration, especially the macrophages and lymphocytes. Furthermore, inflammatory cytokines, growth factors, and angiogenic stimuli, which are released by activated inflammatory cells (e.g., macrophages), can enhance not only the inflammation itself but also the development of VV neovascularization [73]. Some studies suggest that vascular inflammation in atherosclerotic lesions closely associates with cell metabolism-created hypoxia, microvascularization, hemorrhage formation, and plaque rupture [74]. However, the exact mechanisms of the inflammation-induced angiogenesis remain unknown.

3.3. Lipids

The role of lipids in atherosclerosis is an old topic. Several types of lipid complex or lipid-containing substances have been reported in atheromatous lesions, including modified oxidized-LDL, 7-ketocholesterol (7KCh), cholesterol (such as low-density lipoprotein LDL, high-density lipoprotein HDL, and triglyceride), soluble phospholipids, and eicosanoids [75,76]. These lipid complexes or lipid-containing products can be present in the circulation, released from dead foam cells, or exist on the blood cell membrane. High levels of circulating LDL remain a profound risk factor in predicting cardiovascular events. Circulating LDL is an important source of atherosclerotic plaque lipid content and contributes to atherosclerosis progression, such as lipid deposition/foam cell formation and associated inflammatory process [77]. As the disease progresses, lipid-laden foam cells undergo apoptosis and release free cholesterols, leading to the formation of necrotic cores full of lipids [78]. Studies of red blood cell membrane components present another conceivable origin of lipids in atherosclerosis [79]. Taken together, atherosclerotic plaque is recognized as a reservoir of lipid complexes.

VV neovascularization begins at the radial projection at the site of lipid retention [80]. It provides atherosclerotic lesions with blood as well as lipids [81]. Hypoxia may not be the only factor responsible for medial VSMC proliferation or activation due to the restricted hypoxia in intimal lesions [40]. Therefore, experts hypothesize that VV neovascularization may be lipid-dependent. Indeed, intima-borne lipid promotes angiogenesis by activating VSMC PPAR-γ receptors [76]. Conditioned medium from early atheromatous lesions was enriched in oxidized lipid 15-Deoxy-δ-12, 14-prostaglandin J2, and their derivatives. These naturally occurring compounds activate the PPAR-γ pathway in subjacent medial VSMCs [82]. In pace with PPAR-γ activation, the expression of VEGF-A was upregulated in VSMCs, leading to neovascularization. Cholesterol efflux also regulates angiogenesis via the modulation of lipid rafts and VEGFR-2 signaling in ECs. The decline of the lipid rafts results in lower VEGFR-2 contents on the cell membrane, which leads to the down-regulation of VEGFR signaling and culminates in the inhibition of VEGF-stimulated angiogenesis [83]. This might be an entirely new hypothesis to interpret the modulation of the lipid-mediated angiogenic process. These results were all based on the model of dyslipidemia zebrafish, which might be a better model for the study and evaluation of the early development of atherosclerosis. Besides the aforementioned VEGF-dependent mechanism of angiogenesis, the VEGF-independent pathway also contributes to the angiogenesis in vascular disease. Polyunsaturated fatty acid (PUFA), which is prone to oxidation, is capable of activating the Toll-like receptor 2 (TLR2)/MyD88 pathway after oxidation. This leads to the activation of Rac1 to promote NF-κB signaling, causing cell migration and neovascularization [84,85]. Nevertheless, more mechanisms may come to explain VV neovascularization and each mechanism may not be independent but instead may regulate each other.

Growing evidence indicates that the perivascular adipose tissue (PVAT) associates with the inflammatory process in atherosclerosis. PVAT interacts directly with the outer adventitia without fascia or elastic lamina and is capable of conveying signaling molecules (adipokines and cytokines) to the adjacent blood vessels [86]. VV, which penetrate the PVAT, are highly prone to change. Conditioned medium from differentiated murine 3T3-L1 adipocytes concentration-dependently stimulates human saphenous vein and aortic SMC proliferation. There was an about 206% ± 21% increase of SMC proliferation in the vein and 145% ± 9% SMC proliferation increase in the aorta at the highest concentration (100 μL/mL) used, while such an effect was not observed in conditioned medium from premature or undifferentiated adipocytes [87]. Experts concur that adipokines such as visfatin and leptin are the stimuli in SMC proliferation and migration [88]. Compared with conditioned medium from differentiated human subcutaneous and perirenal adipocytes, conditioned medium from differentiated human perivascular adipocytes showed a much stronger ability to induce angiogenesis (elongation and branching) when applied to human coronary artery ECs, consistent with the elevated (two-fold) expression of VEGF in perivascular adipocytes [89]. In advanced stages of atherosclerosis, neovessels were suspected as the conduit for transporting pro/anti-inflammatory mediators into the vascular wall from PVAT. However, since adipocytes are heterogenous in different tissues and even PVAT are biologically and functionally diverse surrounding different blood vessels [90], a detailed relationship between different PVAT locations and properties remain to be tested.

4. Factors Leading to Immature and Fragile Vasa Vasorum

Although VV neovascularization is generally recognized as a compensatory reaction to meet the oxygen and nutritional demand of the inner layer of the vascular wall, intraplaque neovascularization meanwhile gives rise to ensuring plaque destabilization, intraplaque hemorrhage (IPH), atherothrombosis and even ultimate plaque rupture. As mentioned, intraplaque VV are immature, irregular, fragile, and prone to extravasation due to the compromised structural integrity. Different hypotheses have been proposed to explain this immaturity and leakage in varying stages and timescales in atherosclerosis.

4.1. Imbalance of Angiogenic Factors in Proteolytic Environment

Atherosclerotic plaque contains a wide spectrum of proteolytic proteases, including metalloproteinases (*i.e.*, MMPs), serine proteases (e.g., elastase, coagulation factors, plasmin, tissue-type plasminogen activator and urokinase-type plasminogen activator), and cysteine proteases (e.g., cathepsins) [91]. Previous studies have demonstrated their tight correlation to the pathophysiology of atherosclerosis, in particular, concerning the plaque destabilization. The MMP family is involved in intraplaque angiogenesis and plaque instability. Increased expression of MMP-1, -2, -3, and -9 was detected in atherosclerotic plaques [92]. Urokinase-type plasminogen activator receptor (UPAR) expression was 1.4-fold higher in macrophages and 1.5-fold higher in carotid endarterectomies from Caucasian patients with symptomatic carotid stenosis, compared to the control group [93]. In unstable plaques, increased legumain was detected and converted cathepsin L to its mature 25 kDa form, leading to the intraplaque angiogenesis, macrophages apoptosis, and necrotic core formation [94,95].

In human carotid endarterectomy samples, the levels of placental growth factor (PlGF), VEGF, and angiopoietin-1 (Ang-1) were significantly decreased in culprit plaques/hemorrhagic when compared with culprit plaques/non-hemorrhagic, but both were higher than those from the normal control group. Soluble Tie-2 (receptor of Ang-1 and Ang-2) levels were also increased in the hemorrhagic lesions, although Ang-2 levels were similar between hemorrhagic and non-hemorrhagic lesions [96]. These results suggested an angiogenic/anti-angiogenic imbalance in hemorrhagic plaques. Since the normal formation of neovessels requires a precise regulation to maintain the balance between angiogenic and anti-angiogenic factors, the disturbed balance in hemorrhagic plaques may impede the maturity and structural integrity of intraplaque neovessels.

Previous studies revealed a significant increase in plasmin and leucocyte elastase activities in hemorrhagic plaques [97]. These proteases may degrade these angiogenic factors in hemorrhagic plaques, resulting in angiogenic/anti-angiogenic imbalance and potential neovessel immaturity. VEGF promotes the initiation of immature vessels by vasculogenesis or angiogenic sprouting. Paracrine Ang-1 stabilizes the interactions between ECs and their surrounding support cells (SMCs and pericytes) and extracellular matrix (ECM) via binding to the Tie 2 receptor on the EC surface. Autocrine Ang-2, considered as an antagonist for Tie 2, has adverse effects, leading to vascular regression or angiogenic sensitivity (more plastic and destabilized state) [98]. Alteration of Ang-1/Ang-2 influences the normal process of neovessel formation. Although a shift of Ang-1/Ang-2 ratio was observed in several pathological processes, such as brain arteriovenous malformations [99] and tumor microvessel development [100], its role in atherosclerosis remains largely unknown. The imbalance between Ang-1 and Ang-2 in atherosclerosis may be a major deterrent to neovessel maturation. Decreased activity of Ang-1 and the ratio between Ang-1 and Ang-2 levels biased towards Ang-2 were observed in atherosclerotic plaques along with high microvessel content [101]. This is consistent with the observation that plaques with high microvessel density are at a high risk of intraplaque hemorrhage [102]. In addition, the Ang-1/Ang-2 ratio in favor of Ang-2 was also observed in hemorrhagic plaques, indicating an underlying role of angiopoietin/Tie system in microvessel immaturity [96].

Therefore, angiogenesis may depend on a precise balance of positive and negative regulations. The angiogenic and anti-angiogenic factors act in coordination to form well-structured and functional vessels. A disorder of homeostasis in VV neovascularization influences the proliferation and migration of ECs and their surrounding support cells, thereby leading to compromised structural integrity and aberrant neovessel formation. However, angiogenic factors can be regulated at the levels of both expression and proteolytic degradation. It remains unknown how these angiogenic factors are regulated in VV neovascularization during atherogenesis, a possible focus of future studies.

4.2. Further Exacerbation of Neovessel Damage: Iron, Cholesterol Crystal and Proteases

Angiogenic/anti-angiogenic imbalance inherently leads to the extravasation of vessel wall. Iron, cholesterol crystal, and protease activity may cause further exacerbation of neovessel damage, which also facilitates the permeability of intraplaque microvessels. Iron is abundant in the human body, especially in erythrocytes. Differing from normal erythrocytes, erythrocytes in atherosclerotic plaques are prone to undergo rapid lysis to release a large quantity of hemoglobin (Hb) [103]. Extracellular Hb remains susceptible to morphing into ferrihemoglobin via oxidation, and releases heme that contains abundant redox active iron. Redox active iron plays a detrimental role in oxidation reactions *in vivo*, including lipid oxidation. Oxidized LDL from atherosclerosis is cytotoxic to ECs [104,105]. High expression of ferritin and heme oxygenase-1 that control the redox active iron and degraded heme demonstrate a protective compensatory reaction from iron-derived vascular injury [106,107]. Diaspirin cross-linked Hb (DBBF-Hb) and polyethylene glycol (PEG)-conjugated Hb, proposed as blood substitutes, proved to increase arterial microvascular permeability [108]. Therefore, erythrocyte-derived iron may induce vascular damages, establishing a role for heme iron-dependent oxidation in damaging intraplaque immature microvessels. Apart from erythrocyte-derived iron, several other mechanisms, which are not mutually exclusive, have been proposed as underlying causes of vessel injury within plaques, including perforation of microvessels by cholesterol crystals [109] and direct damage induced by protease activity [110].

5. Vasa Vasorum Imaging in Atherosclerosis Plaques

Atherothrombosis resulted from plaque rupture is the direct cause of several acute cardiovascular complications (e.g., stroke, myocardial infarction). Therefore, practical imaging systems for early detection of unstable or even asymptomatic atherosclerotic plaques are urgently needed. Angiographic studies showed that non-obstructive plaques caused approximately 75% of cases with acute coronary occlusion [111]. Therefore, traditional focus on the stenosis of atherosclerotic plaque may be not sufficient to predict vulnerable plaques, thereby forcing us to explore more detailed features of possible culprit plaques, such as the fibrous cap, a lipid-rich necrotic core, signs of inflammation, and VV neovascularization. Visualization of arterial VV and intraplaque neovessels has recently emerged as a new surrogate marker for the early detection of atherosclerotic lesions. Coronary VV neovascularization occurs within the first week of experimental hypercholesterolemia, prior to the development of endothelial dysfunction of the host vessel, suggesting the significance of VV visualization in the identification of atherosclerotic vascular disease in the early stage [16]. Thus, a safe, non-invasive, and affordable imaging technique for the detection of VV has important clinical significance.

5.1. Anatomic Imaging of Vasa Vasorum in Atherosclerosis

Differences in VV structure between normal and atherosclerotic arteries were first detected by autopsy cinematography. The 3D anatomy and tree-like branching architecture of VV are shown in Figure 1. Efforts have been focused on identifying not only diseased and non-diseased arteries, but also stable and unstable plaques among risky populations through anatomic imaging.

Growing evidence confirming the role of VV neovascularization in atherosclerosis is provided first by micro-CT. With micro-CT, increased VV contents in the proximal left anterior descending coronary artery were detected in hypercholesterolemic pigs [48]. VV density was found about two times higher in nonstenotic and noncalcified stenotic plaques when compared with normal and calcified segments [11]. With the limitation of the subject imaging volume, micro-CT is mostly used to scan specimens from autopsy or small animals such as mice. Thus, micro-CT usually applies to retrospective studies or animal experiments, and is not available for humans.

High-speed whole body scanning capability of multi-slice CT demonstrated its capacity of accurate visualization of atherosclerotic plaques in the coronary arteries [112]. Several attempts have been made to improve the resolution of CT in VV visualization. For example, iodinated nanoparticles were used as contrast agents in CT. CT imaging using this compound increased the X-ray absorption at the targeted sites, hence improving the quality of CT images. CT angiography (CTA) is another technique with high spatial and temporal resolution, allowing detailed anatomical delineation of atherosclerotic arteries. CTA scanning of patients with moderate (50%–70%) stenosis of the internal carotid artery showed that plaques derived from patients with neurological symptoms had a higher proportion of VV enhancement than of that in total patients (34% *vs.* 24.1%), which indicated that atherosclerotic patients with enhancing VV were more likely to be symptomatic [113]. This result indicates that CTA imaging of VV may aid in the identification of patients at an increased risk for ischemic stroke within populations with the same degree of stenosis. However, because of the risks associated with radiation exposure, current American Heart Association and American College of Cardiology guidelines do not recommend CTA as a general screening tool in low-risk, asymptomatic patients [114].

Intravascular ultrasound (IVUS) is broadly used to provide high-resolution tomographic images of the lumen and acquire precise measurements of atherosclerotic plaques *in vivo*. However, IVUS imaging systems, which are developed to examine blood flow within the lumen of large arteries, are not designed initially to detect VV morphology [115]. Recently, a porcine experiment demonstrated that the change of IVUS-based vessel wall flow assessment signals paralleled VV density detected by micro-CT, indicating the potential of IVUS estimation of blood flow to quantify VV density [116]. Contrast-enhanced IVUS with contrast enhancement agents is another prominent method used in VV visualization. Contrast agents can increase IVUS echogenicity enhancement in the adventitia of coronary arteries, which is consistent with the enhancement of VV [117]. O'Malley *et al.* [118] presented analyses of human coronary arteries *in vivo*, and demonstrated the feasibility of contrast-enhanced IVUS imaging of VV density and perfusion in atherosclerotic plaques. Further, IVUS with contrast microbubbles tracing neovascularization in non-culprit coronary atherosclerotic plaques demonstrated a significant mean enhancement after intracoronary injection of microbubbles (from 7.1% ± 2.2% to 7.6% ± 2.5%) in the adventitia, which represented the high density of VV in patients with acute coronary syndrome [119]. Other modified techniques, such as contrast-harmonic IVUS and subharmonic contrast IVUS, can visualize contrast agents in adventitial VV [120,121]. Compared with harmonic contrast IVUS, subharmonic (SH20) imaging was even superior to harmonic (H40) imaging in terms of contrast-to-noise and contrast-to-tissue ratio improvement [122]. However, quantitative comparison of harmonic and subharmonic imaging has not been available. Although contrast-enhanced IVUS can provide clear and direct insight into VV in the adventitia, experiments that quantify the neovessels are not available, leading to the limitation of IVUS application in clinical practice. A more accurate index is needed to visualize adventitial VV.

Contrast-enhanced ultrasonography (CEUS), another modality for vascular imaging together with ultrasonographic contrast microbubbles, has developed during the last decade. In a preliminary feasibility study, CEUS enabled the visualization of the adventitial network of VV in human carotid arteries [123]. The enhanced signal was five times higher on average after stimulating atherosclerosis [124,125]. These enhancements correlated with the histological density of intraplaque neovessels. Visualization of VV density by CEUS in an atherosclerotic population also revealed a positive relationship between the abundance of VV and plaque echolucency, a well-accepted marker of high risk lesions [126]. The capability of CEUS in visualizing adventitial VV and intraplaque neovascularization makes it attractive for plaque risk stratification and assessment of anti-atherosclerotic therapy efficacy. Significant linear correlations between CEUS peak video-intensity and histologic VV counting, as well as the cross-sectional area of neovessels were recently reported [127,128]. Video intensity has become a quantitative parameter of CEUS to detect VV and assess the effects of anti-atherosclerotic therapy. Normalized maximal-video intensity enhancement (MVE) in CEUS, which represented the density of VV, demonstrated a positive relationship with plaque volume. A much lower MVE enhancement was observed after four weeks in atorvastatin-treated rabbits (from 0.18 ± 0.08 to 0.16 ± 0.07, $p = 0.11$) than in untreated rabbits (from 0.18 ± 0.08 to 0.25 ± 0.08, $p = 0.001$) [129]. In humans, quantitative CEUS was applied to investigate coronary artery disease patients undergoing lipid-lowering therapy with statins, which parelleled the LDL reduction [130]. All these results inspire the development of a standard diagnostic index for CEUS imaging in quantifying VV density, with which we could identify the populations with unstable plaques and plan the medication. To achieve this goal, large multicenter clinical trials on quantitative CEUS scanning of VV in normal and diseased populations are needed. However, a controversial study indicated that the enhancement of CEUS in carotid atherosclerotic plaques might not always reflect the presence of VV, as verified by the immunochemistry results [131]. Thus, more studies are needed to improve imaging quality and certain clinical standards of CEUS in VV visualization and vulnerable plaques prediction.

Optical coherence tomography (OCT) is an intravascular imaging modality using near-infrared light to generate cross-sectional intravascular images [132]. With its high resolution (10–20 μm), which is 10 times higher than that of IVUS and comparable to that of micro-CT, OCT is widely used for the assessment of coronary atherosclerotic plaques [133]. Under OCT, VV are visualized as a no-signal microchannel within the plaque or the adventitia [134]. The greatest challenge for VV detection under intravascular modalities is the extensive motion artifacts inherently associated with arterial pulsations in addition to other physiological movements. These limitations have been minimized in a recent intensity kurtosis OCT technique, which was developed to visualize VV from carotid arteries *in vivo* [135]. Both the blood flow into VV and dynamic motions of the arterial wall were clearly displayed using this OCT technique. In addition to the earlier time-domain OCT, optical frequency domain imaging (OFDI) was developed as a new-generation OCT that was capable of obtaining A-lines at much higher imaging speeds, facilitating rapid, 3D-pullback imaging during the administration of a non-occlusive flush of an optically transparent media such as Lactated Ringer's or radiocontrast [136]. The laboratory results showed that adventitial VV on OFDI *ex vivo* were clearly displayed and appeared to communicate with the coronary adventitia and media. The results were compatible with histological findings and showed much better resolution when compared with other generations of OCT [137]. More recently, quantification of VV with the 3D OCT method has been applied in both animal and clinical studies. Animal studies conducted on swine suggest significant correlations between the microchannel volume (MCV) count by OCT and the amount of VV by micro-CT [138], which was consistent with the human study [137]. A positive correlation between MCV and plaque volume was also detected from this study [138]. In 2012, international guidelines were formed by the International Working Group for Intravascular OCT Standardization and Validation. OCT imaging modality was recommended as a standard reference in clinical practice [136].

5.2. Molecular Imaging of Vasa Vasorum in Atherosclerosis

The recent recognition that plaque biological features influence the prognosis of atherosclerosis has led to the transition from the sole anatomical assessment to combined anatomic and functional imaging modalities, enabling the application of molecular imaging in VV detection. Molecular imaging, which originates from cancer imaging, is defined as *in vivo* characterization and the measurement of biological processes at the cellular, molecular, whole organ, and whole body levels [139]. Radionuclide tracers or targeted agents with specific binding capacity to molecular targets were used as markers of biological functions in molecular imaging.

Nuclear positron emission tomography (PET) and single-photon emission computed tomography (SPECT) were the first two methods used for molecular imaging. These techniques mostly detected the hypoxia and inflammation levels of atherosclerotic plaques through fluorodeoxyglucose (FDG) uptake or other targets [140,141]. As for the angiogenesis scanning, PET/SPECT with ^{64}Cu-labeled VEGF$_{121}$, ^{111}In-labeled $\alpha v\beta_3$-targeted agent, or other radionuclide tracers have been applied in cancer and post-myocardial infarction neovessel imaging [142–144]. As MMPs participate in intraplaque angiogenesis, MMP inhibitor-based radiotracers bind to activated MMPs and detect angiogenic processes *in vivo*. Several inhibitors have been successfully labeled with ^{123}I, ^{11}C, or ^{18}F for PET imaging, but no animal experiment currently exists [145,146]. Specific uptake of ^{123}I-labelled MMP inhibitors into the plaques was shown in animals on a high-cholesterol diet by planar gamma camera, the radioactivity of which was 2.72-fold of the common artery [147]. Yet, direct visualization of VV neovascularization through PET or SPECT still remains unavailable. Autoradiography, another nuclear technique, can identify angiogenesis in atherosclerotic plaque *ex vivo* with ^{125}I-labeled monoclonal antibodies against fibronectin extra-domain B (ED-B) [148]. More recently, ^{99m}Tc-labeled membrane type 1 MMP monoclonal antibody (^{99m}Tc-MT1-MMP mAb) accumulation, which detects active MMP-2 and MMP-13, was found in atheromatous lesions (4.8 ± 1.9, % injected dose $\times$ body weight/mm$^2 \times 10^2$) and positively correlated with membrane type 1 MMP expression [149]. In conclusion, nuclear neovessel imaging could provide diagnostic imaging capability of vulnerable plaques, and further investigations to improve the modalities are strongly required.

Magnetic Resonance imaging (MRI), by virtue of its ability to characterize various pathological components of atherosclerosis plaques with advantages of high-resolution and radiation avoiding, is another promising modality for studying VV. On traditional anatomical dynamic contrast-enhanced MRI (DCE-MRI), the enhancement of the outer rim of the internal carotid arteries represents VV [150]. With the development of $\alpha v\beta_3$ integrin-targeted gadolinium chelates, MRI molecular imaging emerged. With paramagnetic gadolinium-based nanoparticles, increased angiogenesis was detected as a $26\% \pm 4\%$ and $47\% \pm 5\%$ signal increase over baseline at 15 and 120 min in cholesterolemic rabbits, while only half of the signal augmentation was detected in cholesterol-fed rabbits that received non-targeted nanoparticles. A heterogeneous spatial distribution of neovessels was also observed through molecular imaging [151]. MRI with $\alpha v\beta3$-targeted nanoparticles also showed the ability to assess the therapeutic effect of anti-atherosclerotic agents. After 16 weeks of an appetite suppressant treatment with benfluorex, MR enhancement decreased in treated animals when a steady increase was seen in the untreated group [152]. Gadolinium quantitative MRI of VV reported that the total neovessel area in the matched sections from DCE-MRI correlated with the histological measurement with a high correlation coefficient of 0.80, thereby serving as a quantitative parameter in vascular imaging [153]. In humans, *in vivo* DCE-MRI showed that the transfer constant (K^{trans}) of gadolinium enhancement in the carotid adventitia is a quantitative measurement of the VV extent, a method confirmed by histological measurements on a carotid endarterectomy specimen [154]. K^{trans} represents a kinetic parameter that characterizes the transfer of the contrast agent from plasma to the extravascular space (e.g., adventitia). The transfer therefore depends on VV density. By estimating K^{trans} via DCE-MRI, the transfer of gadolinium into the extravascular space, calculated from dynamic kinetics of tissue enhancement, correlates strongly with macrophage content, neovascularization, and loose matrix areas measured by histology analysis [155]. These studies indicated that adventitial enhancement seen on DCE-MRI with gadolinium chelates can be used to detect VV neovascularization in the process of atherosclerosis, therefore assessing the risk for plaque rupture. However, previous studies show gadolinium associates with nephrogenic systemic fibrosis in patients with reduced renal function [156]. Thus, exploration of more effective contrast enhancement agents with lower toxicity and higher resolution is needed in the future.

CEUS is another tool in molecular imaging. As discussed, CEUS has been employed not only to improve the evaluation of intima-media thickness, but also to highlight wall irregularities, ulcerations, adventitial VV and neovasculature of the atherosclerotic plaque that are often not visible by standard non-invasive ultrasound imaging [157]. Further development of conjugated microbubbles that bind to specific ligands in thrombotic material or neovessels has led to the term "molecular imaging" in CEUS scanning. Microbubbles coupled to the VEGFR may allow for a detection of neovascularization. Using dual ET-1/VEGFsp receptor (DEspR)-targeted microbubbles, CEUS molecular imaging has detected an increased DEspR-expression in carotid artery lesions and expanded VV neovessels in transgenic rats with carotid artery disease [158]. CEUS with VEGFR-2-targeted microbubbles was used to evaluate the response to sorafenib (a drug that inhibits cell proliferation and neovascularization in several tumors) in a mouse model of hepatocellular carcinoma [159]. The amount of bound microbubbles in the tumor quantified by dedicated software was lower in the treatment group through CEUS molecular imaging.

Together, as summarized in Table 1, molecular imaging shows an exciting potential in VV imaging by increasing the quality of resolution. Further studies are needed to modify the existing molecular imaging modalities and targeted agents that are safe, accurate, and easy to detect.

Table 1. Molecular imaging modalities and targets of vasa vasorum in atherosclerosis models.

Imaging Modality	Spatial Resolution	Temporal Resolution	Targets (Reference)	Species	In Vivo Imaging	Histological Validation	Results
Planar gamma camera	cm^3	Hours	^{123}I-labelled MMP inhibitors [147]	Apoe$^{-/-}$ mice	+	+	Signal of ^{123}I-labelled inhibitors into plaques in high cholesterol animals was 2.72-folds of the control
Autoradiograph	μm^3	Milliseconds	ED-B [148]	Apoe$^{-/-}$ mice	−	−	^{125}I-labeled monoclonal antibodies against ED-B identified the angiogenesis in atherosclerotic plaques ex vivo
			99mTc-MT1-MMP mAb [149]	WHHLMI rabbits	+	+	The highest accumulation of ^{99m}Tc-MT1-MMP mAb was found in atheromatous lesions in comparison with stable lesions
MRI	mm^3	Seconds	Integrin αvβ$_3$	Male New Zealand White (NZW) rabbits [151]	+	+	Paramagnetic gadolinium-based nanoparticles showed strong enhancement in atherscletotic lesions that was twice of the non-targeted nanoparticles
				JCR:LA-cp rats [152]	+	+	The enhancement of αvβ3-targeted nanoparticles was preserved in benfluorex treating group
				Humans [153–155]	+	+	Targeted gadolinium compounds detected VV, total area and K^{trans} of the enhancement could be quantitative parameters
CEUS	μm^3	Milliseconds	ET-1/VEGFsp receptor [158]	Tg25 (hCETP) Dahl-S rats	+	+	Expanded VV in transgenic rats with carotid artery disease were detected by targeted microbubbles
			VEGFR-2 [159]	Female nude mice	+	−	VEGFR-2 targeted microbubbles were able to evaluate anti-angiogenic effect of sorafenib

6. Anti- and Pro-Angiogenic Therapies on Vasa Vasorum

6.1. Anti-Angiogenic Therapies

The rupture of neovessels originating from VV may be the main cause of intraplaque hemorrhage in advanced atherosclerosis. It seems logical to speculate that anti-angiogenic strategies can be used to inhibit plaque growth and stabilize existing plaques, although lipid-controlling, anti-inflammation, and invasive angioplasty are among the current main treatments for atherosclerosis. As discussed above, angiogenic factors control neovascularization. Expression regulation of these factors (e.g., Ets-1, Ang-1 receptor, HIF-1α, MMPs) by microRNAs influences EC activation and SMC phenotype switch, thereby decreasing VV neovascularization [160]. In contrast, the effects of angiogenesis inhibitors on atherosclerotic lesions are difficult to classify because the various agents that block angiogenesis do not have uniformed mechanisms of action. Each agent may also have unique effects on different cell types and biochemical pathways that are also present in atherosclerotic lesions. To simplify the understanding of different angiogenic inhibitors, we grouped angiogenic inhibitors into three categories: direct anti-angiogenic molecules (*i.e.*, angiostatics) that are derived from protein proteolysis; inhibitors that target directly or indirectly the angiogenic factors (e.g., VEGF); and others with incompletely characterized mechanisms.

Direct anti-angiogenic compounds, also known as angiostatics, are substances that target ECs and SMCs without affecting endogenous angiogenic factors. Angiostatics were initially identified as tumor-derived factors that inhibit neovascularization of remote metastases of Lewis lung carcinoma (*i.e.*, angiostatin) [161] and hemangioendothelioma (*i.e.*, endostatin) [162]. Endostatin is a fragment from collagen-XVIII proteolysis. In apolipoprotein E-deficient (*Apoe*$^{-/-}$) mice, chronic treatments with endostatin reduced intimal neovascularization and inhibited plaque growth by 85% in atherosclerosis [163]. However, as the plaque intimal SMC contents were similar between control and treated mice in this research, a mechanism for the anti-angiogenic property of endostatin remains incompletely understood. Angiostatin, a proteolytic fragment of plasminogen, blocks the angiogenic potential of atherosclerotic aortas with a parallel reduction of macrophages in the plaques and around VV [164]. Activated macrophages stimulate angiogenesis by recruiting more inflammatory cells to increase angiogenesis further. Angiostatin inhibition interrupts this positive feedback from inflammatory cells and hinders angiogenesis in atherosclerotic plaques. The mechanisms by which endostatin and angiostatin inhibit angiogenesis are not fully understood. Inhibition of EC and SMC proliferation and migration, without affecting endothelial intracellular signaling pathways, seems to play a vital role in this process [165].

Angiogenic factor inhibitors offer another target choice of anti-angiogenic therapy in atherosclerosis. The inhibition of the VEGF signaling pathway by targeting VEGF and VEGFR-1 has been well studied. Bevacizumab is a VEGF-specific antibody that has the capacity to inhibit VV after local delivery by stent in a rabbit atherosclerosis model [166]. Exogenous application of antibodies against VEGFR-1 reduced the size of early and intermediate plaques by 50% and the growth of advanced lesions by ~25% in *Apoe*$^{-/-}$ mice [167]. PlGF is a VEGFR-1 ligand. Deficiency of PlGF inhibited early-stage atherosclerosis. On the other hand, increased adventitial expression of PlGF promoted intimal hyperplasia and VV proliferation [168]. Importantly, the anti-angiogenic property of PlGF antibodies acted only on diseased arteries without affecting healthy vessels [169], offering a great advantage for patient treatment. Other angiogenic factor inhibitors include anti-MMP-2 and anti-MMP-9 antibodies that also have the ability to block endothelial cell tubule formation [170]. MicroRNAs that interfere with the expression of angiogenic factors (e.g., Ets-1, Ang-1 receptor, HIF-1α, MMPs) also decrease VV density in atherosclerotic plaques [160]. Apart from antibodies and microRNAs that act directly on angiogenic factors, indirect agents also play an anti-angiogenic role in VV angiogenesis. Thalidomide is an anti-angiogenic drug that exerts anti-inflammatory and immune-modulatory effects. Treatment with thalidomide preserved VV spatial density by 45% in high-cholesterol, diet-fed atherosclerosic pigs and was only 1.3-fold higher than that of normal pigs when compared with the 2.4-fold increase in the untreated group [171]. Reduced adventitial VV neovascularization and plaque progression after thalidomide treatment were also seen in $Apoe^{-/-}/Ldlr^{-/-}$ double knockout mice [172]. The anti-angiogenic effect of thalidomide in atherosclerosis was accompanied by the inhibition of VEGF expression.

Another group of molecules remain difficult to classify because of their limited study and complicated mechanisms. ET-1 is a vasoconstrictor that has mitogenic activity on SMCs and participates in VV neovascularization during atherogenesis [173]. ET receptor antagonism (ET-A) application in hypercholesterolemic pigs showed that elevated VV density in the hypercholesterolemia group was greatly preserved by ~32% [174]. Fumagillin nanoparticles are also anti-angiogenic agents that target ECs. Treatment of atherosclerosic rabbits with $\alpha v \beta_3$ integrin-targeted paramagnetic nanoparticles together with fumagillin decreased MRI enhancement and reduced the numbers of microvessels [175]. Anti-angiogenic rPAI-1$_{23}$, a truncated isoform of plasminogen activator inhibitor-1 (PAI-1), greatly reduced VV, especially the second order VV, with a 37% reduction in total vessel area and a 43% reduction in vessel length in atherogenic female $ApoB-48^{-/-}/Ldlr^{-/-}$ mice through inhibition of bFGF, suggesting a significant therapeutic potential of this anti-angiogenic protease inhibitor peptide in atherosclerosis [176]. Further study concluded that rPAI-1$_{23}$ caused the regression of adventitial VV in hypercholesterolemic mice by increasing plasmin and MMP activities that degrade perlecan, nidogen, and fibrin in the extracellular milieu. Without a supportive scaffold from these extracellular matrix proteins, ECs may undergo apoptosis, leading to VV regression [177]. The anti-proliferative and anti-inflammatory drug, 3-deazaadenosine (c3Ado), dose-dependently prevents the proliferation and migration of human coronary artery ECs. It also inhibited VV neovascularization along the descending aortas in $Apoe^{-/-}/Ldl^{-/-}$ double knockout mice [178]. Here we summarize this last category of molecules in Table 2.

Table 2. Anti-angiogenic molecules with incompletely characterized mechanisms.

Compounds	Year	Functions	Species	Possible Mechanisms	Results
ET-A	1993 [173], 2002 [174]	Inhibiting ET-1 receptor	Female domestic pigs	Inhibiting mitogenic activity of SMCs	Elevated VV density in hypercholesterolemia pigs were greatly preserved by ~32% after ET-A treatment
Fumagillin nanoparticle	2006 [175]	An anti-angiogenic agent that targets $\alpha v \beta_3$ integrin	Male NZW rabbits	Not investigate	MRI enhancement and the numbers of microvessels are decreased in fumagillin-treated cholesterol-fed rabbits
rPAI-1$_{23}$	2009 [176], 2011 [177]	A truncated isoform of plasminogen activator inhibitor-1 (PAI-1)	Female $ApoB$-48$^{-/-}$/$Ldlr^{-/-}$ mice	Reducing FGF-2 expression. Increasing plasmin and MMP activities on degrading compounds (*i.e.*, perlecan, nidogen, fibrin) that produce supportive scaffold in the extracellular milieu, leading to apoptosis of ECs	A 37% reduction in total vessel area and a 43% reduction in vessel length of the second order VV are observed as a result of apoptosis of ECs
c3Ado	2009 [178]	An anti-proliferative and anti-inflammatory drug	$Apoe^{-/-}$/$Ldl^{-/-}$ double knockout mice	Preventing the proliferation and migration of ECs	VV neovascularization is inhibited dose dependently

6.2. Pro-Angiogenic Therapies

Based on what has been discussed, anti-angiogenic therapies seem to be effective and significant in atherosclerosis medication, at least in animal models. However, a recent report from colorectal cancer patients noted that the anti-VEGF monoclonal antibody bevacizumab showed a higher risk (3.5 additional cases/1000 person-years) of arterial thromboembolic events (e.g., stroke, myocardial infarction, arterial embolism and thrombosis, and angina) despite its anti-angiogenic properties [179]. This observation put into question the risk of angiogenesis inhibitors to atherothrombosis and associated complications. It seems that the role of neovascularization is far more complicated than imagined. A case report from four patients suggested that VV are a source of collateral circulation after carotid artery occlusion secondary to atherosclerotic disease [180]. It has been demonstrated that VSMC-rich lesions are stable because of their high cellular content, whereas acellular lesions with a higher degree of calcification, fibrosis, and lipids are more prone to fracture or rupture [181]. It could be argued that, by enriching the supply of nutrients to the plaque core, neovascularization may increase plaque cellularity, thereby acting as an underlying cause of plaque stabilization.

Studies on HMG-CoA reductase inhibitors support the feasibility of pro-angiogenic therapies in atherosclerosis. Statins, such as atorvastatin and simvastatin, demonstrated beneficial effects in reducing atherosclerotic VV neovascularization independent of lipid lowering [129,182]. While high doses of cerivastatin (2.5 mg/kg/day) blocked angiogenesis, low doses of cerivastatin (0.5 mg/kg/day) induced angiogenesis *in vitro* [183]. In contrast, both high- and low-dose statin therapy blocked plaque progression, indicating that pro-angiogenic effects do not lead to pro-atherosclerotic effects, as we anticipated. The inhibition of VV neovascularization may not be the fundamental strategy for plaque stabilizing in atherosclerosis. More attention may be focused on the normalization and maturation of VV to reduce the risk of VV leakage. As a result, studies in pro-angiogenic therapies have been encouraged in recent years.

Nerve growth factor (NGF) is a potent angiogenic factor that is decreased in atherosclerosis-lesioned arteries [184]. NGF application increased the ratio of large matured vessels ($\geq$20 µm in diameter) from 30% to ~50% compared with the control, whereas VEGF promoted more immature small microvessels (<20 µm) than the control. NGF also enhanced the maturation of VEGF-induced neovessels from 20% to 40% [185]. These studies suggested a therapeutic possibility of pro-angiogenic NGF on atherosclerosis by enhancing VV maturation. bFGF is another predominant angiogenic growth factor that was also required for VV plexus stability in hypercholesterolemic mice [186]. Although it was regarded as a pro-atherogenic factor due to its stimulatory activity on SMC growth [187], recent studies suggested a protective property of bFGF on plaque formation in a hypercholesterolemic rabbit model by reversing endothelial dysfunction and reducing vascular cell adhesion molecule-1 (VCAM-1) expression as well as plaque macrophage content [188]. However, increased endothelial FGF-receptor-2 signaling by EC-selective overexpression of FGF-receptor-2 aggravated atherosclerosis by promoting p21^{Cip1}-mediated EC dysfunction [189]. Therefore the use of bFGF for therapeutic angiogenesis such as ischemic injury may have to be considered due to the possible adverse effects in aggravating atherosclerosis. For example, simvastatin with 1.8 mg/kg/day in rabbits increased the expression of HIF-1α and VEGFR-2 in advanced peri-infarcted myocardium, but blocked the protein expression of HIF-1α, VEGF, and VEGFR-2 in early atherosclerotic arteries. Apart from the dosage of this statin, the stage of atherosclerotic disease may influence the outcome of this statin therapy [190]. Therefore, the stage of atherosclerosis and the microenvironment of plaque should be considered to determine whether a pro-angiogenesis or anti-angiogenesis therapy should be employed.

In conclusion, the role of neovescularization in plaque rupture cannot be simply defined. It is instead an intricate process that may exert various physiological effects in different stages of atherosclerosis. Pro-angiogenic factors that improve the maturation and stabilization of VV and reduce the leakage of these neovessels seem essential in further anti-atherosclerosis studies. The stage of plaque development may be a major determinant of whether we should employ anti-angiogenesis or pro-angiogenesis approaches.

7. Conclusions

VV neovascularization exists in the process of atherosclerosis, which seems like a compensatory reaction in order to provide adequate oxygen and nourishment for atherosclerotic arteries. However, the imbalance between angiogenic and anti-angiogenic factors along with latter damages leads to the dysfunction of ECs and their surrounding supporting cells, resulting in an immature and fragile VV neovasculature with weak integrity. In addition to the VV leakage itself, further stimulation of inflammation and necrosis of atherosclerotic plaques is another cause of VV-triggered intraplaque hemorrhage. It remains unclear if VV play a causative or reactive role in the atherosclerotic process, yet VV assessment has been suspected as an effective marker in the early detection of vulnerable plaques.

Several imaging modalities have been established to visualize VV neovascularization and to identify plaques with a high risk of rupture. Anatomical imaging techniques such as IVUS and OCT provide high-resolution images of VV and atherosclerotic plaques yet fail to recognize the biological features of the tissue. Recent molecular imaging modalities exhibit both the anatomy and pathological function of VV, which benefit from the development of specific target agents. Molecular imaging methods such as DCE-MRI and CEUS are extensively applied in visualizing VV. The results of these studies are encouraging, but problems remain. The toxicity of enhancement agents, the limited resolution of imaging, and some controversial results from different studies all lead to the need of improving the existing imaging modalities and investigating effective, and practical methods that are safe and precise for bedside use.

Considering the role of VV neovascularization in the process of atherosclerosis, anti-angiogenic therapies seem logical to prevent or attenuate the deterioration of this disease. Several studies have proven that angiogenesis inhibitors preserve the density of intraplaque VV in atherosclerosis. However, a higher risk of arterial cardiovascular events is observed in colorectal cancer patients using angiogenic inhibitors. The use of anti-angiogenic therapy as a proper way to treat atherosclerosis and prevent intraplaque hemorrhage remains complicated. The application of pro-angiogenic NGF and bFGF showed the capacity of enhancing the maturation of VV neovessels. Therefore, pro-angiogenesis factors that improve the maturation of VV and reduce the leakage of these neovessels may be the fundamental solution in reducing intraplaque hemorrhage, and may lead to a new direction for the future study of stabilizing vulnerable plaques.

Acknowledgments: The authors thank Chelsea Swallom for her editorial assistance. This study is supported by National Institutes of Health grants HL81090 (GPS).

Author Contributions: All three authors contributed to the writing of this manuscript.

References

1. Mozaffarian, D.; Benjamin, E.J.; Go, A.S.; Arnett, D.K.; Blaha, M.J.; Cushman, M.; de Ferranti, S.; Despres, J.P.; Fullerton, H.J.; Howard, V.J.; *et al.* Heart disease and stroke statistics—2015 update: A report from the American Heart Association. *Circulation* **2015**, *131*, e29–e322. [CrossRef] [PubMed]
2. Davies, M.J.; Richardson, P.D.; Woolf, N.; Katz, D.R.; Mann, J. Risk of thrombosis in human atherosclerotic plaques: Role of extracellular lipid, macrophage, and smooth muscle cell content. *Br. Heart J.* **1993**, *69*, 377–381. [CrossRef] [PubMed]
3. De Boer, O.J.; van der Wal, A.C.; Teeling, P.; Becker, A.E. Leucocyte recruitment in rupture prone regions of lipid-rich plaques: A prominent role for neovascularization? *Cardiovasc. Res.* **1999**, *41*, 443–449. [CrossRef] [PubMed]
4. Staub, D.; Patel, M.B.; Tibrewala, A.; Ludden, D.; Johnson, M.; Espinosa, P.; Coll, B.; Jaeger, K.A.; Feinstein, S.B. Vasa vasorum and plaque neovascularization on contrast-enhanced carotid ultrasound imaging correlates with cardiovascular disease and past cardiovascular events. *Stroke J. Cereb. Circ.* **2010**, *41*, 41–47. [CrossRef]

5. Takano, M.; Mizuno, K.; Okamatsu, K.; Yokoyama, S.; Ohba, T.; Sakai, S. Mechanical and structural characteristics of vulnerable plaques: Analysis by coronary angioscopy and intravascular ultrasound. *J. Am. Coll. Cardiol.* **2001**, *38*, 99–104. [CrossRef] [PubMed]

6. Ritman, E.L.; Lerman, A. The dynamic vasa vasorum. *Cardiovasc. Res.* **2007**, *75*, 649–658. [CrossRef] [PubMed]

7. Koester, W. Endareritis and arteritis. *Berl. Klin. Wochenschr.* **1876**, *13*, 454–455.

8. Paterson, J.C. Vascularization and hemorrhage of the intima of arteriosclerotic coronary arteries. *Arch. Pathol.* **1936**, *22*, 313–324.

9. Patterson, J.C. Capillary rupture with intimal hemorrhage as a causative factor in coronary thrombosis. *Arch. Pathol.* **1938**, *25*, 474–487.

10. Barger, A.C.; Beeuwkes, R., 3rd; Lainey, L.L.; Silverman, K.J. Hypothesis: Vasa vasorum and neovascularization of human coronary arteries. A possible role in the pathophysiology of atherosclerosis. *N. Engl. J. Med.* **1984**, *310*, 175–177. [CrossRef] [PubMed]

11. Gossl, M.; Versari, D.; Hildebrandt, H.A.; Bajanowski, T.; Sangiorgi, G.; Erbel, R.; Ritman, E.L.; Lerman, L.O.; Lerman, A. Segmental heterogeneity of vasa vasorum neovascularization in human coronary atherosclerosis. *JACC Cardiovasc. Imaging* **2010**, *3*, 32–40. [CrossRef] [PubMed]

12. Kwon, H.M.; Sangiorgi, G.; Ritman, E.L.; McKenna, C.; Holmes, D.R., Jr.; Schwartz, R.S.; Lerman, A. Enhanced coronary vasa vasorum neovascularization in experimental hypercholesterolemia. *J. Clin. Investig.* **1998**, *101*, 1551–1556. [CrossRef] [PubMed]

13. Dunmore, B.J.; McCarthy, M.J.; Naylor, A.R.; Brindle, N.P. Carotid plaque instability and ischemic symptoms are linked to immaturity of microvessels within plaques. *J. Vasc. Surg.* **2007**, *45*, 155–159. [CrossRef] [PubMed]

14. Sluimer, J.C.; Kolodgie, F.D.; Bijnens, A.P.; Maxfield, K.; Pacheco, E.; Kutys, B.; Duimel, H.; Frederik, P.M.; van Hinsbergh, V.W.; Virmani, R.; et al. Thin-walled microvessels in human coronary atherosclerotic plaques show incomplete endothelial junctions relevance of compromised structural integrity for intraplaque microvascular leakage. *J. Am. Coll. Cardiol.* **2009**, *53*, 1517–1527. [CrossRef] [PubMed]

15. Khurana, R.; Zhuang, Z.; Bhardwaj, S.; Murakami, M.; de Muinck, E.; Yla-Herttuala, S.; Ferrara, N.; Martin, J.F.; Zachary, I.; Simons, M. Angiogenesis-dependent and independent phases of intimal hyperplasia. *Circulation* **2004**, *110*, 2436–2443. [CrossRef] [PubMed]

16. Herrmann, J.; Lerman, L.O.; Rodriguez-Porcel, M.; Holmes, D.R., Jr.; Richardson, D.M.; Ritman, E.L.; Lerman, A. Coronary vasa vasorum neovascularization precedes epicardial endothelial dysfunction in experimental hypercholesterolemia. *Cardiovasc. Res.* **2001**, *51*, 762–766. [CrossRef] [PubMed]

17. Maiellaro, K.; Taylor, W.R. The role of the adventitia in vascular inflammation. *Cardiovasc. Res.* **2007**, *75*, 640–648. [CrossRef] [PubMed]

18. Clarke, J.A. An X-ray microscopic study of the postnatal development of the vasa vasorum of normal human coronary arteries. *Acta Anat.* **1966**, *64*, 506–516. [CrossRef] [PubMed]

19. Wolinsky, H.; Glagov, S. Nature of species differences in the medial distribution of aortic vasa vasorum in mammals. *Circ. Res.* **1967**, *20*, 409–421. [CrossRef] [PubMed]

20. Schoenenberger, F.; Mueller, A. On the vascularization of the bovine aortic wall. *Helv. Physiol. Pharmacol. Acta* **1960**, *18*, 136–150. [PubMed]

21. Gossl, M.; Rosol, M.; Malyar, N.M.; Fitzpatrick, L.A.; Beighley, P.E.; Zamir, M.; Ritman, E.L. Functional anatomy and hemodynamic characteristics of vasa vasorum in the walls of porcine coronary arteries. *Anat. Rec. Part A Discov. Mol. Cell. Evol. Biol.* **2003**, *272*, 526–537. [CrossRef]

22. Fleiner, M.; Kummer, M.; Mirlacher, M.; Sauter, G.; Cathomas, G.; Krapf, R.; Biedermann, B.C. Arterial neovascularization and inflammation in vulnerable patients: Early and late signs of symptomatic atherosclerosis. *Circulation* **2004**, *110*, 2843–2850. [CrossRef] [PubMed]

23. Bitar, R.; Moody, A.R.; Leung, G.; Symons, S.; Crisp, S.; Butany, J.; Rowsell, C.; Kiss, A.; Nelson, A.; Maggisano, R. In vivo 3D high-spatial-resolution MR imaging of intraplaque hemorrhage. *Radiology* **2008**, *249*, 259–267. [CrossRef] [PubMed]

24. Acoltzin Vidal, C.; Maldonado Villasenor, I.; Rodriguez Cisneros, L.; Muniz Murguia, J.J. Diminished vascular density in the aortic wall. Morphological and functional characteristics of atherosclerosis. *Arch. Cardiol. Mexico* **2004**, *74*, 176–180.

25. Rademakers, T.; Douma, K.; Hackeng, T.M.; Post, M.J.; Sluimer, J.C.; Daemen, M.J.; Biessen, E.A.; Heeneman, S.; van Zandvoort, M.A. Plaque-associated vasa vasorum in aged apolipoprotein E-deficient mice exhibit proatherogenic functional features *in vivo*. *Arterioscler. Thromb. Vasc. Biol.* **2013**, *33*, 249–256. [CrossRef] [PubMed]

26. Gossl, M.; Malyar, N.M.; Rosol, M.; Beighley, P.E.; Ritman, E.L. Impact of coronary vasa vasorum functional structure on coronary vessel wall perfusion distribution. *Am. J. Physiol. Heart Circ. Physiol.* **2003**, *285*, H2019–H2026. [CrossRef] [PubMed]

27. Han, D.G. The innateness of coronary artery: Vasa vasorum. *Med. Hypotheses* **2010**, *74*, 443–444. [CrossRef] [PubMed]

28. Moss, A.J.; Samuelson, P.; Angell, C.; Minken, S.L. Polarographic evaluation of transmural oxygen availabitlity in intact muscular arteries. *J. Atheroscler. Res.* **1968**, *8*, 803–810. [CrossRef] [PubMed]

29. Crawford, D.W.; Back, L.H.; Cole, M.A. *In vivo* oxygen transport in the normal rabbit femoral arterial wall. *J. Clin. Investig.* **1980**, *65*, 1498–1508. [CrossRef] [PubMed]

30. Bratzler, R.L.; Chisolm, G.M.; Colton, C.K.; Smith, K.A.; Lees, R.S. The distribution of labeled low-density lipoproteins across the rabbit thoracic aorta *in vivo*. *Atherosclerosis* **1977**, *28*, 289–307. [CrossRef] [PubMed]

31. Scotland, R.S.; Vallance, P.J.; Ahluwalia, A. Endogenous factors involved in regulation of tone of arterial vasa vasorum: Implications for conduit vessel physiology. *Cardiovasc. Res.* **2000**, *46*, 403–411. [CrossRef] [PubMed]

32. Scotland, R.; Vallance, P.; Ahluwalia, A. Endothelin alters the reactivity of vasa vasorum: Mechanisms and implications for conduit vessel physiology and pathophysiology. *Br. J. Pharmacol.* **1999**, *128*, 1229–1234. [CrossRef] [PubMed]

33. Ohhira, A.; Ohhashi, T. Effects of aortic pressure and vasoactive agents on the vascular resistance of the vasa vasorum in canine isolated thoracic aorta. *J. Physiol.* **1992**, *453*, 233–245. [CrossRef] [PubMed]

34. Vio, A.; Gozzetti, G.; Reggiani, A. Importance of the vasa vasorum in the healing processes of arterial sutures. (Experimental study on the dog). *Boll. Soc. Ital. Biol. Sper.* **1967**, *43*, 88–90. [PubMed]

35. Winternitz, M.C.; Thomas, R.M.; LeCompte, P.M. *The Biology of Arteriosclerosis*; Springfield: Prince George's County, MA, USA, 1938.

36. Ribatti, D.; Levi-Schaffer, F.; Kovanen, P.T. Inflammatory angiogenesis in atherogenesis—A double-edged sword. *Ann. Med.* **2008**, *40*, 606–621. [CrossRef] [PubMed]

37. Williams, J.K.; Armstrong, M.L.; Heistad, D.D. Vasa vasorum in atherosclerotic coronary arteries: Responses to vasoactive stimuli and regression of atherosclerosis. *Circ. Res.* **1988**, *62*, 515–523. [CrossRef] [PubMed]

38. Sano, M.; Sasaki, T.; Hirakawa, S.; Sakabe, J.; Ogawa, M.; Baba, S.; Zaima, N.; Tanaka, H.; Inuzuka, K.; Yamamoto, N.; *et al.* Lymphangiogenesis and angiogenesis in abdominal aortic aneurysm. *PLoS ONE* **2014**, *9*, e89830. [CrossRef] [PubMed]

39. Davie, N.J.; Gerasimovskaya, E.V.; Hofmeister, S.E.; Richman, A.P.; Jones, P.L.; Reeves, J.T.; Stenmark, K.R. Pulmonary artery adventitial fibroblasts cooperate with vasa vasorum endothelial cells to regulate vasa vasorum neovascularization: A process mediated by hypoxia and endothelin-1. *Am. J. Pathol.* **2006**, *168*, 1793–1807. [CrossRef] [PubMed]

40. Bjornheden, T.; Levin, M.; Evaldsson, M.; Wiklund, O. Evidence of hypoxic areas within the arterial wall *in vivo*. *Arterioscler. Thromb. Vasc. Biol.* **1999**, *19*, 870–876. [CrossRef] [PubMed]

41. Nakashima, Y.; Chen, Y.X.; Kinukawa, N.; Sueishi, K. Distributions of diffuse intimal thickening in human arteries: Preferential expression in atherosclerosis-prone arteries from an early age. *Virchows Arch. Int. J. Pathol.* **2002**, *441*, 279–288. [CrossRef]

42. Zemplenyi, T.; Crawford, D.W.; Cole, M.A. Adaptation to arterial wall hypoxia demonstrated *in vivo* with oxygen microcathodes. *Atherosclerosis* **1989**, *76*, 173–179. [CrossRef] [PubMed]

43. Jarvilehto, M.; Tuohimaa, P. Vasa vasorum hypoxia: Initiation of atherosclerosis. *Med. Hypotheses* **2009**, *73*, 40–41. [CrossRef] [PubMed]

44. Den Hartog, J.P. *Strength of Materials*; Dover Publications, Inc.: New York, NY, USA, 1949; p. 323.

45. Bjornheden, T.; Bondjers, G. Oxygen consumption in aortic tissue from rabbits with diet-induced atherosclerosis. *Arteriosclerosis* **1987**, *7*, 238–247. [CrossRef] [PubMed]

46. Sluimer, J.C.; Gasc, J.M.; van Wanroij, J.L.; Kisters, N.; Groeneweg, M.; Sollewijn Gelpke, M.D.; Cleutjens, J.P.; van den Akker, L.H.; Corvol, P.; Wouters, B.G.; *et al.* Hypoxia, hypoxia-inducible transcription factor, and macrophages in human atherosclerotic plaques are correlated with intraplaque angiogenesis. *J. Am. Coll. Cardiol.* **2008**, *51*, 1258–1265. [CrossRef] [PubMed]

47. Kwon, H.M.; Sangiorgi, G.; Ritman, E.L.; Lerman, A.; McKenna, C.; Virmani, R.; Edwards, W.D.; Holmes, D.R.; Schwartz, R.S. Adventitial vasa vasorum in balloon-injured coronary arteries: Visualization and quantitation by a microscopic three-dimensional computed tomography technique. *J. Am. Coll. Cardiol.* **1998**, *32*, 2072–2079. [CrossRef] [PubMed]

48. Gossl, M.; Versari, D.; Mannheim, D.; Ritman, E.L.; Lerman, L.O.; Lerman, A. Increased spatial vasa vasorum density in the proximal LAD in hypercholesterolemia—Implications for vulnerable plaque-development. *Atherosclerosis* **2007**, *192*, 246–252. [CrossRef] [PubMed]

49. Sun, Z. Atherosclerosis and atheroma plaque rupture: Imaging modalities in the visualization of vasa vasorum and atherosclerotic plaques. *Sci. World J.* **2014**, *2014*, 312764.

50. Gossl, M.; Versari, D.; Lerman, L.O.; Chade, A.R.; Beighley, P.E.; Erbel, R.; Ritman, E.L. Low vasa vasorum densities correlate with inflammation and subintimal thickening: Potential role in location–determination of atherogenesis. *Atherosclerosis* **2009**, *206*, 362–368. [CrossRef] [PubMed]

51. Lim, C.S.; Kiriakidis, S.; Sandison, A.; Paleolog, E.M.; Davies, A.H. Hypoxia-inducible factor pathway and diseases of the vascular wall. *J. Vasc. Surg.* **2013**, *58*, 219–230. [CrossRef] [PubMed]

52. Semenza, G.L.; Agani, F.; Booth, G.; Forsythe, J.; Iyer, N.; Jiang, B.H.; Leung, S.; Roe, R.; Wiener, C.; Yu, A. Structural and functional analysis of hypoxia-inducible factor 1. *Kidney Int.* **1997**, *51*, 553–555. [CrossRef] [PubMed]

53. Oikawa, M.; Abe, M.; Kurosawa, H.; Hida, W.; Shirato, K.; Sato, Y. Hypoxia induces transcription factor ETS-1 via the activity of hypoxia-inducible factor-1. *Biochem. Biophys. Res. Commun.* **2001**, *289*, 39–43. [CrossRef] [PubMed]

54. Leung, D.W.; Cachianes, G.; Kuang, W.J.; Goeddel, D.V.; Ferrara, N. Vascular endothelial growth factor is a secreted angiogenic mitogen. *Science* **1989**, *246*, 1306–1309. [CrossRef] [PubMed]

55. Ushio-Fukai, M. VEGF signaling through NADPH oxidase-derived ROS. *Antioxid. Redox Signal.* **2007**, *9*, 731–739. [CrossRef] [PubMed]

56. Shweiki, D.; Itin, A.; Soffer, D.; Keshet, E. Vascular endothelial growth factor induced by hypoxia may mediate hypoxia-initiated angiogenesis. *Nature* **1992**, *359*, 843–845. [CrossRef] [PubMed]

57. Kuwahara, F.; Kai, H.; Tokuda, K.; Shibata, R.; Kusaba, K.; Tahara, N.; Niiyama, H.; Nagata, T.; Imaizumi, T. Hypoxia-inducible factor-1α/vascular endothelial growth factor pathway for adventitial vasa vasorum formation in hypertensive rat aorta. *Hypertension* **2002**, *39*, 46–50. [CrossRef] [PubMed]

58. Joukov, V.; Pajusola, K.; Kaipainen, A.; Chilov, D.; Lahtinen, I.; Kukk, E.; Saksela, O.; Kalkkinen, N.; Alitalo, K. A novel vascular endothelial growth factor, VEGF-C, is a ligand for the Flt4 (VEGFR-3) and KDR (VEGFR-2) receptor tyrosine kinases. *EMBO J.* **1996**, *15*, 290–298. [PubMed]

59. Achen, M.G.; Jeltsch, M.; Kukk, E.; Makinen, T.; Vitali, A.; Wilks, A.F.; Alitalo, K.; Stacker, S.A. Vascular endothelial growth factor D (VEGF-D) is a ligand for the tyrosine kinases VEGF receptor 2 (Flk1) and VEGF receptor 3 (Flt4). *Proc. Natl. Acad. Sci. USA* **1998**, *95*, 548–553. [CrossRef] [PubMed]

60. Kaipainen, A.; Korhonen, J.; Mustonen, T.; van Hinsbergh, V.W.; Fang, G.H.; Dumont, D.; Breitman, M.; Alitalo, K. Expression of the fms-like tyrosine kinase 4 gene becomes restricted to lymphatic endothelium during development. *Proc. Natl. Acad. Sci. USA* **1995**, *92*, 3566–3570. [CrossRef] [PubMed]

61. Kukk, E.; Lymboussaki, A.; Taira, S.; Kaipainen, A.; Jeltsch, M.; Joukov, V.; Alitalo, K. VEGF-C receptor binding and pattern of expression with VEGFR-3 suggests a role in lymphatic vascular development. *Development* **1996**, *122*, 3829–3837. [PubMed]

62. Partanen, T.A.; Arola, J.; Saaristo, A.; Jussila, L.; Ora, A.; Miettinen, M.; Stacker, S.A.; Achen, M.G.; Alitalo, K. VEGF-C and VEGF-D expression in neuroendocrine cells and their receptor, VEGFR-3, in fenestrated blood vessels in human tissues. *FASEB J.* **2000**, *14*, 2087–2096. [CrossRef] [PubMed]

63. Rutanen, J.; Leppanen, P.; Tuomisto, T.T.; Rissanen, T.T.; Hiltunen, M.O.; Vajanto, I.; Niemi, M.; Hakkinen, T.; Karkola, K.; Stacker, S.A.; *et al.* Vascular endothelial growth factor-D expression in human atherosclerotic lesions. *Cardiovasc. Res.* **2003**, *59*, 971–979. [CrossRef] [PubMed]

64. Belgore, F.; Blann, A.; Neil, D.; Ahmed, A.S.; Lip, G.Y. Localisation of members of the vascular endothelial growth factor (VEGF) family and their receptors in human atherosclerotic arteries. *J. Clin. Pathol.* **2004**, *57*, 266–272. [CrossRef] [PubMed]

65. Vuorio, T.; Nurmi, H.; Moulton, K.; Kurkipuro, J.; Robciuc, M.R.; Ohman, M.; Heinonen, S.E.; Samaranayake, H.; Heikura, T.; Alitalo, K.; *et al.* Lymphatic vessel insufficiency in hypercholesterolemic mice alters lipoprotein levels and promotes atherogenesis. *Arterioscler. Thromb. Vasc. Biol.* **2014**, *34*, 1162–1170. [CrossRef] [PubMed]

66. Iwasaka, C.; Tanaka, K.; Abe, M.; Sato, Y. Ets-1 regulates angiogenesis by inducing the expression of urokinase-type plasminogen activator and matrix metalloproteinase-1 and the migration of vascular endothelial cells. *J. Cell. Physiol.* **1996**, *169*, 522–531. [CrossRef] [PubMed]

67. Hashiya, N.; Jo, N.; Aoki, M.; Matsumoto, K.; Nakamura, T.; Sato, Y.; Ogata, N.; Ogihara, T.; Kaneda, Y.; Morishita, R. In vivo evidence of angiogenesis induced by transcription factor Ets-1: Ets-1 is located upstream of angiogenesis cascade. *Circulation* **2004**, *109*, 3035–3041. [CrossRef] [PubMed]

68. Higashida, T.; Kanno, H.; Nakano, M.; Funakoshi, K.; Yamamoto, I. Expression of hypoxia-inducible angiogenic proteins (hypoxia-inducible factor-1α, vascular endothelial growth factor, and E26 transformation-specific-1) and plaque hemorrhage in human carotid atherosclerosis. *J. Neurosurg.* **2008**, *109*, 83–91. [CrossRef] [PubMed]

69. Kitange, G.; Shibata, S.; Tokunaga, Y.; Yagi, N.; Yasunaga, A.; Kishikawa, M.; Naito, S. Ets-1 transcription factor-mediated urokinase-type plasminogen activator expression and invasion in glioma cells stimulated by serum and basic fibroblast growth factors. *Lab. Investig. J. Tech. Methods Pathol.* **1999**, *79*, 407–416.

70. Paumelle, R.; Tulasne, D.; Kherrouche, Z.; Plaza, S.; Leroy, C.; Reveneau, S.; Vandenbunder, B.; Fafeur, V. Hepatocyte growth factor/scatter factor activates the ETS1 transcription factor by a RAS-RAF-MEK-ERK signaling pathway. *Oncogene* **2002**, *21*, 2309–2319. [CrossRef] [PubMed]

71. Langheinrich, A.C.; Kampschulte, M.; Scheiter, F.; Dierkes, C.; Stieger, P.; Bohle, R.M.; Weidner, W. Atherosclerosis, inflammation and lipoprotein glomerulopathy in kidneys of apoE$^{-/-}$/LDL$^{-/-}$ double knockout mice. *BMC Nephrol.* **2010**, *11*. [CrossRef]

72. Kumamoto, M.; Nakashima, Y.; Sueishi, K. Intimal neovascularization in human coronary atherosclerosis: Its origin and pathophysiological significance. *Hum. Pathol.* **1995**, *26*, 450–456. [CrossRef] [PubMed]

73. Yamashita, A.; Shoji, K.; Tsuruda, T.; Furukoji, E.; Takahashi, M.; Nishihira, K.; Tamura, S.; Asada, Y. Medial and adventitial macrophages are associated with expansive atherosclerotic remodeling in rabbit femoral artery. *Histol. Histopathol.* **2008**, *23*, 127–136. [PubMed]

74. Sluimer, J.C.; Daemen, M.J. Novel concepts in atherogenesis: Angiogenesis and hypoxia in atherosclerosis. *J. Pathol.* **2009**, *218*, 7–29. [CrossRef] [PubMed]

75. Brown, A.J.; Dean, R.T.; Jessup, W. Free and esterified oxysterol: Formation during copper-oxidation of low density lipoprotein and uptake by macrophages. *J. Lipid Res.* **1996**, *37*, 320–335. [PubMed]

76. Ho-Tin-Noe, B.; le Dall, J.; Gomez, D.; Louedec, L.; Vranckx, R.; El-Bouchtaoui, M.; Legres, L.; Meilhac, O.; Michel, J.B. Early atheroma-derived agonists of peroxisome proliferator-activated receptor-gamma trigger intramedial angiogenesis in a smooth muscle cell-dependent manner. *Circ. Res.* **2011**, *109*, 1003–1014. [CrossRef] [PubMed]

77. Sahebkar, A.; Watts, G.F. New LDL-cholesterol lowering therapies: Pharmacology, clinical trials, and relevance to acute coronary syndromes. *Clin. Ther.* **2013**, *35*, 1082–1098. [CrossRef] [PubMed]

78. Lusis, A.J. Atherosclerosis. *Nature* **2000**, *407*, 233–241. [CrossRef] [PubMed]

79. Kolodgie, F.D.; Gold, H.K.; Burke, A.P.; Fowler, D.R.; Kruth, H.S.; Weber, D.K.; Farb, A.; Guerrero, L.J.; Hayase, M.; Kutys, R.; *et al.* Intraplaque hemorrhage and progression of coronary atheroma. *N. Engl. J. Med.* **2003**, *349*, 2316–2325. [CrossRef] [PubMed]

80. Tanaka, K.; Nagata, D.; Hirata, Y.; Tabata, Y.; Nagai, R.; Sata, M. Augmented angiogenesis in adventitia promotes growth of atherosclerotic plaque in apolipoprotein E-deficient mice. *Atherosclerosis* **2011**, *215*, 366–373. [CrossRef] [PubMed]

81. Moulton, K.S. Angiogenesis in atherosclerosis: Gathering evidence beyond speculation. *Curr. Opin. Lipidol.* **2006**, *17*, 548–555. [CrossRef] [PubMed]

82. Ricote, M.; Li, A.C.; Willson, T.M.; Kelly, C.J.; Glass, C.K. The peroxisome proliferator-activated receptor-gamma is a negative regulator of macrophage activation. *Nature* **1998**, *391*, 79–82. [CrossRef] [PubMed]

83. Fang, L.; Liu, C.; Miller, Y.I. Zebrafish models of dyslipidemia: Relevance to atherosclerosis and angiogenesis. *Transl. Res. J. Lab. Clin. Med.* **2014**, *163*, 99–108. [CrossRef]

84. Salomon, R.G.; Hong, L.; Hollyfield, J.G. Discovery of carboxyethylpyrroles (CEPs): Critical insights into AMD, autism, cancer, and wound healing from basic research on the chemistry of oxidized phospholipids. *Chem. Res. Toxicol.* **2011**, *24*, 1803–1816. [CrossRef] [PubMed]

85. West, X.Z.; Malinin, N.L.; Merkulova, A.A.; Tischenko, M.; Kerr, B.A.; Borden, E.C.; Podrez, E.A.; Salomon, R.G.; Byzova, T.V. Oxidative stress induces angiogenesis by activating TLR2 with novel endogenous ligands. *Nature* **2010**, *467*, 972–976. [CrossRef] [PubMed]

86. Chatterjee, T.K.; Stoll, L.L.; Denning, G.M.; Harrelson, A.; Blomkalns, A.L.; Idelman, G.; Rothenberg, F.G.; Neltner, B.; Romig-Martin, S.A.; Dickson, E.W.; *et al.* Proinflammatory phenotype of perivascular adipocytes: Influence of high-fat feeding. *Circ. Res.* **2009**, *104*, 541–549. [CrossRef] [PubMed]

87. Barandier, C.; Montani, J.P.; Yang, Z. Mature adipocytes and perivascular adipose tissue stimulate vascular smooth muscle cell proliferation: Effects of aging and obesity. *Am. J. Physiol. Heart Circ. Physiol.* **2005**, *289*, H1807–H1813. [CrossRef] [PubMed]

88. Wang, P.; Xu, T.Y.; Guan, Y.F.; Su, D.F.; Fan, G.R.; Miao, C.Y. Perivascular adipose tissue-derived visfatin is a vascular smooth muscle cell growth factor: Role of nicotinamide mononucleotide. *Cardiovasc. Res.* **2009**, *81*, 370–380. [CrossRef] [PubMed]

89. Manka, D.; Chatterjee, T.K.; Stoll, L.L.; Basford, J.E.; Konaniah, E.S.; Srinivasan, R.; Bogdanov, V.Y.; Tang, Y.; Blomkalns, A.L.; Hui, D.Y.; Weintraub, N.L. Transplanted perivascular adipose tissue accelerates injury-induced neointimal hyperplasia: Role of monocyte chemoattractant protein-1. *Arterioscler. Thromb. Vasc. Biol.* **2014**, *34*, 1723–1730. [CrossRef] [PubMed]

90. Rajsheker, S.; Manka, D.; Blomkalns, A.L.; Chatterjee, T.K.; Stoll, L.L.; Weintraub, N.L. Crosstalk between perivascular adipose tissue and blood vessels. *Curr. Opin. Pharmacol.* **2010**, *10*, 191–196. [CrossRef] [PubMed]

91. Garcia-Touchard, A.; Henry, T.D.; Sangiorgi, G.; Spagnoli, L.G.; Mauriello, A.; Conover, C.; Schwartz, R.S. Extracellular proteases in atherosclerosis and restenosis. *Arterioscler. Thromb. Vasc. Biol.* **2005**, *25*, 1119–1127. [CrossRef] [PubMed]

92. Liu, X.Q.; Mao, Y.; Wang, B.; Lu, X.T.; Bai, W.W.; Sun, Y.Y.; Liu, Y.; Liu, H.M.; Zhang, L.; Zhao, Y.X.; *et al.* Specific matrix metalloproteinases play different roles in intraplaque angiogenesis and plaque instability in rabbits. *PLoS ONE* **2014**, *9*, e107851. [CrossRef] [PubMed]

93. Svensson, P.A.; Olson, F.J.; Hagg, D.A.; Ryndel, M.; Wiklund, O.; Karlstrom, L.; Hulthe, J.; Carlsson, L.M.; Fagerberg, B. Urokinase-type plasminogen activator receptor is associated with macrophages and plaque rupture in symptomatic carotid atherosclerosis. *Int. J. Mol. Med.* **2008**, *22*, 459–464. [PubMed]

94. Mattock, K.L.; Gough, P.J.; Humphries, J.; Burnand, K.; Patel, L.; Suckling, K.E.; Cuello, F.; Watts, C.; Gautel, M.; Avkiran, M.; *et al.* Legumain and cathepsin-L expression in human unstable carotid plaque. *Atherosclerosis* **2010**, *208*, 83–89. [CrossRef] [PubMed]

95. Li, W.; Kornmark, L.; Jonasson, L.; Forssell, C.; Yuan, X.M. Cathepsin L is significantly associated with apoptosis and plaque destabilization in human atherosclerosis. *Atherosclerosis* **2009**, *202*, 92–102. [CrossRef] [PubMed]

96. Le Dall, J.; Ho-Tin-Noe, B.; Louedec, L.; Meilhac, O.; Roncal, C.; Carmeliet, P.; Germain, S.; Michel, J.B.; Houard, X. Immaturity of microvessels in haemorrhagic plaques is associated with proteolytic degradation of angiogenic factors. *Cardiovasc. Res.* **2010**, *85*, 184–193.

97. Leclercq, A.; Houard, X.; Philippe, M.; Ollivier, V.; Sebbag, U.; Meilhac, O.; Michel, J.B. Involvement of intraplaque hemorrhage in atherothrombosis evolution via neutrophil protease enrichment. *J. Leukoc. Biol.* **2007**, *82*, 1420–1429. [CrossRef] [PubMed]

98. Maisonpierre, P.C.; Suri, C.; Jones, P.F.; Bartunkova, S.; Wiegand, S.J.; Radziejewski, C.; Compton, D.; McClain, J.; Aldrich, T.H.; Papadopoulos, N.; *et al.* Angiopoietin-2, a natural antagonist for Tie2 that disrupts *in vivo* angiogenesis. *Science* **1997**, *277*, 55–60. [CrossRef] [PubMed]

99. Hashimoto, T.; Lam, T.; Boudreau, N.J.; Bollen, A.W.; Lawton, M.T.; Young, W.L. Abnormal balance in the angiopoietin-tie2 system in human brain arteriovenous malformations. *Circ. Res.* **2001**, *89*, 111–113. [CrossRef] [PubMed]

100. Anagnostopoulos, A.; Eleftherakis-Papaiakovou, V.; Kastritis, E.; Tsionos, K.; Bamias, A.; Meletis, J.; Dimopoulos, M.A.; Terpos, E. Serum concentrations of angiogenic cytokines in Waldenstrom macroglobulinaemia: The ration of angiopoietin-1 to angiopoietin-2 and angiogenin correlate with disease severity. *Br. J. Haematol.* **2007**, *137*, 560–568. [CrossRef] [PubMed]

101. Post, S.; Peeters, W.; Busser, E.; Lamers, D.; Sluijter, J.P.; Goumans, M.J.; de Weger, R.A.; Moll, F.L.; Doevendans, P.A.; Pasterkamp, G.; *et al.* Balance between angiopoietin-1 and angiopoietin-2 is in favor of angiopoietin-2 in atherosclerotic plaques with high microvessel density. *J. Vasc. Res.* **2008**, *45*, 244–250. [CrossRef] [PubMed]

102. Chistiakov, D.A.; Orekhov, A.N.; Bobryshev, Y.V. Contribution of neovascularization and intraplaque haemorrhage to atherosclerotic plaque progression and instability. *Acta Physiol.* **2015**, *213*, 539–553. [CrossRef]

103. Nagy, E.; Eaton, J.W.; Jeney, V.; Soares, M.P.; Varga, Z.; Galajda, Z.; Szentmiklosi, J.; Mehes, G.; Csonka, T.; Smith, A.; *et al.* Red cells, hemoglobin, heme, iron, and atherogenesis. *Arterioscler. Thromb. Vasc. Biol.* **2010**, *30*, 1347–1353. [CrossRef] [PubMed]

104. Balla, J.; Jacob, H.S.; Balla, G.; Nath, K.; Eaton, J.W.; Vercellotti, G.M. Endothelial-cell heme uptake from heme proteins: Induction of sensitization and desensitization to oxidant damage. *Proc. Natl. Acad. Sci. USA* **1993**, *90*, 9285–9289. [CrossRef] [PubMed]

105. Potor, L.; Banyai, E.; Becs, G.; Soares, M.P.; Balla, G.; Balla, J.; Jeney, V. Atherogenesis may involve the prooxidant and proinflammatory effects of ferryl hemoglobin. *Oxid. Med. Cell. Longev.* **2013**, *2013*. [CrossRef]

106. Juckett, M.B.; Balla, J.; Balla, G.; Jessurun, J.; Jacob, H.S.; Vercellotti, G.M. Ferritin protects endothelial cells from oxidized low density lipoprotein *in vitro*. *Am. J. Pathol.* **1995**, *147*, 782–789. [PubMed]

107. Lee, F.Y.; Lee, T.S.; Pan, C.C.; Huang, A.L.; Chau, L.Y. Colocalization of iron and ceroid in human atherosclerotic lesions. *Atherosclerosis* **1998**, *138*, 281–288. [CrossRef] [PubMed]

108. Baldwin, A.L. Modified hemoglobins produce venular interendothelial gaps and albumin leakage in the rat mesentery. *Am. J. Physiol.* **1999**, *277*, H650–H659. [PubMed]

109. Abela, G.S.; Aziz, K.; Vedre, A.; Pathak, D.R.; Talbott, J.D.; Dejong, J. Effect of cholesterol crystals on plaques and intima in arteries of patients with acute coronary and cerebrovascular syndromes. *Am. J. Cardiol.* **2009**, *103*, 959–968. [CrossRef] [PubMed]

110. Kaartinen, M.; Penttila, A.; Kovanen, P.T. Mast cells accompany microvessels in human coronary atheromas: Implications for intimal neovascularization and hemorrhage. *Atherosclerosis* **1996**, *123*, 123–131. [CrossRef] [PubMed]

111. Ambrose, J.A.; Tannenbaum, M.A.; Alexopoulos, D.; Hjemdahl-Monsen, C.E.; Leavy, J.; Weiss, M.; Borrico, S.; Gorlin, R.; Fuster, V. Angiographic progression of coronary artery disease and the development of myocardial infarction. *J. Am. Coll. Cardiol.* **1988**, *12*, 56–62. [CrossRef] [PubMed]

112. Hyafil, F.; Cornily, J.C.; Feig, J.E.; Gordon, R.; Vucic, E.; Amirbekian, V.; Fisher, E.A.; Fuster, V.; Feldman, L.J.; Fayad, Z.A. Noninvasive detection of macrophages using a nanoparticulate contrast agent for computed tomography. *Nat. Med.* **2007**, *13*, 636–641. [CrossRef] [PubMed]

113. Romero, J.M.; Pizzolato, R.; Atkinson, W.; Meader, A.; Jaimes, C.; Lamuraglia, G.; Jaff, M.R.; Buonanno, F.; Delgado Almandoz, J.; Gonzalez, R.G. Vasa vasorum enhancement on computerized tomographic angiography correlates with symptomatic patients with 50% to 70% carotid artery stenosis. *Stroke J. Cereb. Circ.* **2013**, *44*, 3344–3349. [CrossRef]

114. Sadeghi, M.M.; Glover, D.K.; Lanza, G.M.; Fayad, Z.A.; Johnson, L.L. Imaging atherosclerosis and vulnerable plaque. *J. Nucl. Med.* **2010**, *51*, 51S–65S. [CrossRef] [PubMed]

115. Li, W.; van der Steen, A.F.; Lancee, C.T.; Cespedes, I.; Bom, N. Blood flow imaging and volume flow quantitation with intravascular ultrasound. *Ultrasound Med. Biol.* **1998**, *24*, 203–214. [CrossRef] [PubMed]

116. Moritz, R.; Eaker, D.R.; Anderson, J.L.; Kline, T.L.; Jorgensen, S.M.; Lerman, A.; Ritman, E.L. IVUS detection of vasa vasorum blood flow distribution in coronary artery vessel wall. *JACC Cardiovasc. Imaging* **2012**, *5*, 935–940. [CrossRef] [PubMed]

117. Papaioannou, T.G.; Vavuranakis, M.; Androulakis, A.; Lazaros, G.; Kakadiaris, I.; Vlaseros, I.; Naghavi, M.; Kallikazaros, I.; Stefanadis, C. *In-vivo* imaging of carotid plaque neoangiogenesis with contrast-enhanced harmonic ultrasound. *Int. J. Cardiol.* **2009**, *134*, e110–e112. [CrossRef] [PubMed]

118. O'Malley, S.M.; Vavuranakis, M.; Naghavi, M.; Kakadiaris, I.A. Intravascular ultrasound-based imaging of vasa vasorum for the detection of vulnerable atherosclerotic plaque. *Med. Image Comput. Comput. Assist. Interv. MICCAI* **2005**, *8 Pt 1*, 343–351.

119. Vavuranakis, M.; Kakadiaris, I.A.; O'Malley, S.M.; Papaioannou, T.G.; Sanidas, E.A.; Naghavi, M.; Carlier, S.; Tousoulis, D.; Stefanadis, C. A new method for assessment of plaque vulnerability based on vasa vasorum imaging, by using contrast-enhanced intravascular ultrasound and differential image analysis. *Int. J. Cardiol.* **2008**, *130*, 23–29. [CrossRef] [PubMed]

120. Goertz, D.E.; Frijlink, M.E.; Tempel, D.; van Damme, L.C.; Krams, R.; Schaar, J.A.; Ten Cate, F.J.; Serruys, P.W.; de Jong, N.; van der Steen, A.F. Contrast harmonic intravascular ultrasound: A feasibility study for vasa vasorum imaging. *Investig. Radiol.* **2006**, *41*, 631–638. [CrossRef]

121. Goertz, D.E.; Frijlink, M.E.; Tempel, D.; Bhagwandas, V.; Gisolf, A.; Krams, R.; de Jong, N.; van der Steen, A.F. Subharmonic contrast intravascular ultrasound for vasa vasorum imaging. *Ultrasound Med. Biol.* **2007**, *33*, 1859–1872. [CrossRef] [PubMed]

122. Goertz, D.E.; Frijlink, M.E.; de Jong, N.; van der Steen, A.F. Nonlinear intravascular ultrasound contrast imaging. *Ultrasound Med. Biol.* **2006**, *32*, 491–502. [CrossRef] [PubMed]

123. Magnoni, M.; Coli, S.; Marrocco-Trischitta, M.M.; Melisurgo, G.; de Dominicis, D.; Cianflone, D.; Chiesa, R.; Feinstein, S.B.; Maseri, A. Contrast-enhanced ultrasound imaging of periadventitial vasa vasorum in human carotid arteries. *Eur. J. Echocardiogr.* **2009**, *10*, 260–264. [CrossRef] [PubMed]

124. Shah, F.; Balan, P.; Weinberg, M.; Reddy, V.; Neems, R.; Feinstein, M.; Dainauskas, J.; Meyer, P.; Goldin, M.; Feinstein, S.B. Contrast-enhanced ultrasound imaging of atherosclerotic carotid plaque neovascularization: A new surrogate marker of atherosclerosis? *Vasc. Med.* **2007**, *12*, 291–297. [CrossRef] [PubMed]

125. Schinkel, A.F.; Krueger, C.G.; Tellez, A.; Granada, J.F.; Reed, J.D.; Hall, A.; Zang, W.; Owens, C.; Kaluza, G.L.; Staub, D.; et al. Contrast-enhanced ultrasound for imaging vasa vasorum: Comparison with histopathology in a swine model of atherosclerosis. *Eur. J. Echocardiogr.* **2010**, *11*, 659–664. [CrossRef] [PubMed]

126. Coli, S.; Magnoni, M.; Sangiorgi, G.; Marrocco-Trischitta, M.M.; Melisurgo, G.; Mauriello, A.; Spagnoli, L.; Chiesa, R.; Cianflone, D.; Maseri, A. Contrast-enhanced ultrasound imaging of intraplaque neovascularization in carotid arteries: Correlation with histology and plaque echogenicity. *J. Am. Coll. Cardiol.* **2008**, *52*, 223–230. [CrossRef] [PubMed]

127. Lee, S.C.; Carr, C.L.; Davidson, B.P.; Ellegala, D.; Xie, A.; Ammi, A.; Belcik, T.; Lindner, J.R. Temporal characterization of the functional density of the vasa vasorum by contrast-enhanced ultrasonography maximum intensity projection imaging. *JACC Cardiovasc. Imaging* **2010**, *3*, 1265–1272. [CrossRef] [PubMed]

128. Moguillansky, D.; Leng, X.; Carson, A.; Lavery, L.; Schwartz, A.; Chen, X.; Villanueva, F.S. Quantification of plaque neovascularization using contrast ultrasound: A histologic validation. *Eur. Heart J.* **2011**, *32*, 646–653. [CrossRef] [PubMed]

129. Tian, J.; Hu, S.; Sun, Y.; Yu, H.; Han, X.; Cheng, W.; Ban, X.; Zhang, S.; Yu, B.; Jang, I.K. Vasa vasorum and plaque progression, and responses to atorvastatin in a rabbit model of atherosclerosis: Contrast-enhanced ultrasound imaging and intravascular ultrasound study. *Heart* **2013**, *99*, 48–54. [CrossRef] [PubMed]

130. Deyama, J.; Nakamura, T.; Takishima, I.; Fujioka, D.; Kawabata, K.; Obata, J.E.; Watanabe, K.; Watanabe, Y.; Saito, Y.; Mishina, H.; et al. Contrast-enhanced ultrasound imaging of carotid plaque neovascularization is useful for identifying high-risk patients with coronary artery disease. *Circ. J.* **2013**, *77*, 1499–1507. [CrossRef] [PubMed]

131. Vavuranakis, M.; Sigala, F.; Vrachatis, D.A.; Papaioannou, T.G.; Filis, K.; Kavantzas, N.; Kalogeras, K.I.; Massoura, C.; Toufektzian, L.; Kariori, M.G.; et al. Quantitative analysis of carotid plaque vasa vasorum by CEUS and correlation with histology after endarterectomy. *VASA Z. Gefasskrankh.* **2013**, *42*, 184–195. [CrossRef]

132. Kubo, T.; Tanaka, A.; Ino, Y.; Kitabata, H.; Shiono, Y.; Akasaka, T. Assessment of coronary atherosclerosis using optical coherence tomography. *J. Atheroscler. Thromb.* **2014**, *21*, 895–903. [CrossRef] [PubMed]

133. Kume, T.; Akasaka, T.; Kawamoto, T.; Watanabe, N.; Toyota, E.; Neishi, Y.; Sukmawan, R.; Sadahira, Y.; Yoshida, K. Assessment of coronary intima—Media thickness by optical coherence tomography: Comparison with intravascular ultrasound. *Circ. J.* **2005**, *69*, 903–907. [CrossRef] [PubMed]

134. Kitabata, H.; Tanaka, A.; Kubo, T.; Takarada, S.; Kashiwagi, M.; Tsujioka, H.; Ikejima, H.; Kuroi, A.; Kataiwa, H.; Ishibashi, K.; *et al.* Relation of microchannel structure identified by optical coherence tomography to plaque vulnerability in patients with coronary artery disease. *Am. J. Cardiol.* **2010**, *105*, 1673–1678. [CrossRef] [PubMed]

135. Cheng, K.H.; Sun, C.; Vuong, B.; Lee, K.K.; Mariampillai, A.; Marotta, T.R.; Spears, J.; Montanera, W.J.; Herman, P.R.; Kiehl, T.R.; *et al.* Endovascular optical coherence tomography intensity kurtosis: Visualization of vasa vasorum in porcine carotid artery. *Biomed. Opt. Express* **2012**, *3*, 388–399. [CrossRef] [PubMed]

136. Tearney, G.J.; Regar, E.; Akasaka, T.; Adriaenssens, T.; Barlis, P.; Bezerra, H.G.; Bouma, B.; Bruining, N.; Cho, J.M.; Chowdhary, S.; *et al.* Consensus standards for acquisition, measurement, and reporting of intravascular optical coherence tomography studies: A report from the International Working Group for Intravascular Optical Coherence Tomography Standardization and Validation. *J. Am. Coll. Cardiol.* **2012**, *59*, 1058–1072. [CrossRef] [PubMed]

137. Nishimiya, K.; Matsumoto, Y.; Takahashi, J.; Uzuka, H.; Odaka, Y.; Nihei, T.; Hao, K.; Tsuburaya, R.; Ito, K.; Shimokawa, H. *In vivo* visualization of adventitial vasa vasorum of the human coronary artery on optical frequency domain imaging. Validation study. *Circ. J.* **2014**, *78*, 2516–2518. [CrossRef] [PubMed]

138. Aoki, T.; Rodriguez-Porcel, M.; Matsuo, Y.; Cassar, A.; Kwon, T.G.; Franchi, F.; Gulati, R.; Kushwaha, S.S.; Lennon, R.J.; Lerman, L.O.; *et al.* Evaluation of coronary adventitial vasa vasorum using 3D optical coherence tomography—Animal and human studies. *Atherosclerosis* **2015**, *239*, 203–208. [CrossRef] [PubMed]

139. Dobrucki, L.W.; Sinusas, A.J. PET and SPECT in cardiovascular molecular imaging. *Nat. Rev. Cardiol.* **2010**, *7*, 38–47. [CrossRef] [PubMed]

140. Tawakol, A.; Migrino, R.Q.; Bashian, G.G.; Bedri, S.; Vermylen, D.; Cury, R.C.; Yates, D.; LaMuraglia, G.M.; Furie, K.; Houser, S.; *et al. In vivo* ^{18}F-fluorodeoxyglucose positron emission tomography imaging provides a noninvasive measure of carotid plaque inflammation in patients. *J. Am. Coll. Cardiol.* **2006**, *48*, 1818–1824. [CrossRef] [PubMed]

141. Folco, E.J.; Sheikine, Y.; Rocha, V.Z.; Christen, T.; Shvartz, E.; Sukhova, G.K.; di Carli, M.F.; Libby, P. Hypoxia but not inflammation augments glucose uptake in human macrophages: Implications for imaging atherosclerosis with [18]Fluorine-labeled 2-deoxy-D-glucose positron emission tomography. *J. Am. Coll. Cardiol.* **2011**, *58*, 603–614. [CrossRef] [PubMed]

142. Rodriguez-Porcel, M.; Cai, W.; Gheysens, O.; Willmann, J.K.; Chen, K.; Wang, H.; Chen, I.Y.; He, L.; Wu, J.C.; Li, Z.B.; *et al.* Imaging of VEGF receptor in a rat myocardial infarction model using PET. *J. Nucl. Med.* **2008**, *49*, 667–673. [CrossRef] [PubMed]

143. Meoli, D.F.; Sadeghi, M.M.; Krassilnikova, S.; Bourke, B.N.; Giordano, F.J.; Dione, D.P.; Su, H.; Edwards, D.S.; Liu, S.; Harris, T.D.; *et al.* Noninvasive imaging of myocardial angiogenesis following experimental myocardial infarction. *J. Clin. Investig.* **2004**, *113*, 1684–1691. [CrossRef] [PubMed]

144. Janssen, M.L.; Oyen, W.J.; Dijkgraaf, I.; Massuger, L.F.; Frielink, C.; Edwards, D.S.; Rajopadhye, M.; Boonstra, H.; Corstens, F.H.; Boerman, O.C. Tumor targeting with radiolabeled $\alpha_v\beta_3$ integrin binding peptides in a nude mouse model. *Cancer Res.* **2002**, *62*, 6146–6151. [PubMed]

145. Kopka, K.; Breyholz, H.J.; Wagner, S.; Law, M.P.; Riemann, B.; Schroer, S.; Trub, M.; Guilbert, B.; Levkau, B.; Schober, O.; *et al.* Synthesis and preliminary biological evaluation of new radioiodinated MMP inhibitors for imaging MMP activity *in vivo. Nucl. Med. Biol.* **2004**, *31*, 257–267. [CrossRef] [PubMed]

146. Furumoto, S.; Takashima, K.; Kubota, K.; Ido, T.; Iwata, R.; Fukuda, H. Tumor detection using ^{18}F-labeled matrix metalloproteinase-2 inhibitor. *Nucl.Med. Biol.* **2003**, *30*, 119–125. [CrossRef] [PubMed]

147. Schafers, M.; Riemann, B.; Kopka, K.; Breyholz, H.J.; Wagner, S.; Schafers, K.P.; Law, M.P.; Schober, O.; Levkau, B. Scintigraphic imaging of matrix metalloproteinase activity in the arterial wall *in vivo. Circulation* **2004**, *109*, 2554–2559. [CrossRef] [PubMed]

148. Matter, C.M.; Schuler, P.K.; Alessi, P.; Meier, P.; Ricci, R.; Zhang, D.; Halin, C.; Castellani, P.; Zardi, L.; Hofer, C.K.; *et al.* Molecular imaging of atherosclerotic plaques using a human antibody against the extra-domain B of fibronectin. *Circ. Res.* **2004**, *95*, 1225–1233. [CrossRef] [PubMed]

149. Kuge, Y.; Takai, N.; Ogawa, Y.; Temma, T.; Zhao, Y.; Nishigori, K.; Ishino, S.; Kamihashi, J.; Kiyono, Y.; Shiomi, M.; *et al.* Imaging with radiolabelled anti-membrane type 1 matrix metalloproteinase (MT1-MMP) antibody: Potentials for characterizing atherosclerotic plaques. *Eur. J. Nucl. Med. Mol. Imaging* **2010**, *37*, 2093–2104. [CrossRef] [PubMed]

150. Aoki, S.; Aoki, K.; Ohsawa, S.; Nakajima, H.; Kumagai, H.; Araki, T. Dynamic MR imaging of the carotid wall. *J. Magn. Reson. Imaging JMRI* **1999**, *9*, 420–427. [CrossRef]

151. Winter, P.M.; Morawski, A.M.; Caruthers, S.D.; Fuhrhop, R.W.; Zhang, H.; Williams, T.A.; Allen, J.S.; Lacy, E.K.; Robertson, J.D.; Lanza, G.M.; et al. Molecular imaging of angiogenesis in early-stage atherosclerosis with $\alpha_v\beta_3$-integrin-targeted nanoparticles. *Circulation* **2003**, *108*, 2270–2274. [CrossRef] [PubMed]

152. Cai, K.; Caruthers, S.D.; Huang, W.; Williams, T.A.; Zhang, H.; Wickline, S.A.; Lanza, G.M.; Winter, P.M. MR molecular imaging of aortic angiogenesis. *JACC Cardiovasc. Imaging* **2010**, *3*, 824–832. [CrossRef] [PubMed]

153. Kerwin, W.; Hooker, A.; Spilker, M.; Vicini, P.; Ferguson, M.; Hatsukami, T.; Yuan, C. Quantitative magnetic resonance imaging analysis of neovasculature volume in carotid atherosclerotic plaque. *Circulation* **2003**, *107*, 851–856. [CrossRef] [PubMed]

154. Kerwin, W.S.; Oikawa, M.; Yuan, C.; Jarvik, G.P.; Hatsukami, T.S. MR imaging of adventitial vasa vasorum in carotid atherosclerosis. *Magn. Reson. Med.* **2008**, *59*, 507–514. [CrossRef] [PubMed]

155. Sun, J.; Song, Y.; Chen, H.; Kerwin, W.S.; Hippe, D.S.; Dong, L.; Chen, M.; Zhou, C.; Hatsukami, T.S.; Yuan, C. Adventitial perfusion and intraplaque hemorrhage: A dynamic contrast-enhanced MRI study in the carotid artery. *Stroke J. Cereb. Circ.* **2013**, *44*, 1031–1036. [CrossRef]

156. Grobner, T. Gadolinium—A specific trigger for the development of nephrogenic fibrosing dermopathy and nephrogenic systemic fibrosis? *Nephrol. Dial. Transpl.* **2006**, *21*, 1104–1108. [CrossRef]

157. Feinstein, S.B. Contrast ultrasound imaging of the carotid artery vasa vasorum and atherosclerotic plaque neovascularization. *J. Am. Coll. Cardiol.* **2006**, *48*, 236–243. [CrossRef] [PubMed]

158. Decano, J.L.; Moran, A.M.; Ruiz-Opazo, N.; Herrera, V.L. Molecular imaging of vasa vasorum neovascularization via DEspR-targeted contrast-enhanced ultrasound micro-imaging in transgenic atherosclerosis rat model. *Mol. Imaging Biol. MIB* **2011**, *13*, 1096–1106. [CrossRef]

159. Baron Toaldo, M.; Salvatore, V.; Marinelli, S.; Palama, C.; Milazzo, M.; Croci, L.; Venerandi, L.; Cipone, M.; Bolondi, L.; Piscaglia, F. Use of VEGFR-2 targeted ultrasound contrast agent for the early evaluation of response to sorafenib in a mouse model of hepatocellular carcinoma. *Mol. Imaging Biol. MIB* **2015**, *17*, 29–37. [CrossRef]

160. Araldi, E.; Chamorro-Jorganes, A.; van Solingen, C.; Fernandez-Hernando, C.; Suarez, Y. Therapeutic potential of modulating microRNAs in atherosclerotic vascular disease. *Curr. Vasc. Pharmacol.* **2013**, in press.

161. O'Reilly, M.S.; Holmgren, L.; Shing, Y.; Chen, C.; Rosenthal, R.A.; Moses, M.; Lane, W.S.; Cao, Y.; Sage, E.H.; Folkman, J. Angiostatin: A novel angiogenesis inhibitor that mediates the suppression of metastases by a Lewis lung carcinoma. *Cell* **1994**, *79*, 315–328. [CrossRef] [PubMed]

162. O'Reilly, M.S.; Boehm, T.; Shing, Y.; Fukai, N.; Vasios, G.; Lane, W.S.; Flynn, E.; Birkhead, J.R.; Olsen, B.R.; Folkman, J. Endostatin: An endogenous inhibitor of angiogenesis and tumor growth. *Cell* **1997**, *88*, 277–285. [CrossRef] [PubMed]

163. Moulton, K.S.; Heller, E.; Konerding, M.A.; Flynn, E.; Palinski, W.; Folkman, J. Angiogenesis inhibitors endostatin or TNP-470 reduce intimal neovascularization and plaque growth in apolipoprotein E-deficient mice. *Circulation* **1999**, *99*, 1726–1732. [CrossRef] [PubMed]

164. Moulton, K.S.; Vakili, K.; Zurakowski, D.; Soliman, M.; Butterfield, C.; Sylvin, E.; Lo, K.M.; Gillies, S.; Javaherian, K.; Folkman, J. Inhibition of plaque neovascularization reduces macrophage accumulation and progression of advanced atherosclerosis. *Proc. Natl. Acad. Sci. USA* **2003**, *100*, 4736–4741. [CrossRef] [PubMed]

165. Eriksson, K.; Magnusson, P.; Dixelius, J.; Claesson-Welsh, L.; Cross, M.J. Angiostatin and endostatin inhibit endothelial cell migration in response to FGF and VEGF without interfering with specific intracellular signal transduction pathways. *FEBS Lett.* **2003**, *536*, 19–24. [CrossRef] [PubMed]

166. Stefanadis, C.; Toutouzas, K.; Stefanadi, E.; Kolodgie, F.; Virmani, R.; Kipshidze, N. First experimental application of bevacizumab-eluting PC coated stent for inhibition of vasa vasorum of atherosclerotic plaque: Angiographic results in a rabbit atheromatic model. *Hell. J. Cardiol. HJC* **2006**, *47*, 7–10.

167. Luttun, A.; Tjwa, M.; Moons, L.; Wu, Y.; Angelillo-Scherrer, A.; Liao, F.; Nagy, J.A.; Hooper, A.; Priller, J.; de Klerck, B.; et al. Revascularization of ischemic tissues by PlGF treatment, and inhibition of tumor angiogenesis, arthritis and atherosclerosis by anti-Flt1. *Nat. Med.* **2002**, *8*, 831–840. [PubMed]

168. Khurana, R.; Moons, L.; Shafi, S.; Luttun, A.; Collen, D.; Martin, J.F.; Carmeliet, P.; Zachary, I.C. Placental growth factor promotes atherosclerotic intimal thickening and macrophage accumulation. *Circulation* **2005**, *111*, 2828–2836. [CrossRef] [PubMed]

169. Fischer, C.; Jonckx, B.; Mazzone, M.; Zacchigna, S.; Loges, S.; Pattarini, L.; Chorianopoulos, E.; Liesenborghs, L.; Koch, M.; de Mol, M.; *et al.* Anti-PlGF inhibits growth of VEGF(R)-inhibitor-resistant tumors without affecting healthy vessels. *Cell* **2007**, *131*, 463–475. [CrossRef] [PubMed]

170. Johnson, M.D.; Kim, H.R.; Chesler, L.; Tsao-Wu, G.; Bouck, N.; Polverini, P.J. Inhibition of angiogenesis by tissue inhibitor of metalloproteinase. *J. Cell. Physiol.* **1994**, *160*, 194–202. [CrossRef] [PubMed]

171. Gossl, M.; Herrmann, J.; Tang, H.; Versari, D.; Galili, O.; Mannheim, D.; Rajkumar, S.V.; Lerman, L.O.; Lerman, A. Prevention of vasa vasorum neovascularization attenuates early neointima formation in experimental hypercholesterolemia. *Basic Res. Cardiol.* **2009**, *104*, 695–706. [CrossRef] [PubMed]

172. Kampschulte, M.; Gunkel, I.; Stieger, P.; Sedding, D.G.; Brinkmann, A.; Ritman, E.L.; Krombach, G.A.; Langheinrich, A.C. Thalidomide influences atherogenesis in aortas of $ApoE^{-/-}/LDLR^{-/-}$ double knockout mice: A nano-CT study. *Int. J. Cardiovasc. Imaging* **2014**, *30*, 795–802. [CrossRef] [PubMed]

173. Dashwood, M.R.; Barker, S.G.; Muddle, J.R.; Yacoub, M.H.; Martin, J.F. [125I]-endothelin-1 binding to vasa vasorum and regions of neovascularization in human and porcine blood vessels: A possible role for endothelin in intimal hyperplasia and atherosclerosis. *J. Cardiovasc. Pharmacol.* **1993**, *22*, S343–S347. [CrossRef] [PubMed]

174. Herrmann, J.; Best, P.J.; Ritman, E.L.; Holmes, D.R.; Lerman, L.O.; Lerman, A. Chronic endothelin receptor antagonism prevents coronary vasa vasorum neovascularization in experimental hypercholesterolemia. *J. Am. Coll. Cardiol.* **2002**, *39*, 1555–1561. [CrossRef] [PubMed]

175. Winter, P.M.; Neubauer, A.M.; Caruthers, S.D.; Harris, T.D.; Robertson, J.D.; Williams, T.A.; Schmieder, A.H.; Hu, G.; Allen, J.S.; Lacy, E.K.; *et al.* Endothelial $\alpha_v\beta_3$ integrin-targeted fumagillin nanoparticles inhibit angiogenesis in atherosclerosis. *Arterioscler. Thromb. Vasc. Biol.* **2006**, *26*, 2103–2109. [CrossRef] [PubMed]

176. Drinane, M.; Mollmark, J.; Zagorchev, L.; Moodie, K.; Sun, B.; Hall, A.; Shipman, S.; Morganelli, P.; Simons, M.; Mulligan-Kehoe, M.J. The antiangiogenic activity of $rPAI-1_{23}$ inhibits vasa vasorum and growth of atherosclerotic plaque. *Circ. Res.* **2009**, *104*, 337–345. [CrossRef] [PubMed]

177. Mollmark, J.; Ravi, S.; Sun, B.; Shipman, S.; Buitendijk, M.; Simons, M.; Mulligan-Kehoe, M.J. Antiangiogenic activity of $rPAI-1_{23}$ promotes vasa vasorum regression in hypercholesterolemic mice through a plasmin-dependent mechanism. *Circ. Res.* **2011**, *108*, 1419–1428. [CrossRef] [PubMed]

178. Langheinrich, A.C.; Sedding, D.G.; Kampschulte, M.; Moritz, R.; Wilhelm, J.; Haberbosch, W.G.; Ritman, E.L.; Bohle, R.M. 3-Deazaadenosine inhibits vasa vasorum neovascularization in aortas of $ApoE^{-/-}/LDLR^{-/-}$ double knockout mice. *Atherosclerosis* **2009**, *202*, 103–110. [CrossRef] [PubMed]

179. Tsai, H.T.; Marshall, J.L.; Weiss, S.R.; Huang, C.Y.; Warren, J.L.; Freedman, A.N.; Fu, A.Z.; Sansbury, L.B.; Potosky, A.L. Bevacizumab use and risk of cardiovascular adverse events among elderly patients with colorectal cancer receiving chemotherapy: A population-based study. *Ann. Oncol.* **2013**, *24*, 1574–1579. [CrossRef] [PubMed]

180. Colon, G.P.; Deveikis, J.P.; Dickinson, L.D. Revascularization of occluded internal carotid arteries by hypertrophied vasa vasorum: Report of four cases. *Neurosurgery* **1999**, *45*, 634–637. [CrossRef] [PubMed]

181. Shanahan, C.M.; Weissberg, P.L. Smooth muscle cell phenotypes in atherosclerotic lesions. *Curr. Opin. Lipidol.* **1999**, *10*, 507–513. [CrossRef] [PubMed]

182. Wilson, S.H.; Herrmann, J.; Lerman, L.O.; Holmes, D.R., Jr.; Napoli, C.; Ritman, E.L.; Lerman, A. Simvastatin preserves the structure of coronary adventitial vasa vasorum in experimental hypercholesterolemia independent of lipid lowering. *Circulation* **2002**, *105*, 415–418. [CrossRef] [PubMed]

183. Urbich, C.; Dernbach, E.; Zeiher, A.M.; Dimmeler, S. Double-edged role of statins in angiogenesis signaling. *Circ. Res.* **2002**, *90*, 737–744. [CrossRef] [PubMed]

184. Chaldakov, G.N.; Stankulov, I.S.; Fiore, M.; Ghenev, P.I.; Aloe, L. Nerve growth factor levels and mast cell distribution in human coronary atherosclerosis. *Atherosclerosis* **2001**, *159*, 57–66. [CrossRef] [PubMed]

185. Asanome, A.; Kawabe, J.; Matsuki, M.; Kabara, M.; Hira, Y.; Bochimoto, H.; Yamauchi, A.; Aonuma, T.; Takehara, N.; Watanabe, T.; *et al.* Nerve growth factor stimulates regeneration of perivascular nerve, and induces the maturation of microvessels around the injured artery. *Biochem. Biophys. Res. Commun.* **2014**, *443*, 150–155. [CrossRef] [PubMed]

186. Mollmark, J.I.; Park, A.J.; Kim, J.; Wang, T.Z.; Katzenell, S.; Shipman, S.L.; Zagorchev, L.G.; Simons, M.; Mulligan-Kehoe, M.J. Fibroblast growth factor-2 is required for vasa vasorum plexus stability in hypercholesterolemic mice. *Arterioscler. Thromb. Vasc. Biol.* **2012**, *32*, 2644–2651. [CrossRef] [PubMed]

187. Lindner, V.; Lappi, D.A.; Baird, A.; Majack, R.A.; Reidy, M.A. Role of basic fibroblast growth factor in vascular lesion formation. *Circ. Res.* **1991**, *68*, 106–113. [CrossRef] [PubMed]

188. Six, I.; Mouquet, F.; Corseaux, D.; Bordet, R.; Letourneau, T.; Vallet, B.; Dosquet, C.C.; Dupuis, B.; Jude, B.; Bertrand, M.E.; *et al.* Protective effects of basic fibroblast growth factor in early atherosclerosis. *Growth Factors* **2004**, *22*, 157–167. [CrossRef] [PubMed]

189. Che, J.; Okigaki, M.; Takahashi, T.; Katsume, A.; Adachi, Y.; Yamaguchi, S.; Matsunaga, S.; Takeda, M.; Matsui, A.; Kishita, E.; *et al.* Endothelial FGF receptor signaling accelerates atherosclerosis. *Am. J. Physiol. Heart Circ. Physiol.* **2011**, *300*, H154–H161. [CrossRef] [PubMed]

190. Shen, W.; Shi, H.M.; Fan, W.H.; Luo, X.P.; Jin, B.; Li, Y. The effects of simvastatin on angiogenesis: Studied by an original model of atherosclerosis and acute myocardial infarction in rabbit. *Mol. Biol. Rep.* **2011**, *38*, 3821–3828. [CrossRef] [PubMed]

Permissions

The contributors of this book come from diverse backgrounds, making this book a truly international effort. This book will bring forth new frontiers with its revolutionizing research information and detailed analysis of the nascent developments around the world.

We would like to thank all the contributing authors for lending their expertise to make the book truly unique. They have played a crucial role in the development of this book. Without their invaluable contributions this book wouldn't have been possible. They have made vital efforts to compile up to date information on the varied aspects of this subject to make this book a valuable addition to the collection of many professionals and students.

This book was conceptualized with the vision of imparting up-to-date information and advanced data in this field. To ensure the same, a matchless editorial board was set up. Every individual on the board went through rigorous rounds of assessment to prove their worth. After which they invested a large part of their time researching and compiling the most relevant data for our readers.

The editorial board has been involved in producing this book since its inception. They have spent rigorous hours researching and exploring the diverse topics which have resulted in the successful publishing of this book. They have passed on their knowledge of decades through this book. To expedite this challenging task, the publisher supported the team at every step. A small team of assistant editors was also appointed to further simplify the editing procedure and attain best results for the readers.

Apart from the editorial board, the designing team has also invested a significant amount of their time in understanding the subject and creating the most relevant covers. They scrutinized every image to scout for the most suitable representation of the subject and create an appropriate cover for the book.

The publishing team has been an ardent support to the editorial, designing and production team. Their endless efforts to recruit the best for this project, has resulted in the accomplishment of this book. They are a veteran in the field of academics and their pool of knowledge is as vast as their experience in printing. Their expertise and guidance has proved useful at every step. Their uncompromising quality standards have made this book an exceptional effort. Their encouragement from time to time has been an inspiration for everyone.

The publisher and the editorial board hope that this book will prove to be a valuable piece of knowledge for researchers, students, practitioners and scholars across the globe.

List of Contributors

Jean-Baptiste Michel
UMR 1148, Inserm & Paris University, X. Bichat University Hospital, 75018 Paris, France

José Luis Martin-Ventura
IIS-Fundation Jimenez-Diaz, Autonoma University of Madrid and CIBERCV, 28040 Madrid, Spain

Lei Wang
Cyrus Tang Hematology Center, Cyrus Tang Medical Institute, Soochow University, Suzhou 215123, China

Chaojun Tang
Cyrus Tang Hematology Center, Cyrus Tang Medical Institute, Soochow University, Suzhou 215123, China
Collaborative Innovation Center of Hematology of Jiangsu Province, Soochow University, Suzhou 215123, China
National Clinical Research Center for Hematologic Diseases, the First Affiliated Hospital of Soochow University, Suzhou 215123, China

Silvia Lee
Department of Advanced Clinical and Translational Cardiovascular Imaging, Harry Perkins Institute of Medical Research, Murdoch 6150, Australia
Department of Microbiology, Pathwest Laboratory Medicine, Murdoch 6150, Australia

Benjamin Bartlett
Department of Advanced Clinical and Translational Cardiovascular Imaging, Harry Perkins Institute of Medical Research, Murdoch 6150, Australia
School of Medicine, University of Western Australia, Nedlands 6009, Australia

Girish Dwivedi
Department of Advanced Clinical and Translational Cardiovascular Imaging, Harry Perkins Institute of Medical Research, Murdoch 6150, Australia
School of Medicine, University of Western Australia, Nedlands 6009, Australia
Department of Cardiology, Fiona Stanley Hospital, Murdoch 6150, Australia

Rachel Nicoll, Pranvera Ibrahimi and Michael Henein
Department of Public Health and Clinical Medicine, Umea University and Heart Centre, Umea SE-901-87, Sweden

Ying Zhao
Department of Ultrasound, Beijing Anzhen Hospital, Capital Medical University, Beijing 100029, China

Gunilla Olivecrona
Department of Medical Biosciences, Umea University, Umea SE-901-87, Sweden

Peiqiu Cao, Haitao Pan, Jiao Guo and Zhengquan Su
Key Research Center of Liver Regulation for Hyperlipemia SATCM/Class III, Laboratory of Metabolism SATCM, Guangdong TCM Key Laboratory for Metabolic Diseases, Guangdong Pharmaceutical University, Guangzhou 510006, China

Tiancun Xiao
Inorganic Chemistry Laboratory, University of Oxford, South Parks Road, Oxford OX1 3QR, UK
Guangzhou Boxabio Ltd., D-106 Guangzhou International Business Incubator, Guangzhou 510530, China

Ting Zhou
Guangzhou Boxabio Ltd., D-106 Guangzhou International Business Incubator, Guangzhou 510530, China

Slaven Pikija, Johannes Sebastian Mutzenbach and Helmut F. Novak
Department of Neurology, Christian Doppler Medical Center, Paracelsus Medical University, 5020 Salzburg, Austria

Jozef Magdic
Department of Neurology, Univerzitetni Klinični Center, 2000 Maribor, Slovenia

Vladimir Trkulja
Department for Pharmacology, School of Medicine, University of Zagreb, 10000 Zagreb, Croatia

Peter Unterkreuter
Department of Neurology, Bezirkskrankenhaus Lienz, 9900 Lienz, Austria

Friedrich Weymayr
Division of Neuroradiology, Christian Doppler Medical Center, Paracelsus Medical University, 5020 Salzburg, Austria

Larissa Hauer
Department of Psychiatry, Christian Doppler Medical Center, Paracelsus Medical University, 5020 Salzburg, Austria

Johann Sellner
Department of Neurology, Christian Doppler Medical Center, Paracelsus Medical University, 5020 Salzburg, Austria
Department of Neurology, Klinikum rechts der Isar, Technische Universität, 81675 München, Germany
Institute of Linguistics, University of Salzburg, 5020 Salzburg, Austria

Eugenio Picano
Biomedicine Department, NU School of Medicine, Astana 010000, Kazakistan

Marco Paterni
CNR (Consiglio Nazionale Ricerche), Institute of Clinical Physiology, 56124 Pisa, Italy

Olga Kruszelnicka and Jadwiga Nessler
Department of Coronary Artery Disease and Heart Failure, Jagiellonian University Medical College and John Paul II Hospital, 80 Prądnicka, 31-202 Cracow, Poland

Jolanta Świerszcz, Bernadeta Chyrchel and Andrzej Surdacki
Second Department of Cardiology, Jagiellonian University Medical College and University Hospital, 17 Kopernika, 31-501 Cracow, Poland

Jacek Bednarek
Department of Electrocardiology, John Paul II Hospital, 80 Prądnicka, 31-202 Cracow, Poland

Irfan Zeb
Department of Medicine, Bronx-Lebanon Hospital Center, 1650 Grand Concourse, Bronx, NY 10457, USA

Matthew Budoff
Department of Cardiology, Los Angeles Biomedical Research Institute at Harbor-UCLA Medical Center, Torrance, CA 90502, USA

Pier-Luc Tardif, Maxime Abran and Frédéric Lesage
Département de Génie Électrique et Institut de Génie Biomédical, École Polytechnique de Montréal, Montreal, QC H3T 1J4, Canada
Montreal Heart Institute, Montreal, QC H1T 1C8, Canada

Alexandre Castonguay and Joël Lefebvre
Département de Génie Électrique et Institut de Génie Biomédical, École Polytechnique de Montréal, Montreal, QC H3T 1J4, Canada

Barbara E. Stähli, Nolwenn Merlet, Teodora Mihalache-Avram, Pascale Geoffroy, Mélanie Mecteau and David Busseuil
Montreal Heart Institute, Montreal, QC H1T 1C8, Canada

Feng Ni and Abedelnasser Abulrob
National Research Council Canada (NRCC), Montreal, QC H3A 1A3, Canada

Marie-Jeanne Bertrand, Éric Rhéaume, Philippe L'Allier and Jean-Claude Tardif
Montreal Heart Institute, Montreal, QC H1T 1C8, Canada
Département de Médecine, Université de Montréal, Montreal, QC H3C 3J7, Canada

Joachim Eckert, Marco Schmidt, Annett Magedanz, Thomas Voigtländer and Axel Schmermund
Cardioangiologisches Centrum Bethanien, Im Prüfling 23, D-60389 Frankfurt, Germany

Shoichi Ehara, Kenji Matsumoto and Kenei Shimada
Department of Cardiovascular Medicine, Osaka City University Graduate School of Medicine, Osaka 545-8585, Japan

Fisnik Jashari, Gani Bajraktari, Per Wester and Michael Y. Henein
Department of Public Health and Clinical Medicine, Umeå University, Umeå 901 87, Sweden

Jian Guo, Yang Li, Jie Dong, Han Yan and Gu-Yan Zheng
Department of Human Population Genetics, Institute of Molecular Medicine, Peking University, Beijing 100871, China

Yi-Hong Ren and Zhijun Sun
Department of Cardiovascular, PLA General Hospital, Beijing 100853, China

Yujun Xu and Dao Wen Wang
The Institute of Hypertension and Department of Internal Medicine, Tongji Hospital, Tongji Medical College, Huazhong University of Science and Technology, Wuhan 430074, China

Jie Du
Beijing Anzhen Hospital, Capital Medical University, The Key Laboratory of Remodeling-Related Cardiovascular Diseases, Ministry of Education, Beijing Collaborative Innovation Center for Cardiovascular Disorders, Beijing Institute of Heart, Lung & Blood Vessel Disease, Beijing 100029, China

Xiao-Li Tian
Department of Human Population Genetics, Institute of Molecular Medicine, Peking University, Beijing 100871, China
Department of Human Population Genetics, Human Aging Research Institute and School of Life Science, Nanchang University, Nanchang 330031, China

Junyan Xu and Xiaotong Lu
Second Clinical Medical College, Zhujiang Hospital and Southern Medical University, Guangzhou 510280, China

Guo-Ping Shi
Second Clinical Medical College, Zhujiang Hospital and Southern Medical University, Guangzhou 510280, China
Department of Medicine, Brigham and Women's Hospital and Harvard Medical School, Boston, MA 02115, USA

Index